The Book of Calm

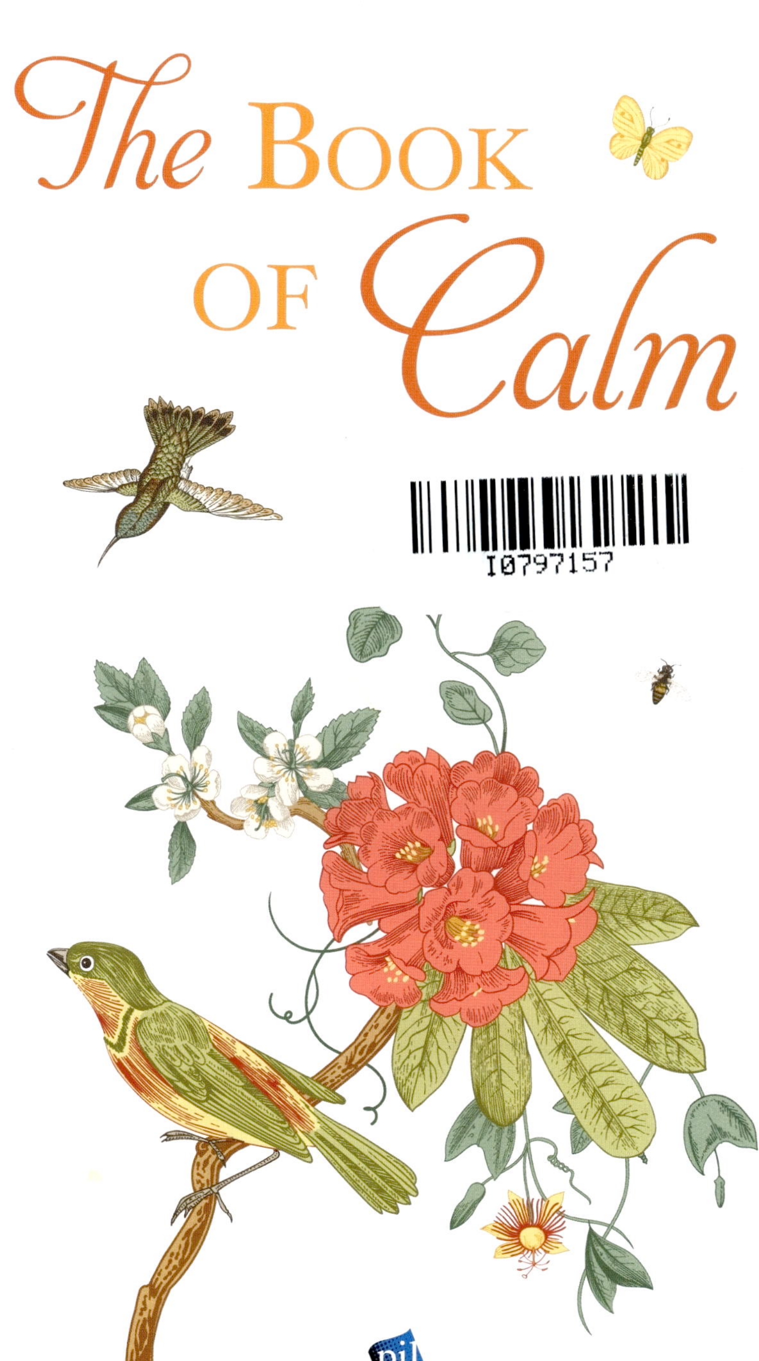

pil
Publications International, Ltd.

Images from Shutterstock.com

Louis Weber, CEO
Publications International, Ltd.
5250 Old Orchard Road, Suite 500
Skokie, IL 60077

ISBN: 978-1-63938-815-8

Manufactured in China.

8 7 6 5 4 3 2 1

Table of Contents

Introduction

A state of calm is within your reach. Release your stress and worries and cultivate a mindset of serenity with this collection. In this book, you'll discover a selection of uplifting reflections, mantras, and quotations, along with practical guidance about various forms of meditation, including breath meditation, art meditation, and movement meditation.

The Book of Calm can be read from front to back, or you can turn to a specific section that captures your interest. The chapter on "Breathing and Meditation" talks about the basics of meditation and mindfulness, while "Types of Meditation" offers further options like the body scan meditation, gazing meditation, and more. The third chapter offers more than fifty calming mantras and meditations, so that you can browse through to discover which ones resonate with you. "Calming Movements" discusses practices like Tai Chi and progressive muscle relaxation, while "The Calming Effects of Nature" takes you outside, where you can appreciate the beauty and sounds of nature, whether you're hiking in the wilderness or wandering through a garden. The final chapter includes information on the roles that art appreciation and creation, sounds, music, and scents can play in helping us achieve a state of calm.

You don't need to be tense, stressed out, or anxious. With practical tips, soothing reflections, and inspiring quotes, **The Book of Calm** can show the way.

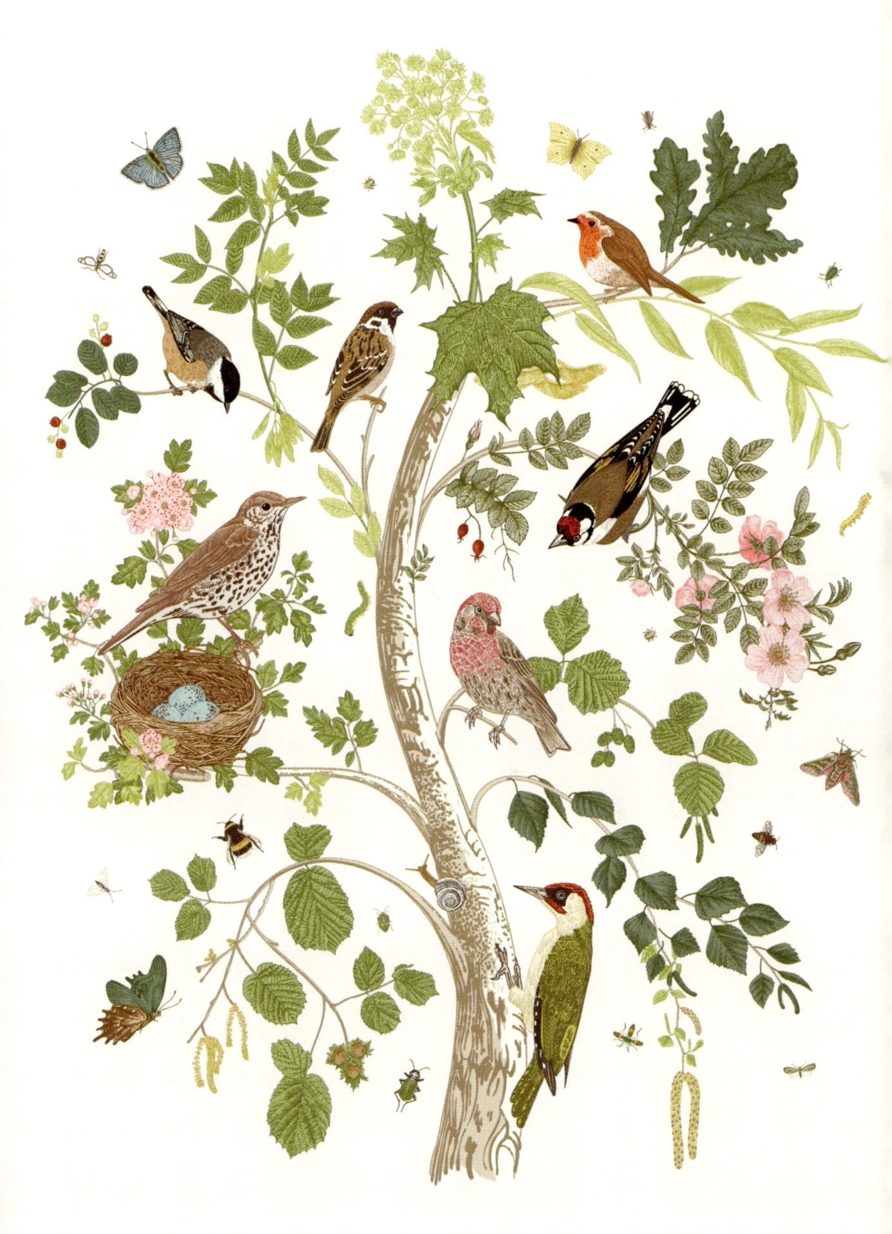

Breathing and Meditation

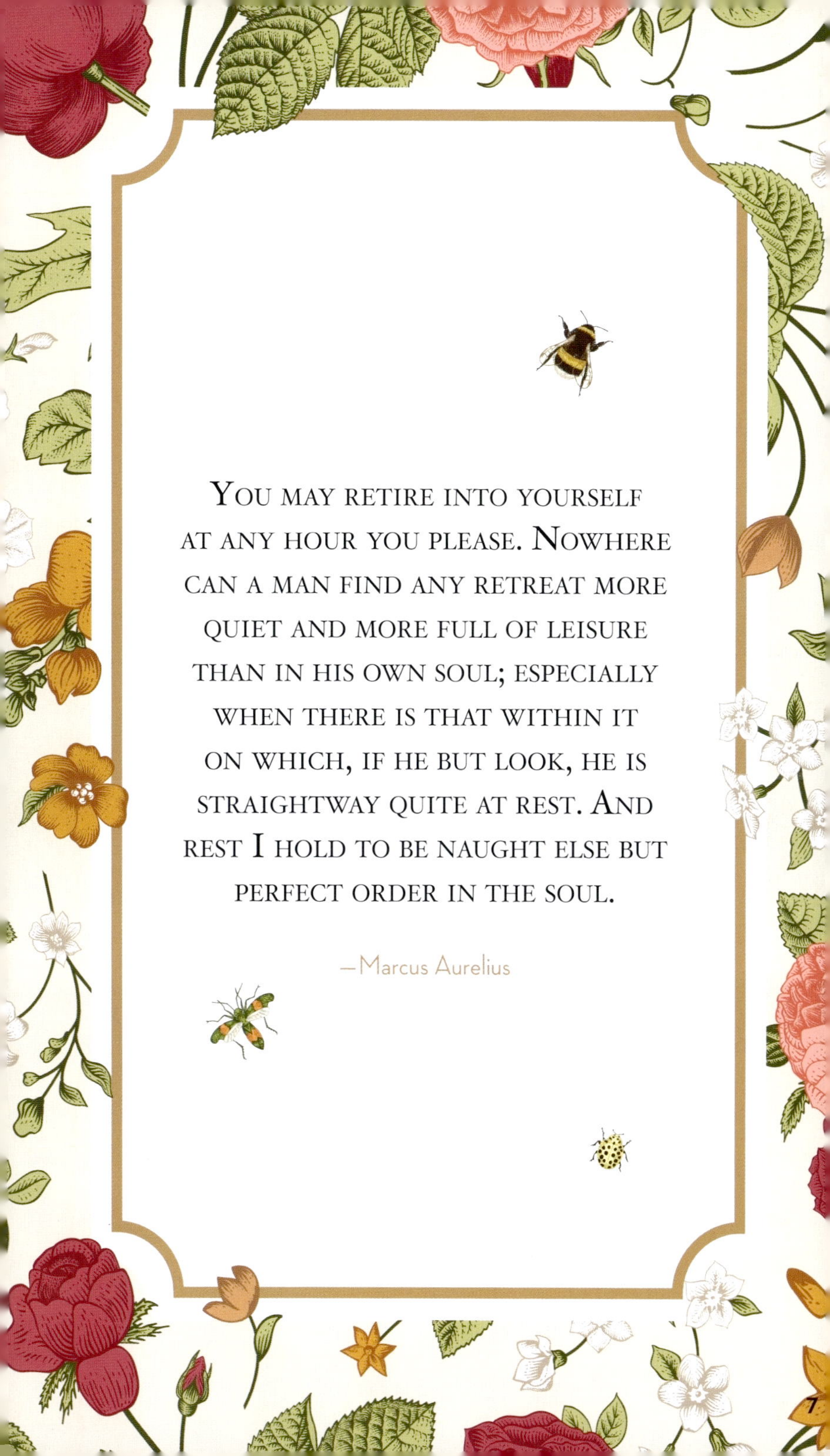

You may retire into yourself at any hour you please. Nowhere can a man find any retreat more quiet and more full of leisure than in his own soul; especially when there is that within it on which, if he but look, he is straightway quite at rest. And rest I hold to be naught else but perfect order in the soul.

—Marcus Aurelius

What Is Meditation?

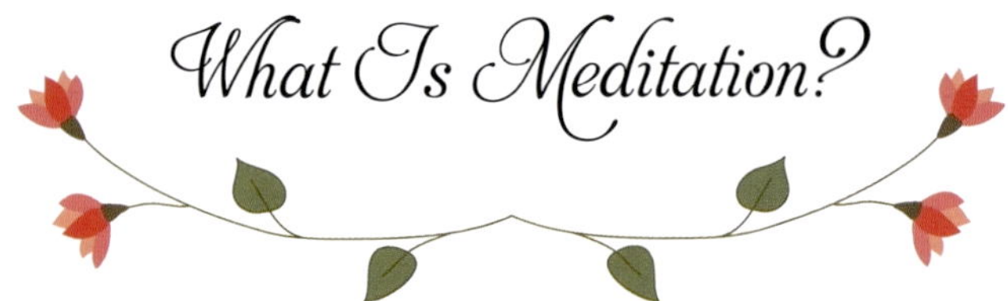

Meditation actively trains the mind to cultivate awareness, focus, and clarity. This is primarily done through focused attention. Left to its own devices, the mind can bombard a person with an uncontrolled waterfall of thoughts. Meditation can help turn this waterfall into a steadier, more manageable stream. Like any other form of exercise, meditation comes more easily with time and practice.

Over the millennia and around the world, people have meditated with a variety of intentions and methods. For some, meditation is part of their religious practice or spiritual journey. It is disciplined devotion that brings the practitioner closer to the divine. To other people, it is entirely secular. Meditation may be done in movement or stillness, with sound or in silence, over hours or minutes.

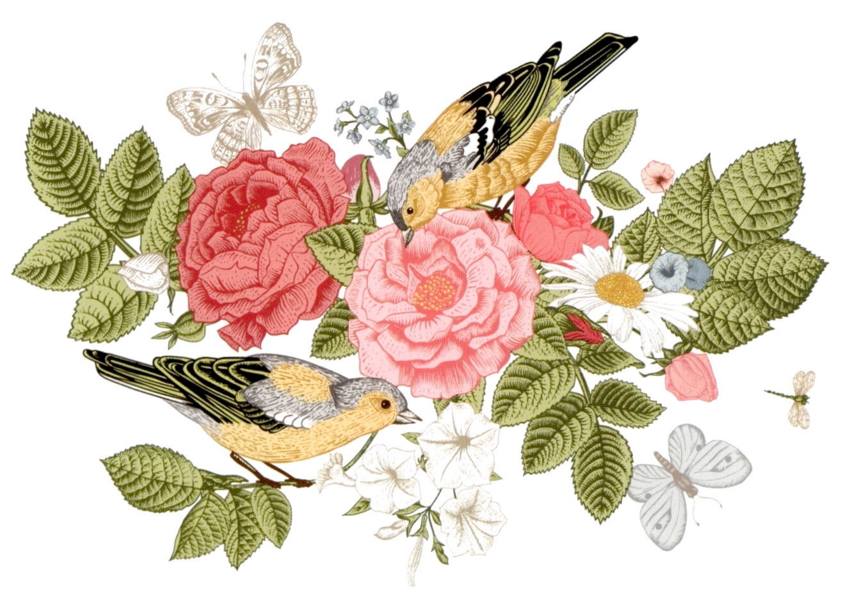

By all means use
sometimes to be alone.
Salute thyself: see what
thy soul doth wear.
Dare to look in thy chest;
for 'tis thine own;
And tumble up and down
what thou find'st there.
Who cannot rest till he
good fellows find,
He breaks up house, turns
out of doors his mind.

—George Herbert

Why Meditate?

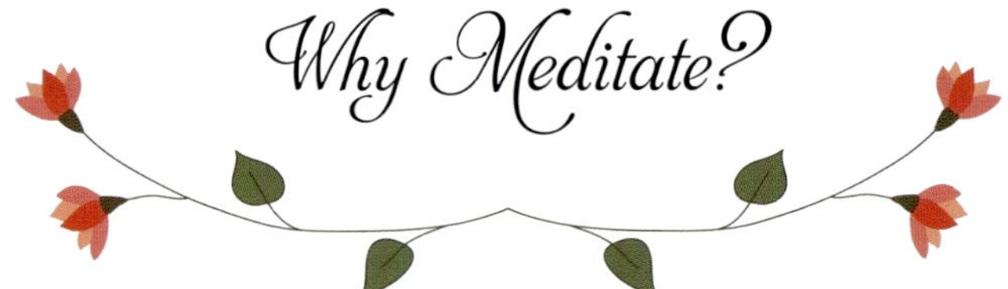

A number of benefits can come from meditating. Depending on the meditation technique you use, you might see more of some benefits over others. Research so far has suggested:

- Meditation increases your ability to concentrate. It can improve your memory and thought processes.
- It helps preserve your brain as it ages, resulting in less gray matter loss.
- It helps with stress-related illnesses such as anxiety, depression, irritable bowel syndrome, and insomnia.
- It may help reduce the severity of menopausal symptoms, including hot flashes, muscle and joint pain, and changes in sleep and mood.
- It might reduce asthma symptoms.
- It can reduce your blood pressure.
- It can help fight the habit of rumination, or prolonged focus on negative or distressing thoughts.
- It may help reduce inflammation and pain.
- It causes changes in the areas of the brain that regulate emotion.
- It may help treat addiction by causing changes in the parts of the brain that deal with self-control.
- It can help increase compassion, felt for both yourself and others.

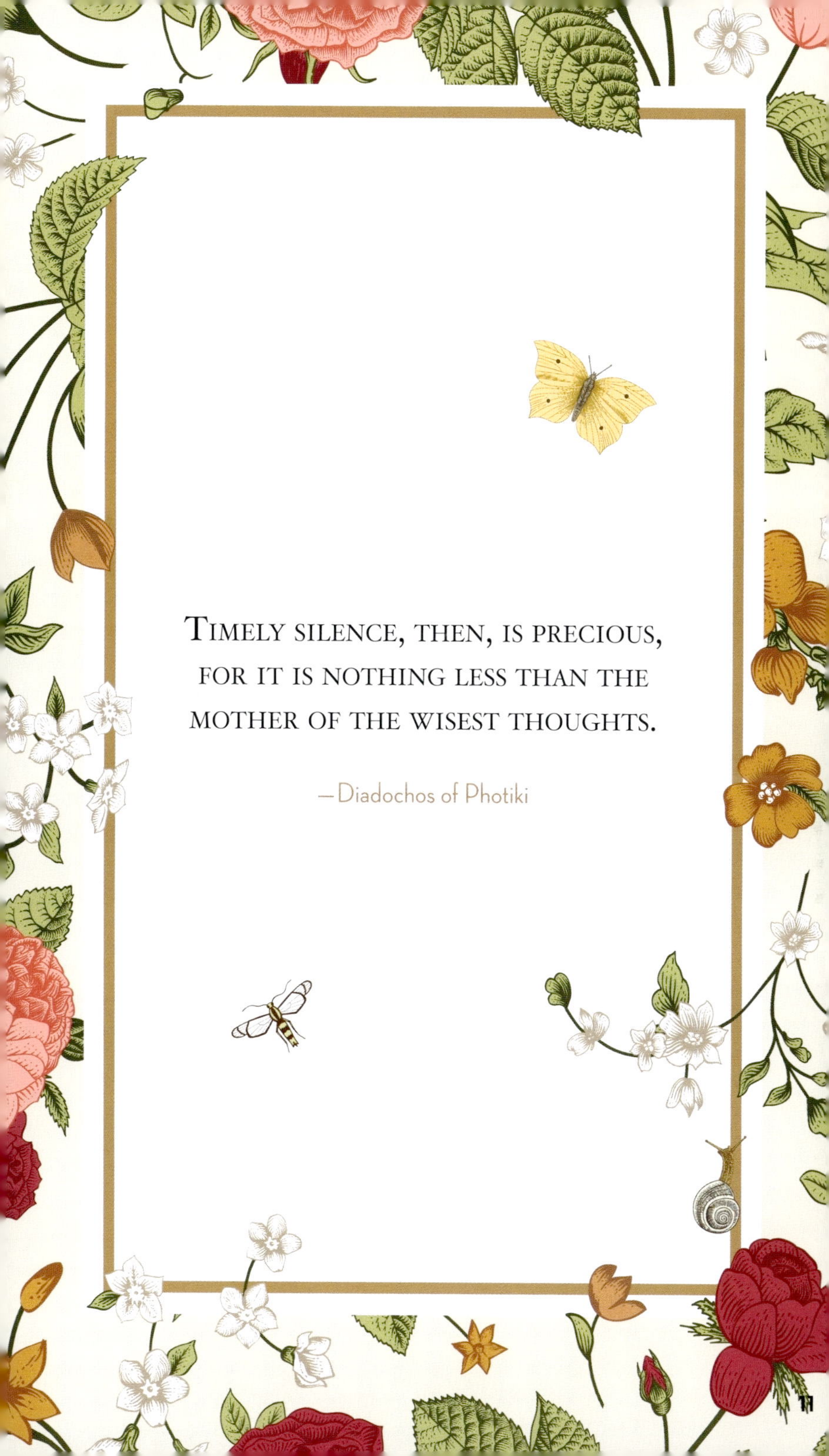

TIMELY SILENCE, THEN, IS PRECIOUS, FOR IT IS NOTHING LESS THAN THE MOTHER OF THE WISEST THOUGHTS.

—Diadochos of Photiki

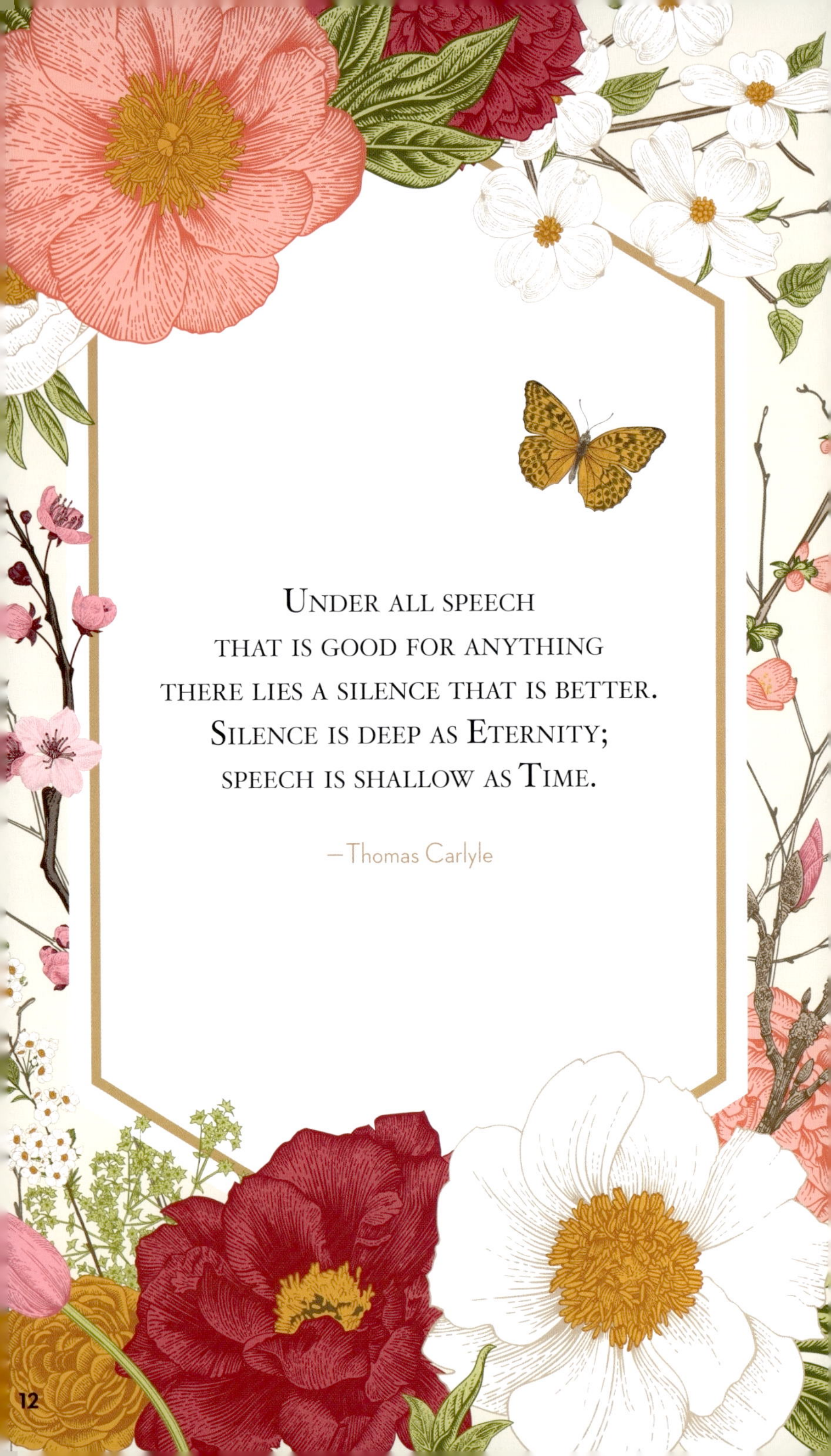

Under all speech
that is good for anything
there lies a silence that is better.
Silence is deep as Eternity;
speech is shallow as Time.

—Thomas Carlyle

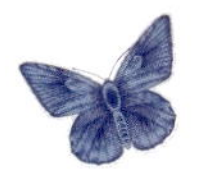

Breathing Meditation

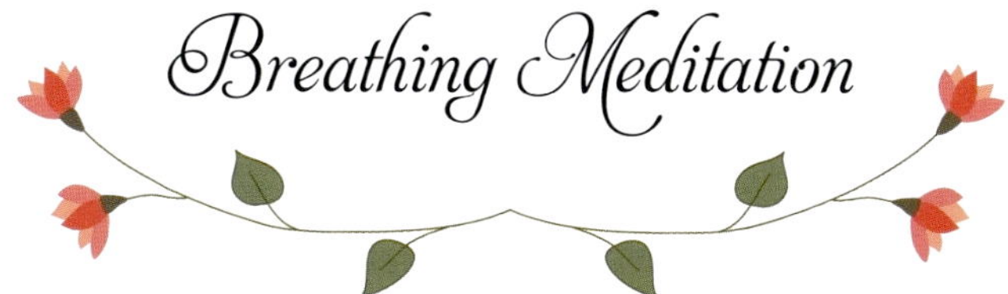

Meditative breathing is a great entry point for a meditation beginner. It's a challenge to practice, but it's simple to learn. Breath exercises can be just part of a larger practice, such as Vipassana or Zazen. They can also be the whole heart and soul of a practice.

Time

The length of your breathing practice depends on the method you use and what you're using it for.

Posture

You can sit or stand in a comfortable position, or hold another pose when doing a movement meditation.

Remember

Your mind will wander, and that's ok. That's part of what you're working on with this type of meditation. When your mind wanders or becomes fixed on a topic, acknowledge that it has. Then gently bring your attention back to your breath.

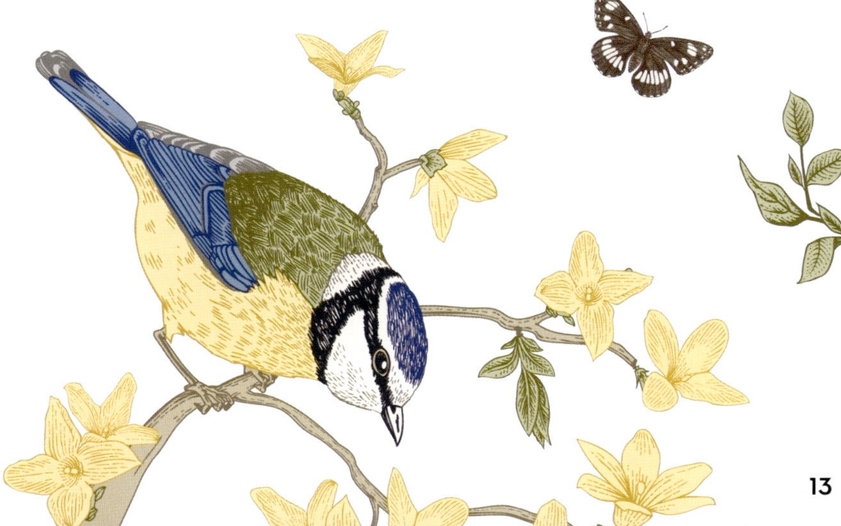

Breath Awareness

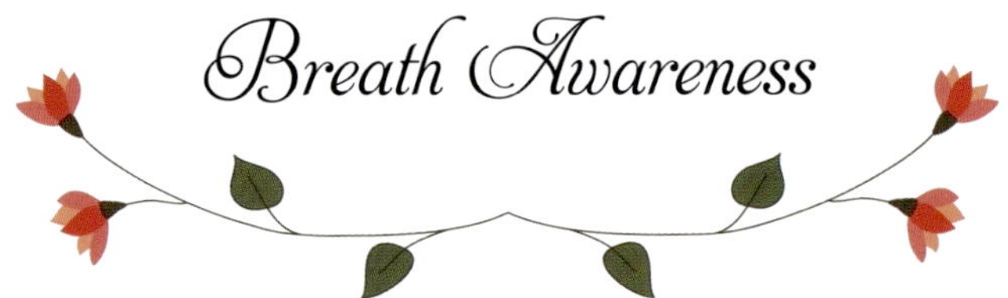

Spend a few minutes with simple breath awareness to ground yourself before beginning another meditation practice, or spend a longer time with it as a mindfulness exercise.

All you have to do is bring your attention to your breath. Breathe naturally; there's no need to lengthen or shorten your inhales or exhales.

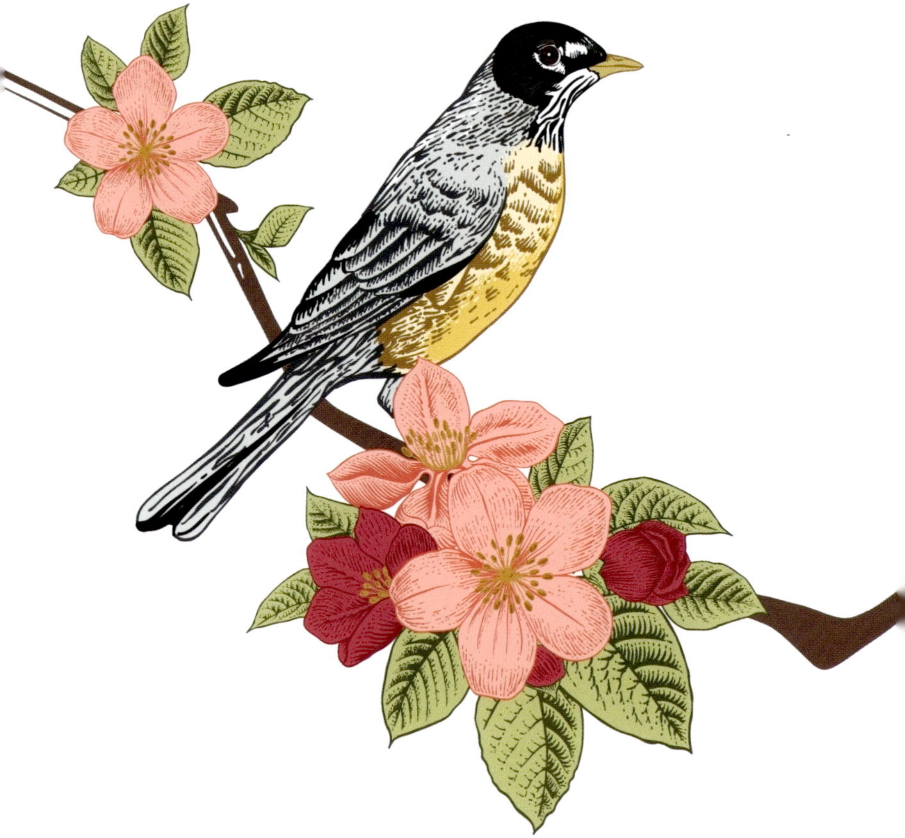

A bhikkhu, having gone to the forest, or to the foot of a tree, or to an empty, solitary place, sits down cross-legged, keeping his body erect, and directs his mindfulness. Then only with keen mindfulness he breathes in and only with keen mindfulness he breathes out. Breathing in a long breath, he knows, "I breathe in a long breath"; breathing out a long breath, he knows, "I breathe out a long breath"; breathing in a short breath, he knows, "I breathe in a short breath"; breathing out a short breath, he knows, "I breathe out a short breath."

—Gautama Buddha

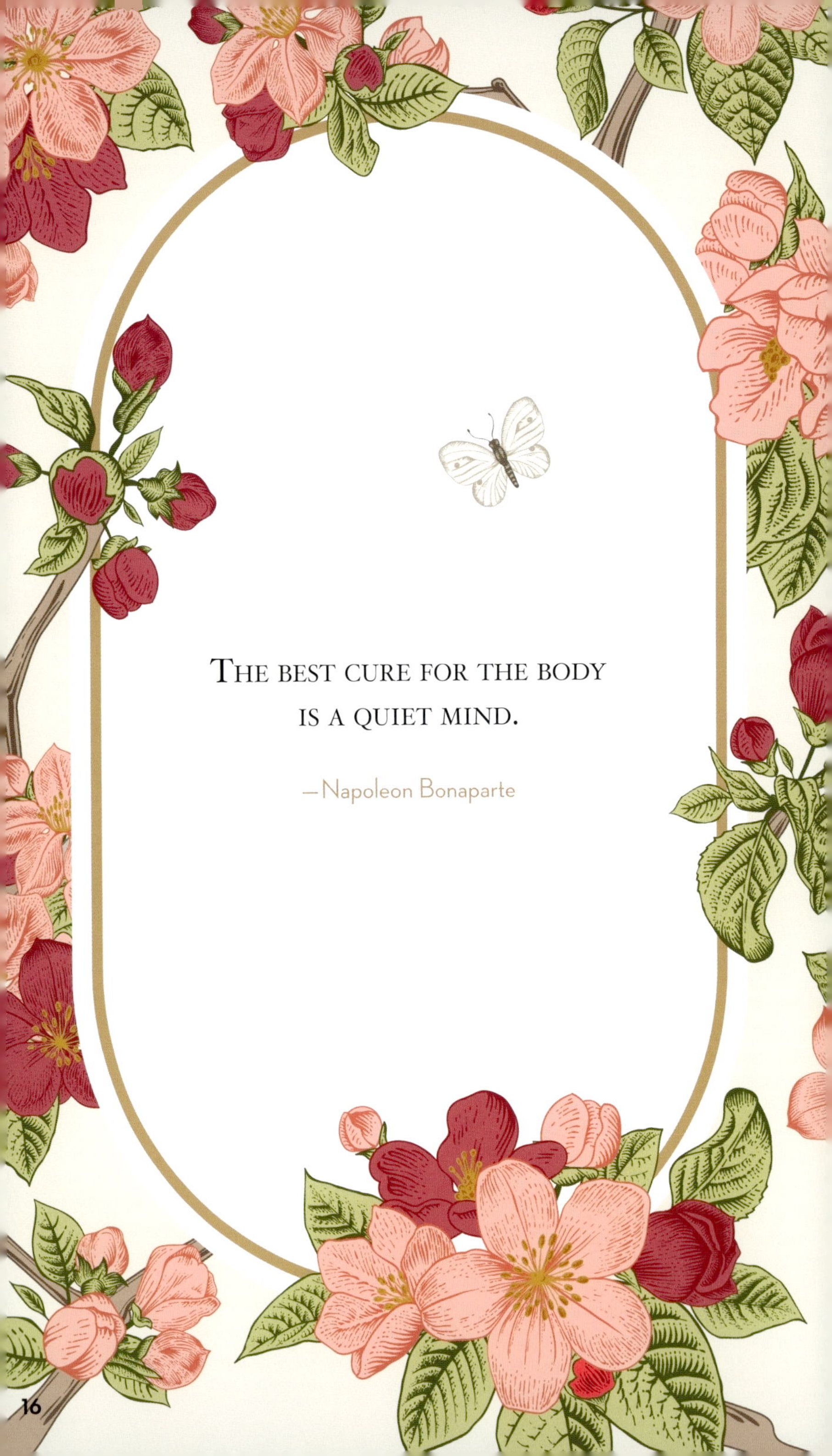

THE BEST CURE FOR THE BODY
IS A QUIET MIND.

—Napoleon Bonaparte

Belly Breathing

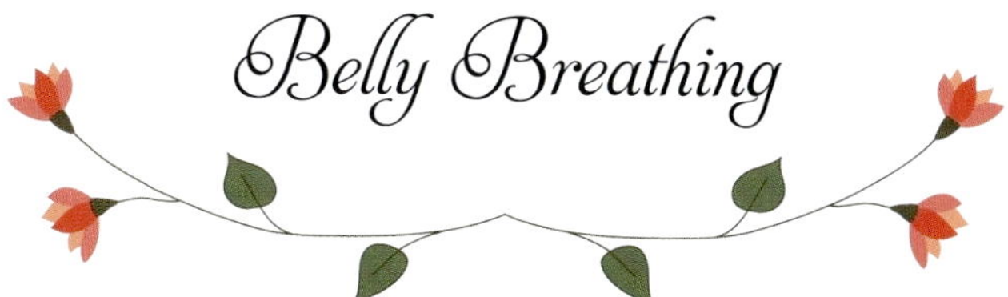

This is a good technique to use throughout your practice. It involves deliberate control of your diaphragm, the muscle located just below the lungs. Contracting the diaphragm makes space for the lungs to expand and take in air. The diaphragm relaxes as you exhale.

To prepare, place one palm flat against your chest. Place the other palm just below your ribs, the location of your diaphragm. Inhale slowly, letting your belly expand out as the diaphragm contracts. Your chest should remain more or less unchanged. Then exhale slowly. Let your belly come back down as the diaphragm relaxes. Again, your chest should remain more or less unchanged.

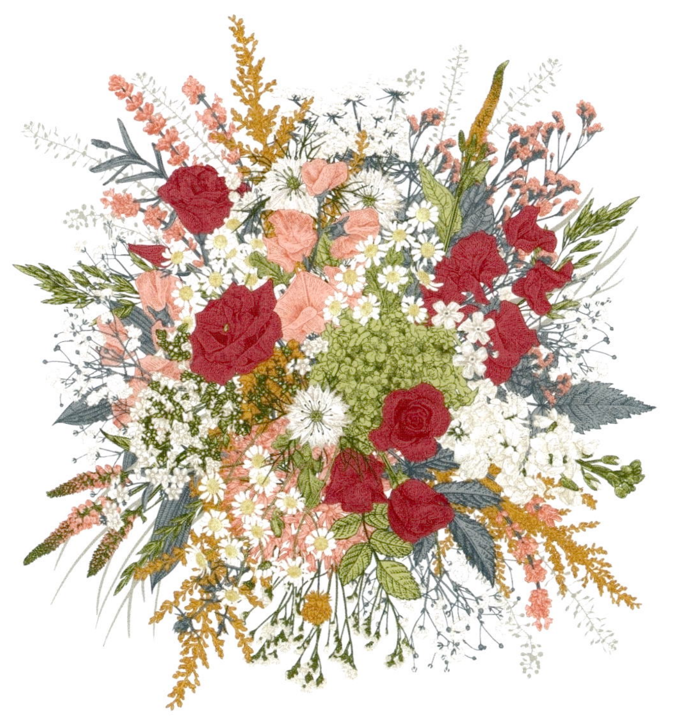

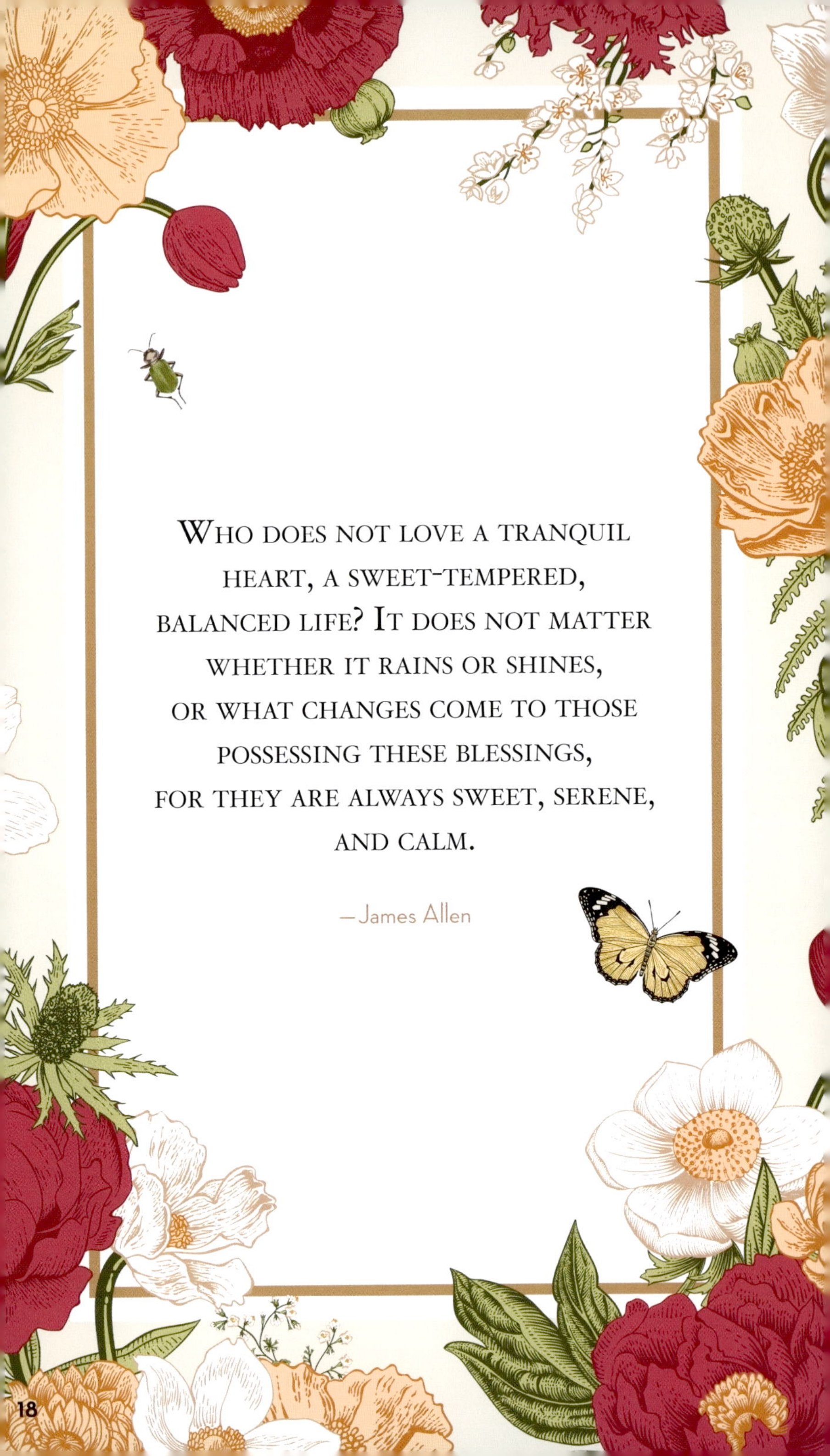

WHO DOES NOT LOVE A TRANQUIL HEART, A SWEET-TEMPERED, BALANCED LIFE? IT DOES NOT MATTER WHETHER IT RAINS OR SHINES, OR WHAT CHANGES COME TO THOSE POSSESSING THESE BLESSINGS, FOR THEY ARE ALWAYS SWEET, SERENE, AND CALM.

—James Allen

Breath Counting

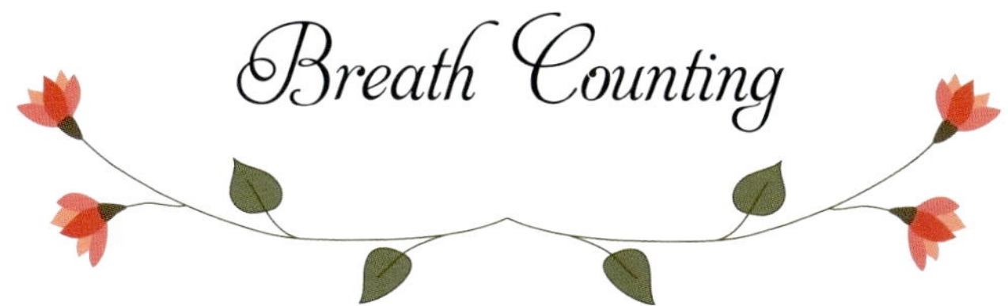

Use this to help ground yourself if your mind has been wandering uncontrollably during a meditation session, or if you just need a moment of focus and clarity during the day.

Count each inhale and exhale (inhale 1, exhale 2, inhale 3, exhale 4, and so on) until you reach 6. Then start again from 1.

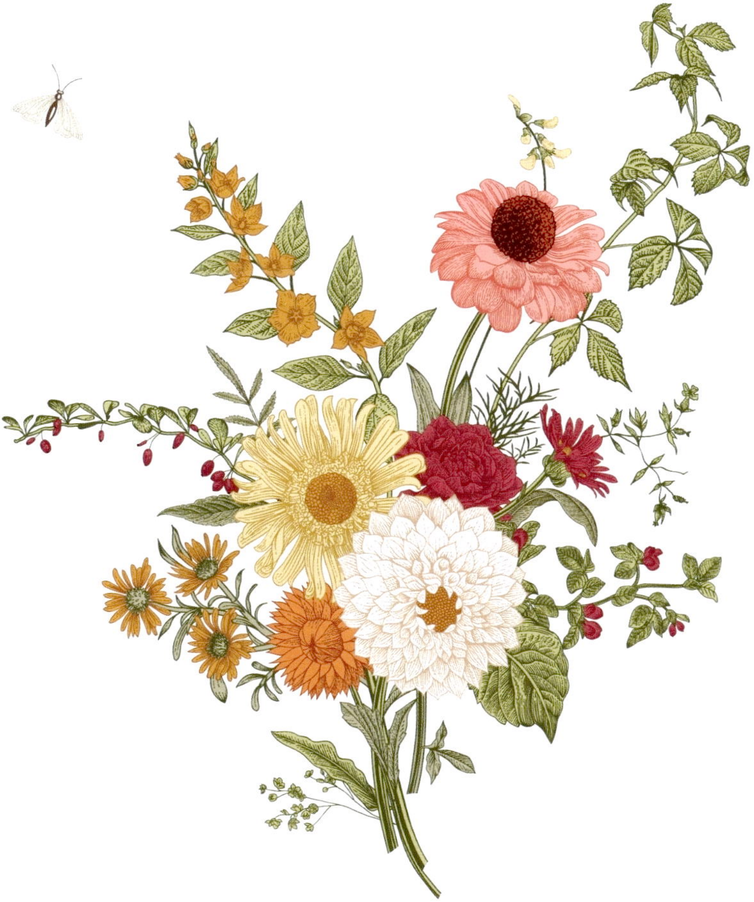

WE MUST TRY TO KEEP THE MIND IN TRANQUILITY. FOR JUST AS THE EYE WHICH CONSTANTLY SHIFTS ITS GAZE, NOW TURNING TO THE RIGHT OR TO THE LEFT, NOW INCESSANTLY PEERING UP AND DOWN, CANNOT SEE DISTINCTLY WHAT LIES BEFORE IT, BUT THE SIGHT MUST BE FIXED FIRMLY ON THE OBJECT IN VIEW IF ONE WOULD MAKE HIS VISION OF IT CLEAR, SO TOO MAN'S MIND WHEN DISTRACTED BY HIS COUNTLESS WORLDLY CARES CANNOT FOCUS ITSELF DISTINCTLY ON THE TRUTH.

—Basil of Caesarea

4-7-8 Breathing

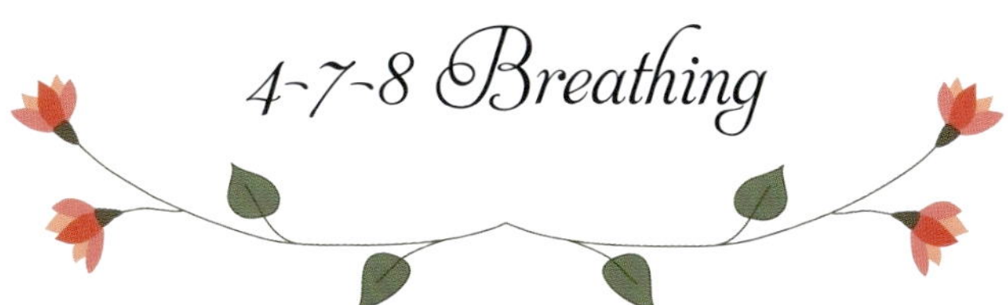

A few cycles of this exercise can help calm your nerves. Some insomniacs also find it helps them fall asleep.

Inhale through your nose for a count of 4, filling your lungs. Pause for a count of 7. Exhale through your mouth for a count of 8, emptying your lungs. Then repeat the cycle.

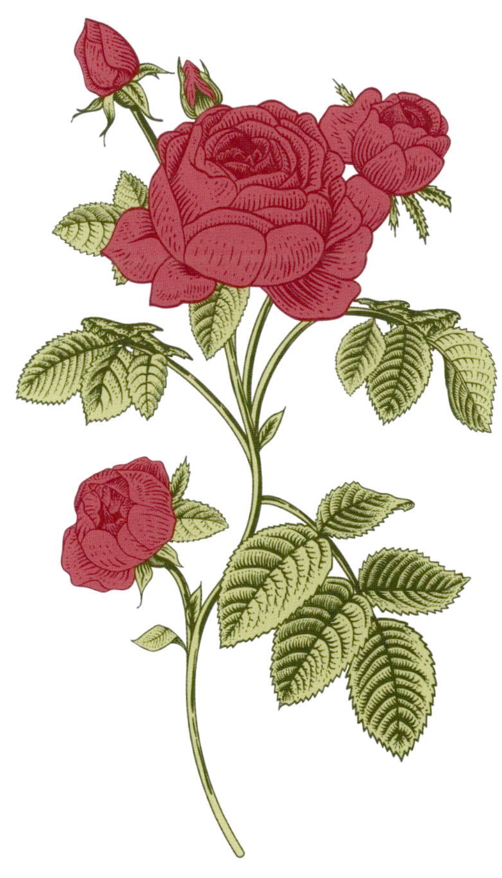

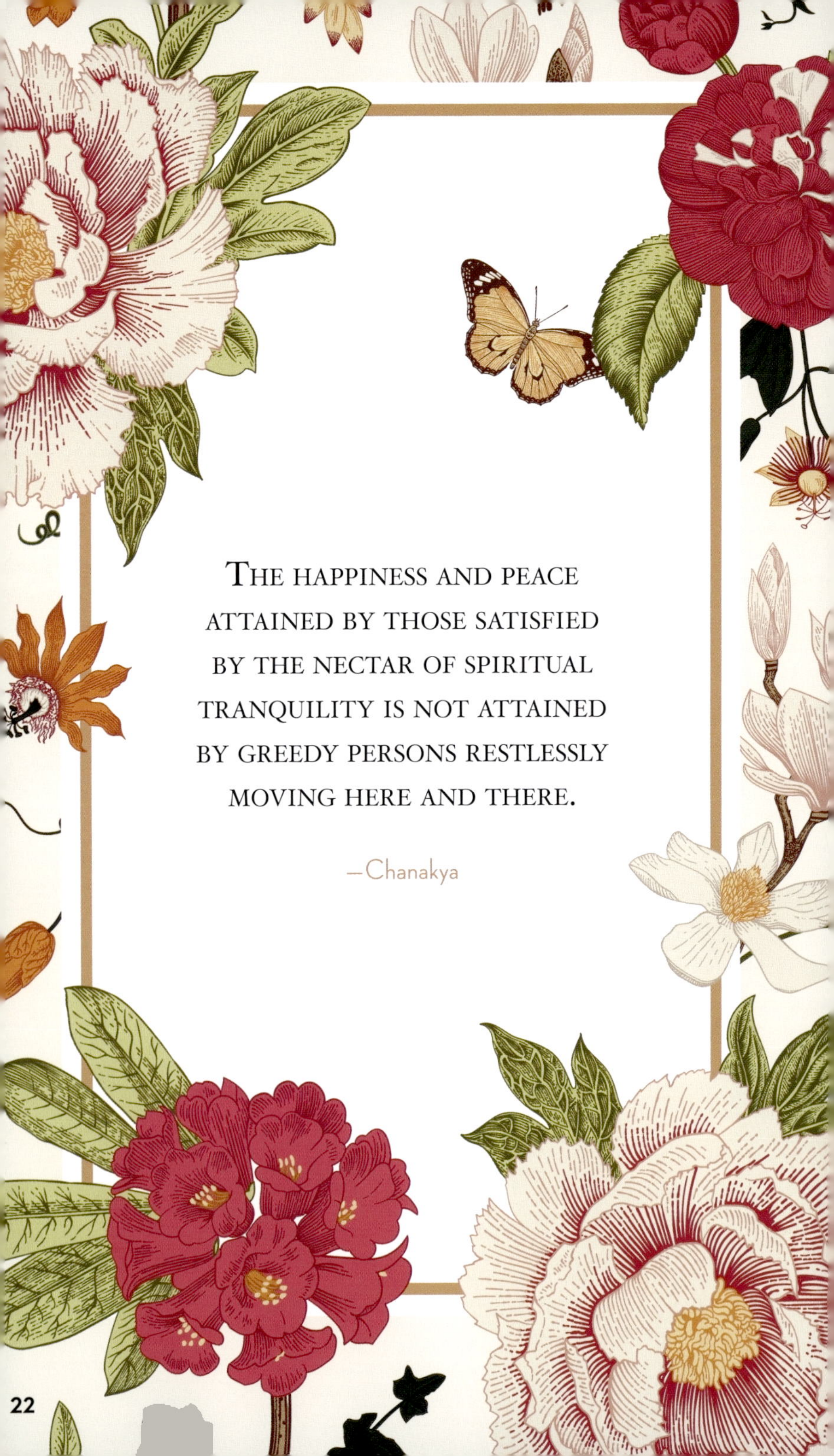

THE HAPPINESS AND PEACE ATTAINED BY THOSE SATISFIED BY THE NECTAR OF SPIRITUAL TRANQUILITY IS NOT ATTAINED BY GREEDY PERSONS RESTLESSLY MOVING HERE AND THERE.

—Chanakya

4-Count Breathing

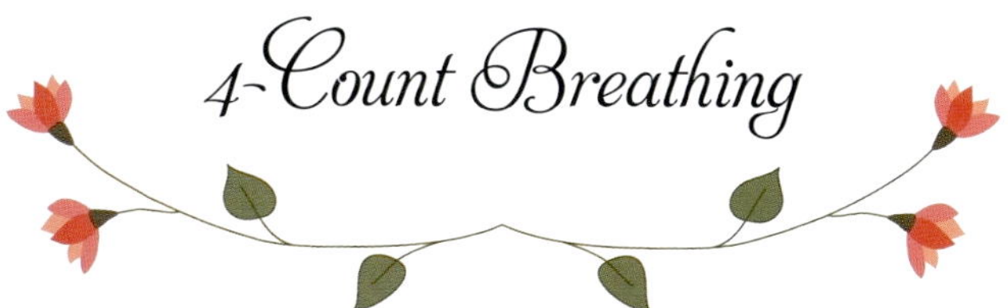

Use this exercise as a stand-alone meditation or as part of a larger practice.

Inhale for a count of 4. Pause for a count of 4. Exhale for a count of 4. Pause for a count of 4. Then repeat the cycle.

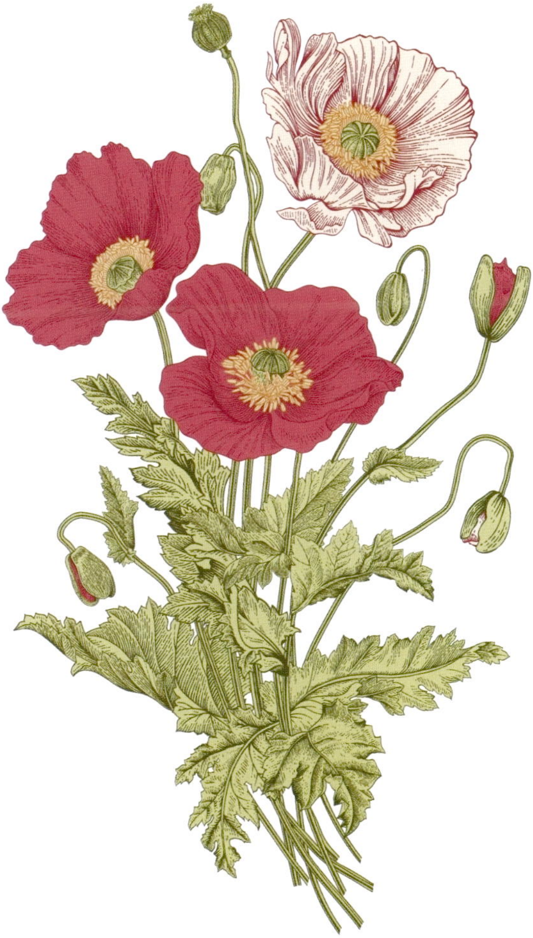

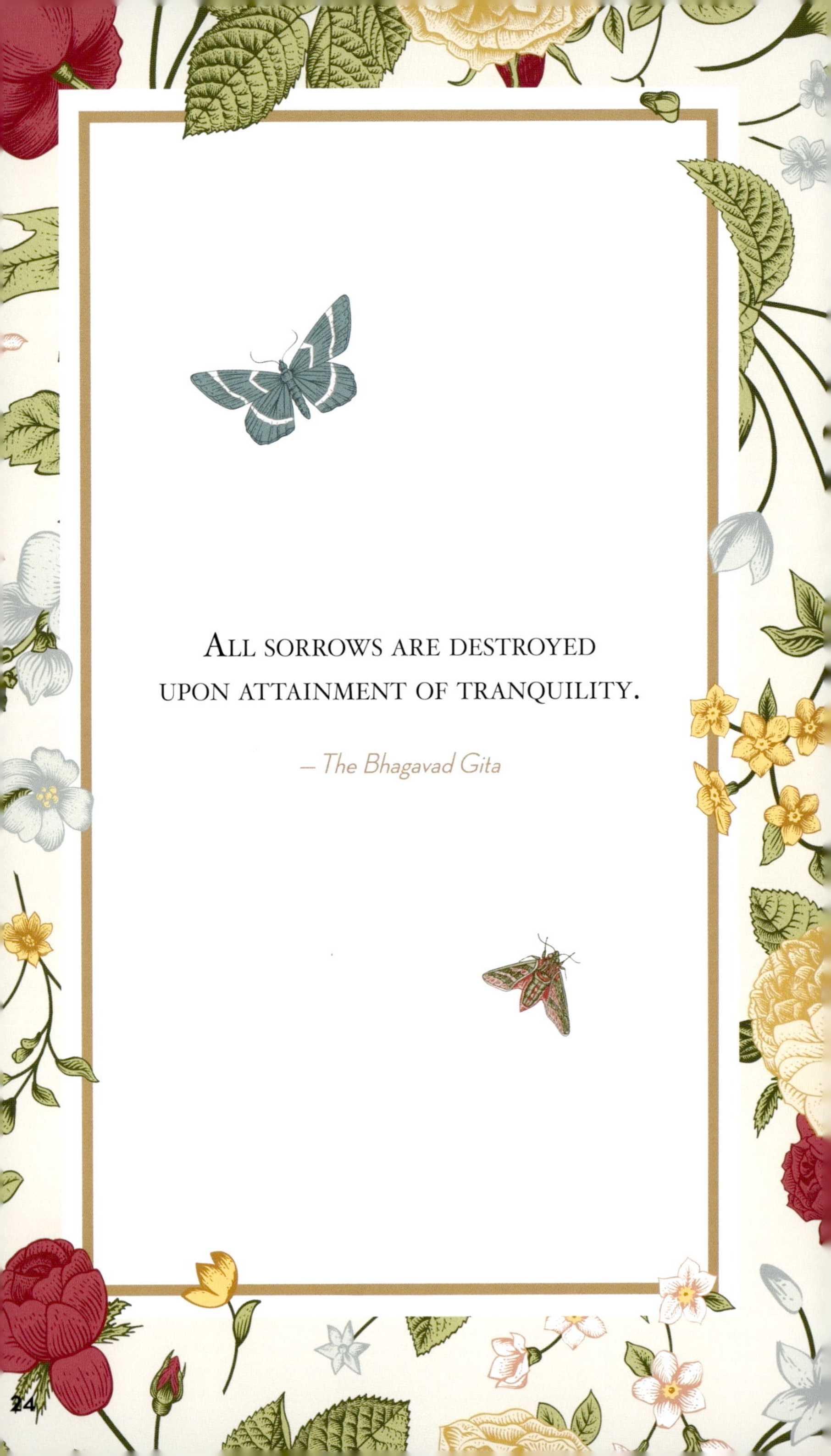

All sorrows are destroyed upon attainment of tranquility.

— The Bhagavad Gita

Bellows Breath

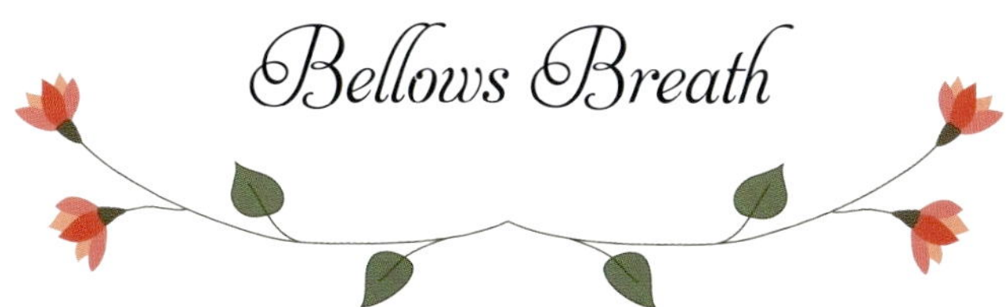

Bring energy to your body and alertness to your mind with this stimulating technique. Start small with this exercise, with each inhale/exhale cycle lasting a full second. Increase the speed of the cycles gradually, as your comfort allows.

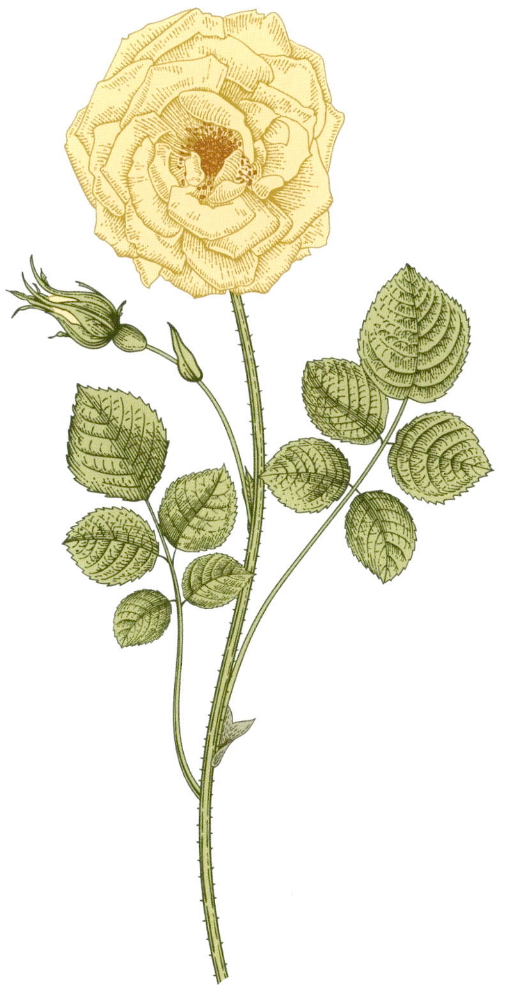

Step 1

Inhale and exhale sharply through the nose in quick succession for 10 seconds. Breathe from the diaphragm, as in belly breathing.

Step 2

Rest for 30 seconds, breathing naturally.

Step 3

Return to your quick bellows breath for 20 seconds. Then rest for another 30 seconds.

Step 4

Return to bellows breath for 30 seconds. Then breathe naturally.

Vipassana

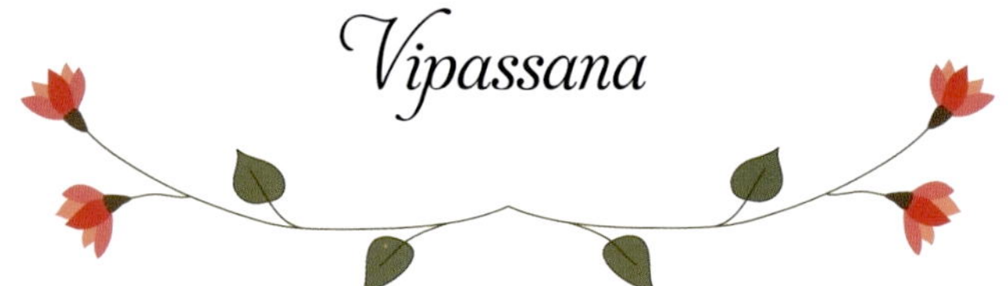

Vipassana is the oldest form of meditation in Buddhism, and over the millennia it has spread from India to the world. The word *vipassana* can be roughly translated as, "to see into something clearly," or "to see in a special way." Many people have used the rough English translation of "insight," which describes the driving intention of the meditation. Practicing Vipassana is meant to help you reach balance within yourself and understand the true nature of reality. You build this awareness and understanding up over the course of years.

Vipassana can be described as both gentle and thorough, as it gradually and patiently strives toward full-awareness of yourself, the world, and reality in general. The practice uses elements of mindfulness, noting, and breathing meditations to do this.

Time

As a beginner, you can start with 5 or 10 minutes. As you become more comfortable, you can extend that time. Some people practice Vipassana for hours, and meditation retreats lasting more than a week are found in many places.

Posture

Sit in a comfortable position. Legs may be crossed or in a lotus position if you're on the floor or a cushion. If you're sitting in a chair, position yourself so your feet are flat on the floor if you can. Support yourself with cushions behind your back, under your knees, or elsewhere as needed. Keep your back comfortably straight, eyes closed.

REMEMBER

Your mind will wander, and that's ok. When it wanders, acknowledge that it has. Then gently bring your attention back to the breath.

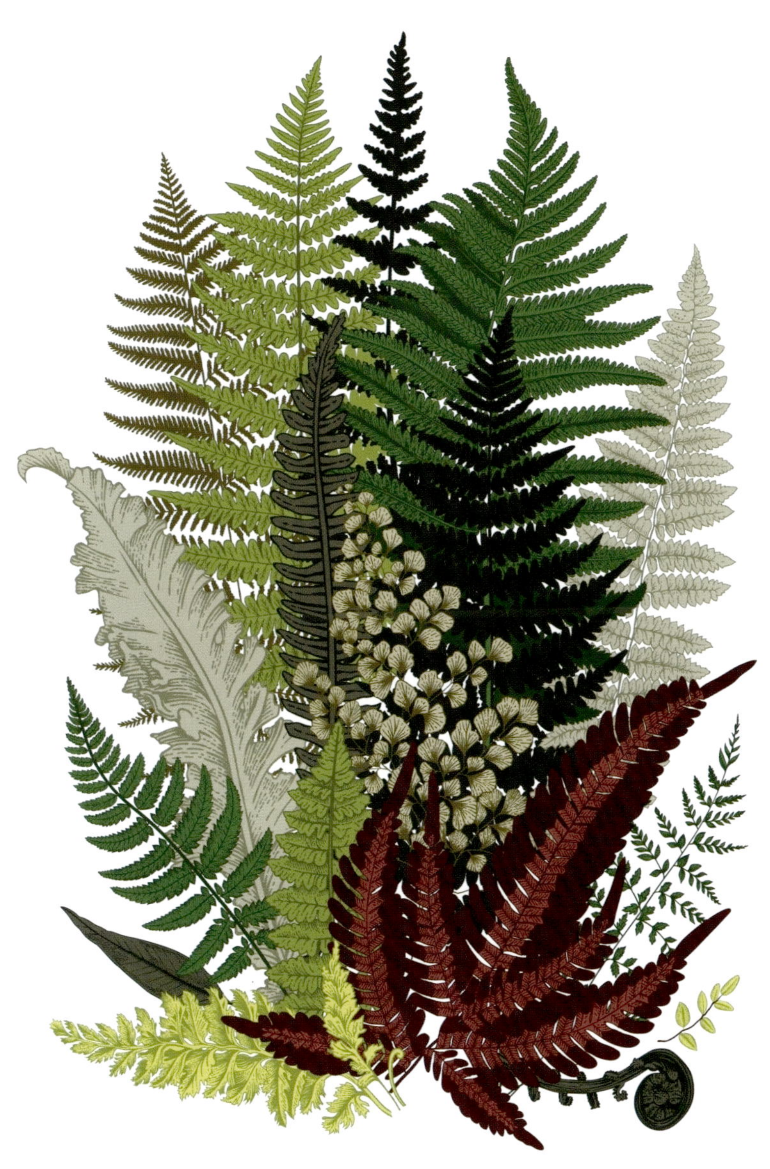

Step 1

Take a few deep breaths to ground yourself. Then return to normal breathing.

Step 2

Bring your focus to the feeling of the air as it moves through your nostrils with each inhale and exhale.

Step 3

Move your attention to your abdomen, feeling the belly move out as you inhale, and in as you exhale. If it helps, repeat "rising" in your mind as you inhale, and "falling" as you exhale.

Step 4

Note any sounds, smells, tastes, or physical sensations you experience. Label your experience of them ("hearing," "smelling," "tasting," "touching") and let them go.

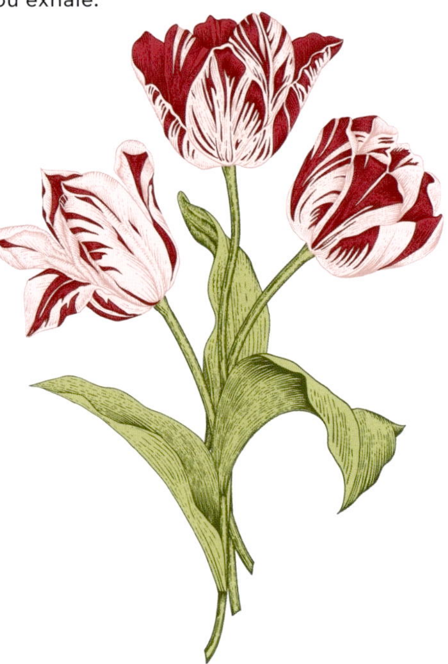

Step 5

As thoughts and emotions come up, note that you are "thinking," "feeling," then let them go.

If you can empty your
mind of all thoughts
your heart will embrace the
tranquility of peace.
Watch the workings of
all of creation,
but contemplate their
return to the source.
All creatures in the universe
return to the point where
they began. Returning to
the source is tranquility
because we submit to Heaven's
mandate. Returning to
Heaven's mandate is called being
constant. Knowing the constant
is called "enlightenment."

—Lao-tzu

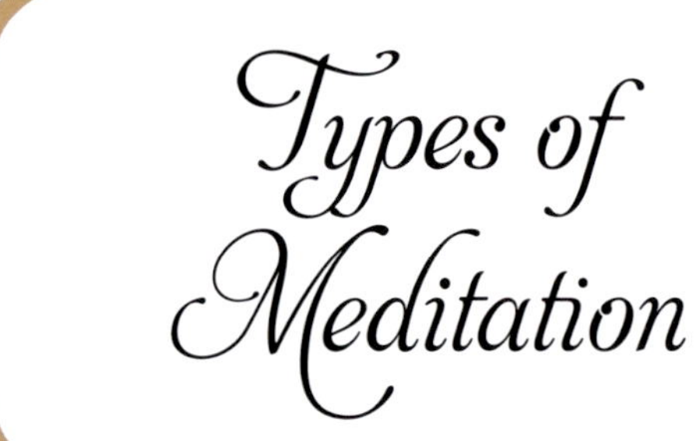

Types of Meditation

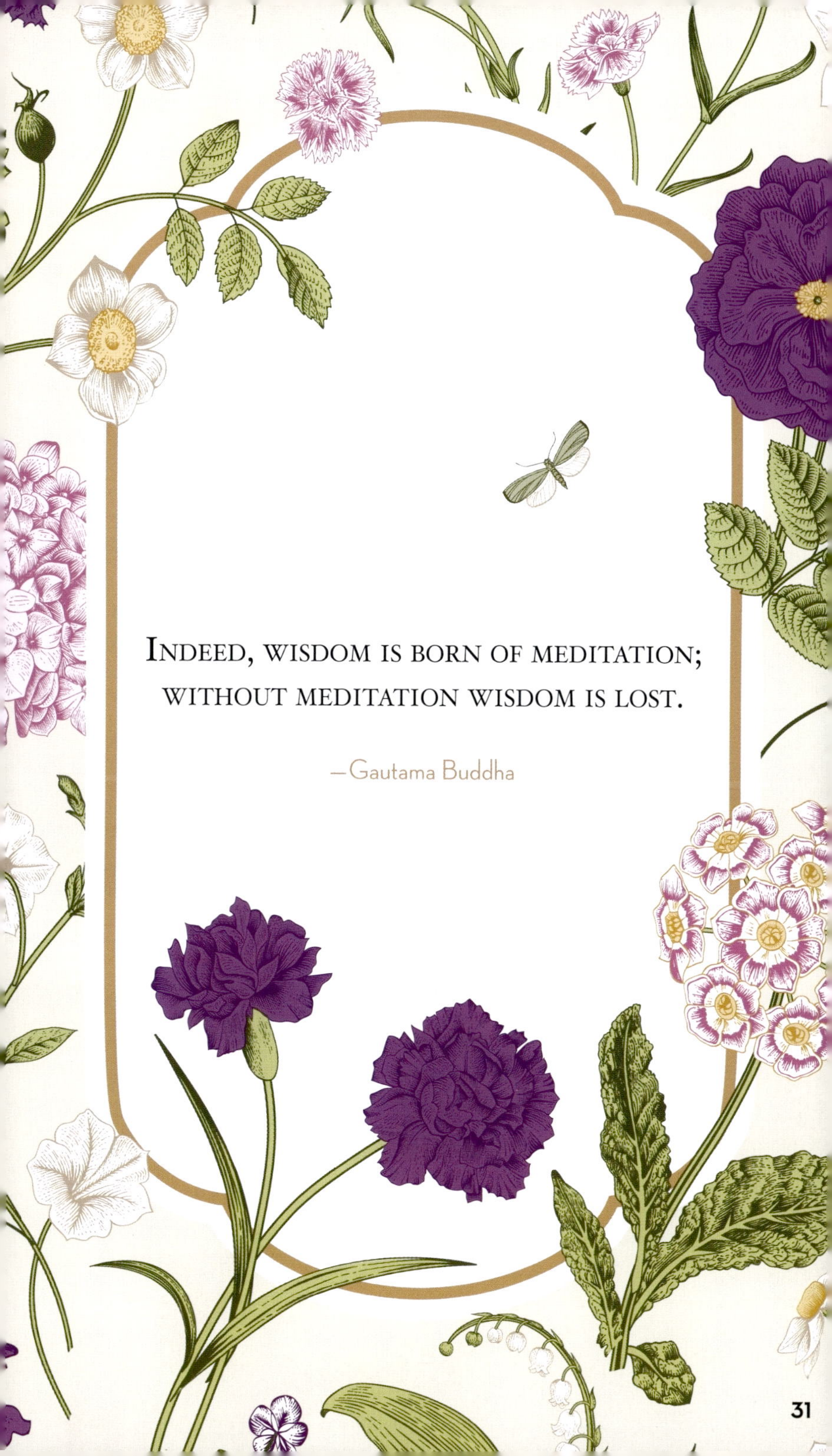

Indeed, wisdom is born of meditation;
without meditation wisdom is lost.

—Gautama Buddha

Meditation Guidelines

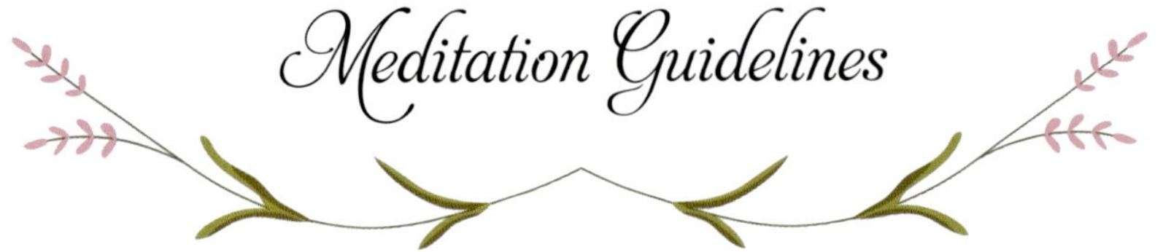

As simple as meditation sometimes seems, putting it into practice can be a challenge. Keep the ideas below in mind as you begin your practice. They can help make the start a little easier. The goal of meditation is simple and singular: to meditate. That's it. There is no need to worry about anything else as you practice.

Meditation does not need to be perfect. It is continual practice. Everyone has easier days and more difficult days. Be kind to yourself—to try is really to succeed. Your mind will wander. When it does, take a moment to notice what it is that has distracted you. Then gently bring your attention back to the focus of your meditation. Let thoughts and emotions come and go. Don't try to suppress or remove them. Acknowledge them when they appear, and then let them go.

Wear comfortable clothing. Yoga leggings or loose pants, fitted tank or oversized sweater—whatever keeps you comfortable, wear that. Soft fabrics are a good idea, as are outfits that allow freedom of movement. No method works for everyone. Each of us has a unique brain and body. Find what works for your brain and body. Experiment and explore to discover what is best for you.

Decide how long you want to meditate before you begin. Start small, perhaps with a 3- to 4-minute meditation. As you become more comfortable with the practice, you can increase the time. A timer can make a huge difference. You don't want to keep breaking your concentration to look at your watch. Set an alarm on your phone or even use an egg timer.

Make meditation a routine. As much as possible, meditate at the same time and in the same place each time you practice. This makes it easier to keep the practice up over time. How often you meditate matters more than how long you meditate. Set aside time to practice at least a couple of days a week. Work toward practicing every day if you can, even if it's only for a few minutes at a time.

Meditation involves your entire self, positive and negative. Difficult emotions surface as easily as positive ones. If you have trouble with negative thoughts as you meditate, perhaps try talking with a professional who is either a counselor or an expert in that form of meditation.

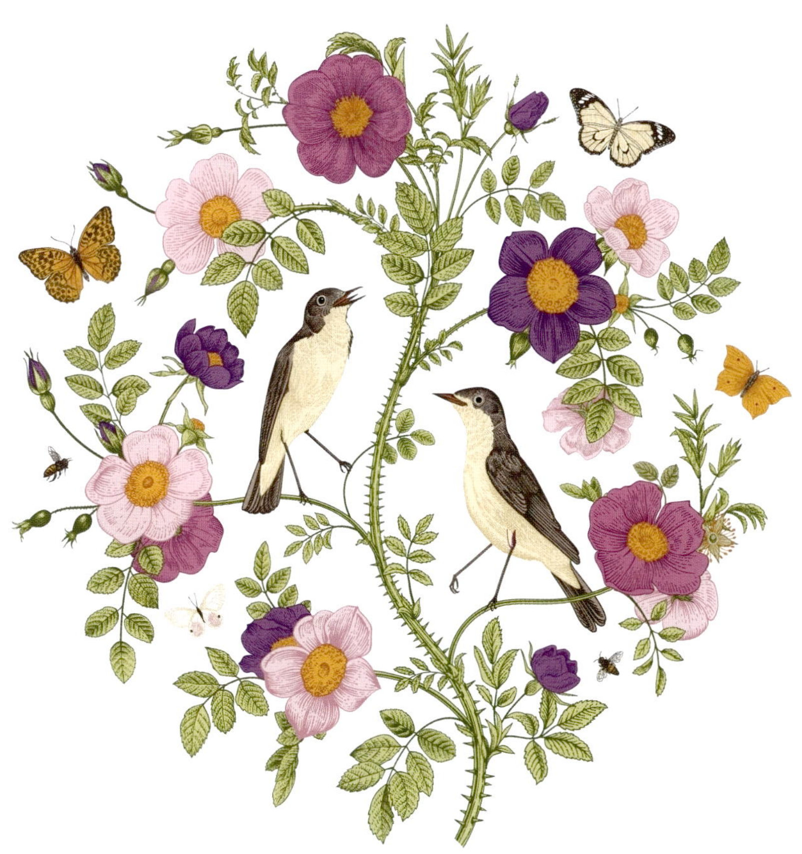

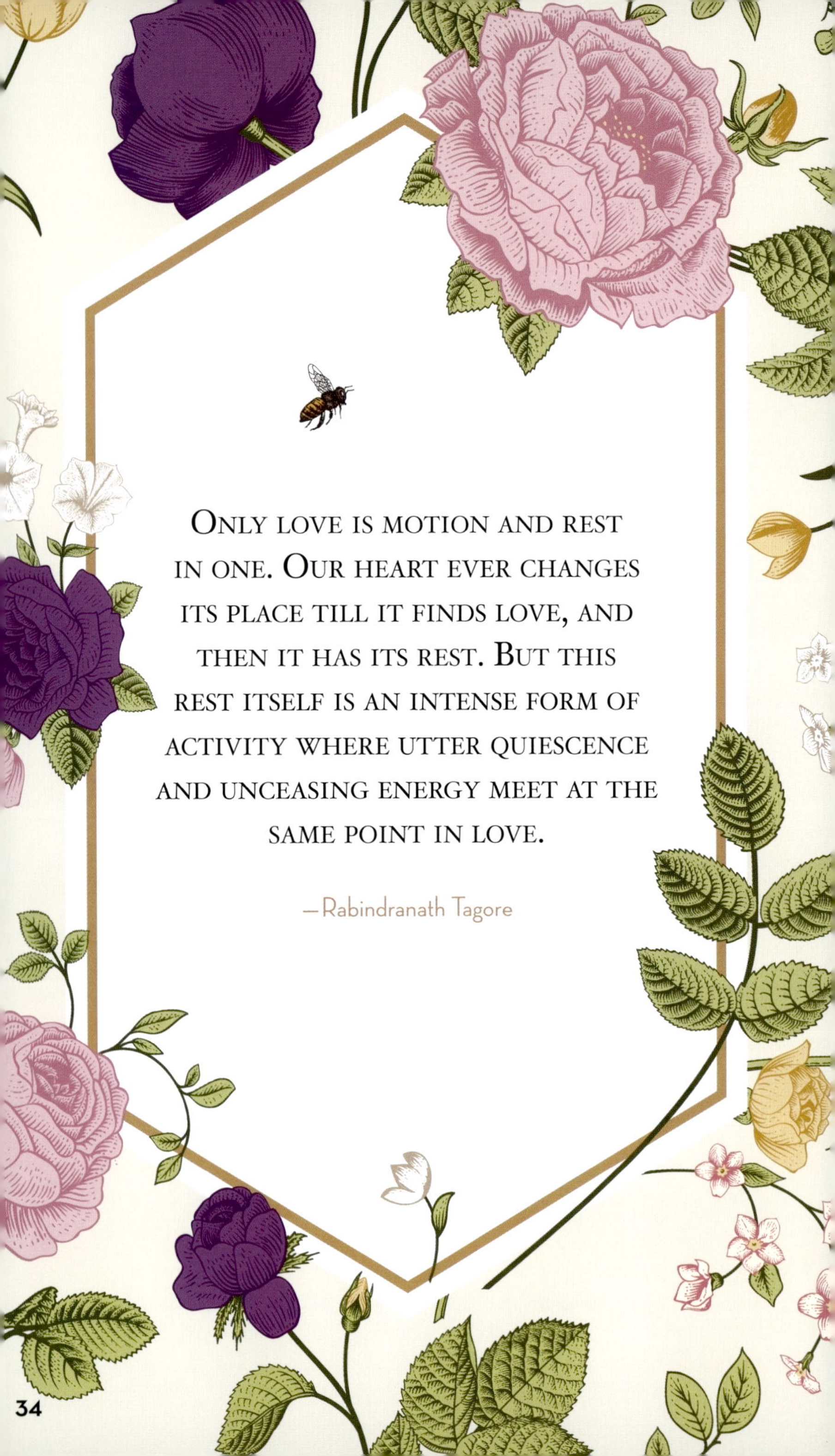

Only love is motion and rest in one. Our heart ever changes its place till it finds love, and then it has its rest. But this rest itself is an intense form of activity where utter quiescence and unceasing energy meet at the same point in love.

—Rabindranath Tagore

Scents and Senses

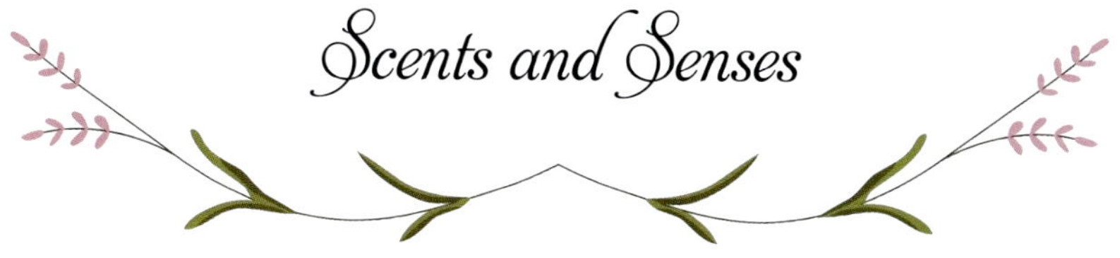

A scent can affect your mood, even when you're not consciously paying attention to it. With this in mind, you can change the atmosphere of your meditation space dramatically by adding certain scents. Incense, essential oils, candles, and a variety of other sources are just a few examples of how to accomplish this.

Neroli

A product of bitter orange blossoms, neroli oil is used to inspire cheerfulness, enthusiasm, mental clarity, and creativity.

Benzoin

The scent, produced by benzoin resin, can produce a feeling of stability, comfort, and groundedness.

Cardamom

Cardamom's spicy smell is known to increase blood flow to the brain. It can also bring greater alertness, clarity, self-worth, and inspiration.

Cedarwood

This scent actually comes from a juniper tree, not cedar. Its scent can help a person access inner strength and self-reliance, as well as better judgement skills.

Bitter Orange

While bitter orange flowers produce neroli, the fruit's rind produces bitter orange oil. This and other citrus scents are uplifting, and they can bring relaxation and patience.

Vetiver

This comes from vetiver grass. Its scent combats mental fatigue and anxiety. It can also improve a person's breathing during sleep.

Lavender

The flowers of the lavender plant are as pleasing to the eye as they are to the nose. Lavender is well-known for its relaxing smell.

Sandalwood

The sandalwood tree produces a heady-scented wood. The smell can reduce anxiety even as it increases alertness.

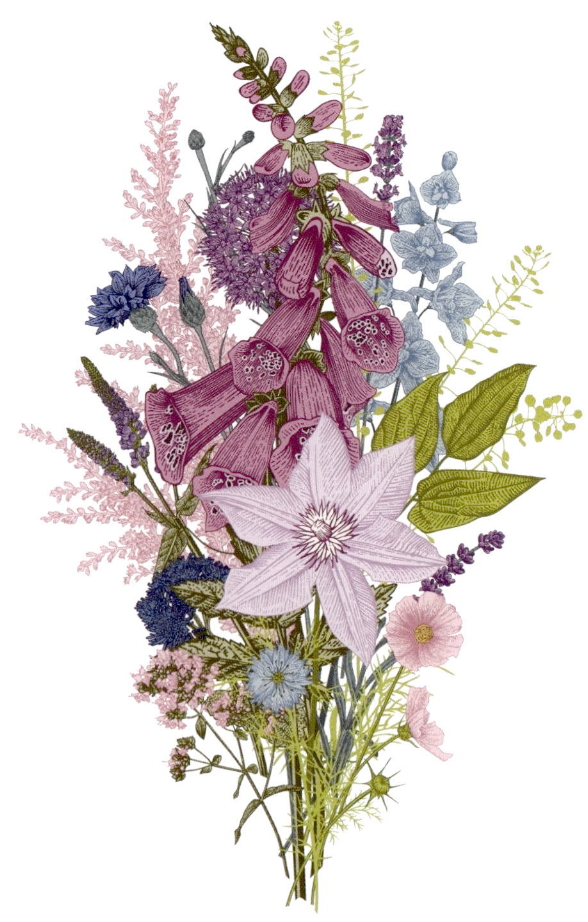

Sweet oil,
the fragrance of the gods.

—Lahar

Body Scan Meditation

Body scan meditation is a kind of mindfulness with razor-sharp focus on the body. Emotions—from anxiety to fear to joy—have physical symptoms. Delight can make us feel lighter, deep sadness can cause tightness in the chest, and stress can be a literal pain in the neck. With a body scan, you take stock of these symptoms and the emotions behind them.

The intent of this meditation is simply to notice, not to judge. In the words of Paul McCartney, let it be.

Time

A thorough body scan can take as long as 45 minutes. If you're pressed for time, you can try a quick 5-minute or 10-minute scan instead.

Posture

Because it can take awhile to complete a body scan, make sure you're comfortable. Most people lie down. Pillows under the knees, neck, or upper back can help reduce pain and keep your body relaxed. If you're worried about falling asleep, you can sit up on a cushion or a chair.

Remember

Your mind will wander, and that's ok. When it does, acknowledge that it has, then gently bring your attention back to the part of your body where you left off.

Step 1
Take a few deep breaths. Breathe in through the nose and out through the mouth.

Step 2
Notice the heaviness of your body. Where does your body come in contact with the floor, bed, or other object beneath you? Feel the pressure at those points.

Step 3
Bring your attention to one toe. Notice every physical sensation you're experiencing with that toe. Is it cold? Warm? Is there pressure or tightness of any kind? What else do you notice?

Step 4
Do the same to the next toe, then the next. When you've gone through all the toes, move on to the soles of your feet, the tops of your feet, your ankles, all the way up to the top of your head. When you reach a spot that is experiencing tension, breathe into that area. Feel your lungs fill as you inhale, and imagine the oxygen and energy passing through the muscles as you exhale, releasing the tension.

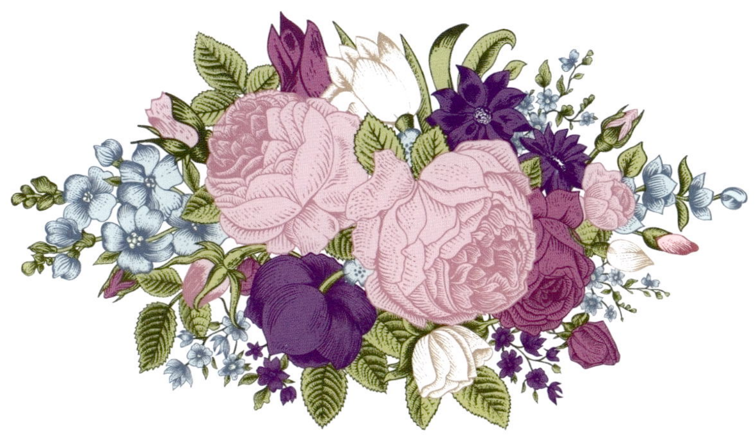

Chakra Meditation

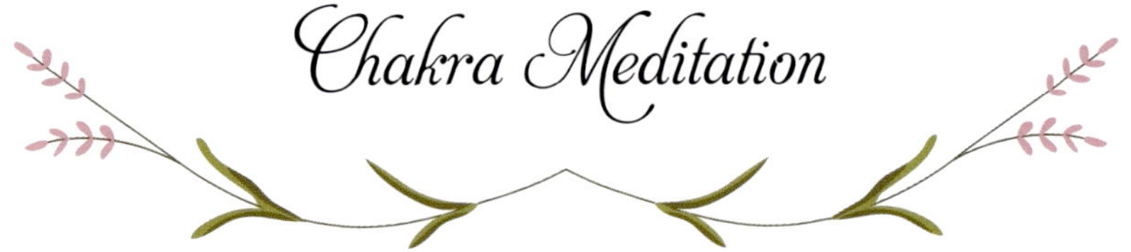

Chakra is Sanskrit for "wheel." Chakras are believed by some to be the points where the metaphysical self connects to the physical self. The chakras spin, moving energy through the body. When one or more chakras are blocked, others spin faster to compensate. This imbalance then causes difficulties.

Chakra meditation focuses on the seven most important chakras, which are located along the spine and at the top of your head. Some practitioners go through certain body postures, hand positions, and mantras as they meditate. Others—especially beginners—can simply stay seated.

Time

Beginners may have sessions lasting 10 to 15 minutes. More seasoned practitioners often meditate for at least 30 minutes.

Posture

Sit in a comfortable position. Legs may be crossed or in a lotus position if you're on the floor or a cushion. If you're sitting in a chair, position yourself so your feet are flat on the floor if you can. Support yourself with cushions behind your back, under your knees, or elsewhere as needed. Keep your back comfortably straight, gaze down or eyes closed.

Remember

Your mind will wander, and that's ok. When it wanders or becomes fixed on a topic, acknowledge that it has. Then gently bring your attention back to your visualization.

Step 1

Take a few deep breaths. Breathe in through the nose and out through the mouth.

Step 2

Bring your focus to your root chakra, located at the base of your spine. Visualize a ball of energy there, gently glowing red. Imagine your breath flowing into it, making it bigger and brighter.

Step 3

Move to your sacral chakra, just below the navel. Visualize a ball of orange energy. Breathe into it until it matches the size and brightness of your root chakra.

Step 4

Do the same with your solar plexus chakra in your abdomen, below your sternum (which glows yellow), heart (green), throat (blue), third eye (indigo), and finally the crown (violet or white).

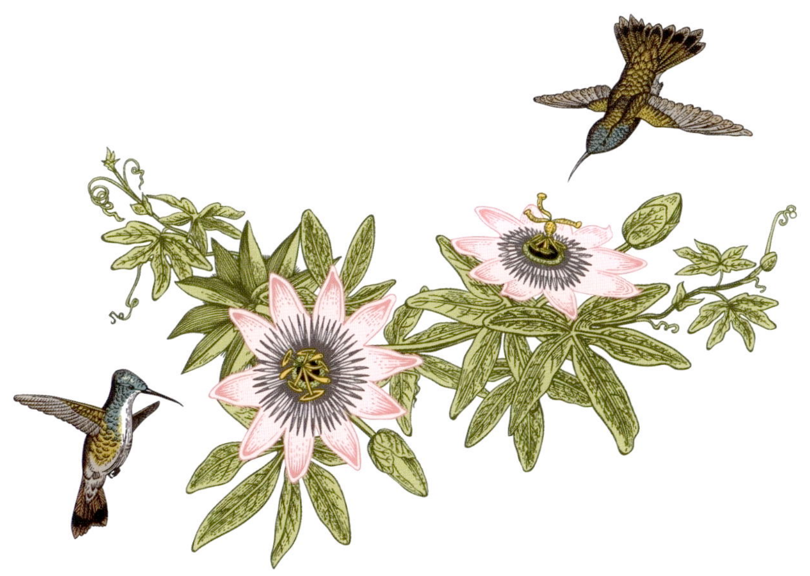

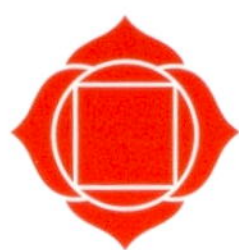

The first chakra is the root chakra, located at the base of the spine. Like the strong foundation of a pyramid, the root chakra represents stability and basic sustenance. Its color is red.

The second is the sacral chakra, named for its location above the sacrum. The sacrum is the largest vertebra and the one that connects with both sides of your pelvis. This chakra is orange and represents creativity as an integrated part of your mind and energy.

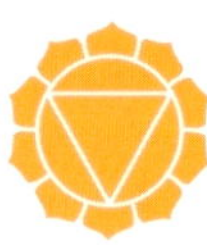

The third, the solar plexus chakra, is found below the sternum. It's named after the radiating cluster of nerves sometimes also called the celiac plexus. This chakra is yellow and associated with both physical digestion and the metaphorical digestion of new ideas.

The fourth, the heart chakra, is associated with circulation, but also with the understanding of the heart as the "emotional brain" of the body. This chakra is green.

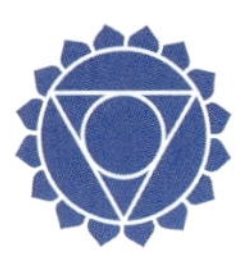

The fifth, the throat chakra, is associated with communication and with hormones because of its location among the thyroid, pituitary, and other glands. This chakra is blue.

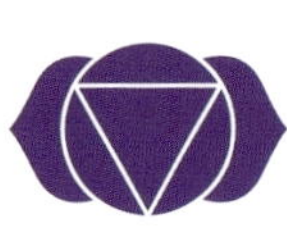

The sixth, the third eye chakra, is the most well-known chakra in the popular imagination. It represents insight, clarity, and intuition or psychic ability. A clear sixth chakra is said to allow you to see your place within the fabric of the universe. This chakra is indigo.

The seventh, the crown chakra, is both the top of the head and the upper limit of human existence. This chakra is violet.

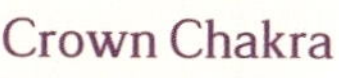
Crown Chakra

Third Eye Chakra

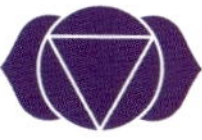

Throat Chakra

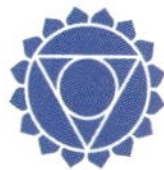

Heart Chakra

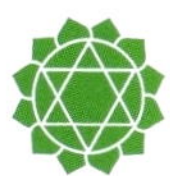

Solar Plexus Chakra

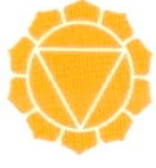

Sacral Chakra

Root Chakra

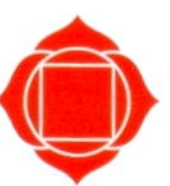

I TEACH NO MODE OF AWAKENING THE CENTRES, BECAUSE RIGHT IMPULSE, STEADY REACTION TO HIGHER IMPULSIONS, AND THE PRACTICAL RECOGNITION OF THE SOURCES OF INSPIRATION, WILL AUTOMATICALLY AND SAFELY SWING THE CENTRES INTO NEEDED AND APPROPRIATE ACTIVITY.

—Alice Bailey

Gazing Meditation

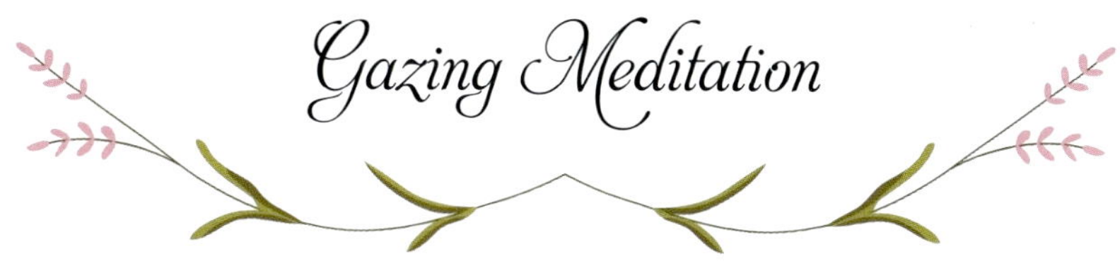

This practice is sometimes used in Hatha Yoga, where it's called Trataka, but gazing meditation is by no means limited to yogis. It's an excellent method to try if you have trouble keeping your mind focused in other forms of meditation. Gazing meditation involves focusing on a physical object in front of you, such as a candle.

Time

When you first try this meditation, start with 5 to 10 minutes. As you become more comfortable with the practice, you can increase the time.

Posture

Sit in a comfortable position. Legs may be crossed or in a lotus position if you're on the floor or a cushion. If you're sitting in a chair, position yourself so your feet are flat on the floor if you can. Support yourself with cushions behind your back, under your knees, or elsewhere as needed. Keep your back comfortably straight.

Remember

Your mind will wander, and that's ok. When it wanders or becomes fixed on a topic, acknowledge that it has. Then gently bring your attention back to the flame or other object of focus.

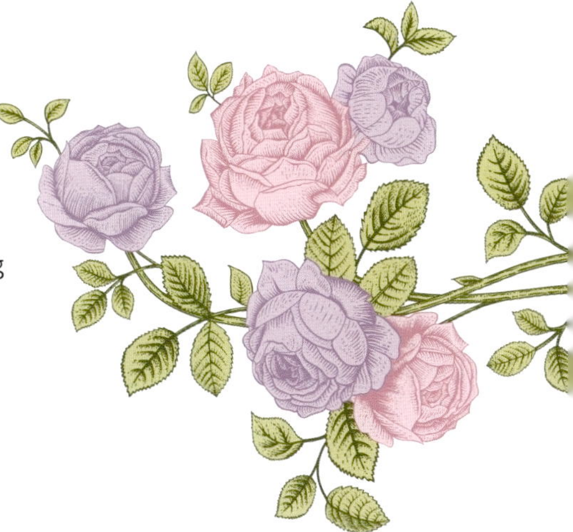

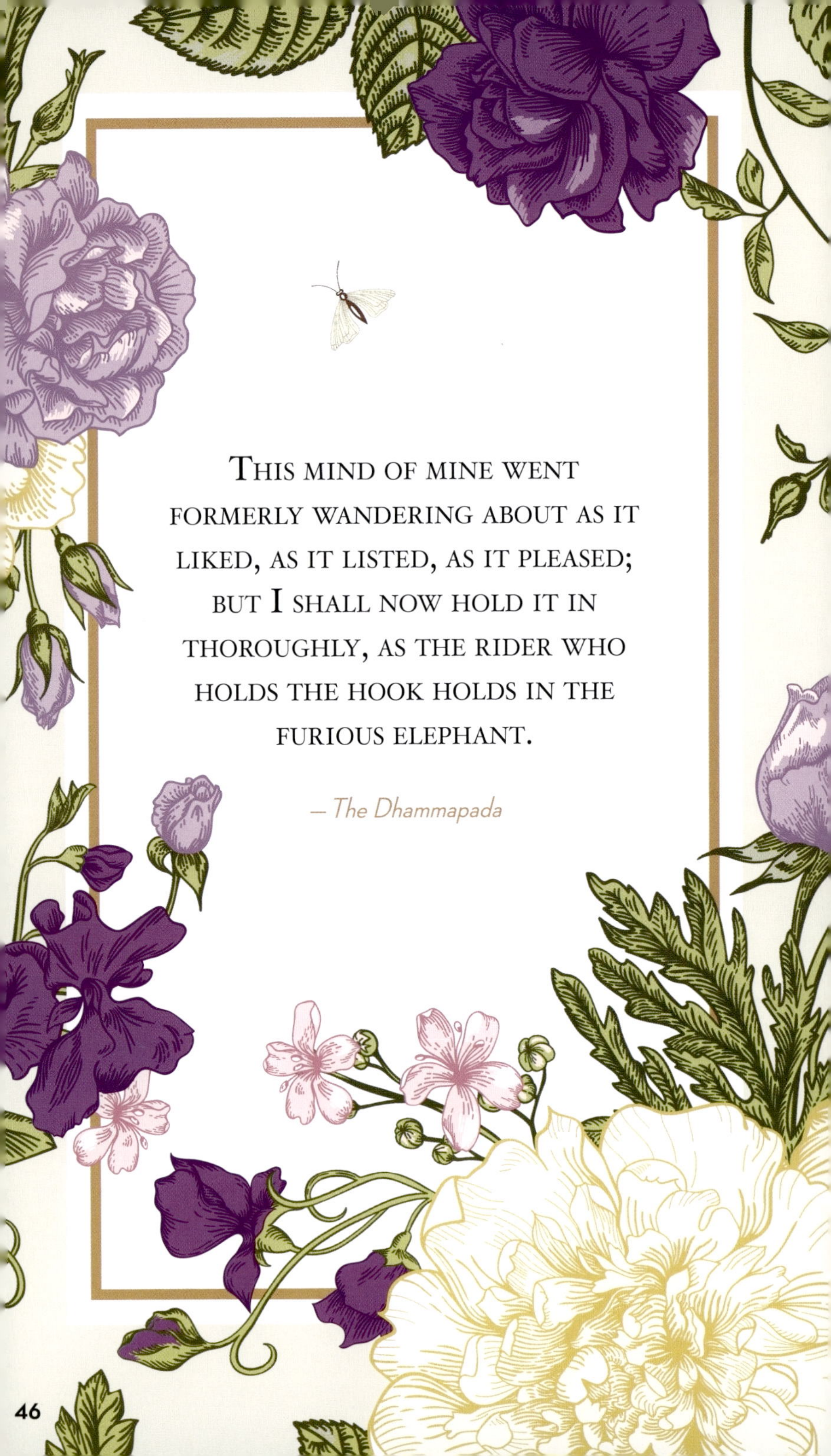

THIS MIND OF MINE WENT FORMERLY WANDERING ABOUT AS IT LIKED, AS IT LISTED, AS IT PLEASED; BUT I SHALL NOW HOLD IT IN THOROUGHLY, AS THE RIDER WHO HOLDS THE HOOK HOLDS IN THE FURIOUS ELEPHANT.

— The Dhammapada

Step 1
Place a candle on a level surface that is free of anything flammable. The candle should sit a couple of feet from you, at about eye level. Darken the room, if you wish to.

Step 2
Close your eyes and take a few deep breaths. Focus on each inhale and exhale. Then return to natural breathing.

Step 3
Open your eyes and focus on the candle's flame. Try to blink as little as possible. It helps to open your eyes a little wider than usual. If you notice the flame blurring in your vision, consciously bring it back into focus.

Step 4
If the eyes begin to feel strained, close them for a moment to let them rest. You can also cover your eyes with cupped hands. Then return to gazing at the flame.

Step 5
When you are ready, close your eyes and bring the image of the flame up in your mind's eye. Hold it there and concentrate on it, just as you did with your eyes open.

Step 6
If your mind becomes still and the mental image of the flame fades, you can let the image go and remain simply in stillness.

Heartbeat Meditation

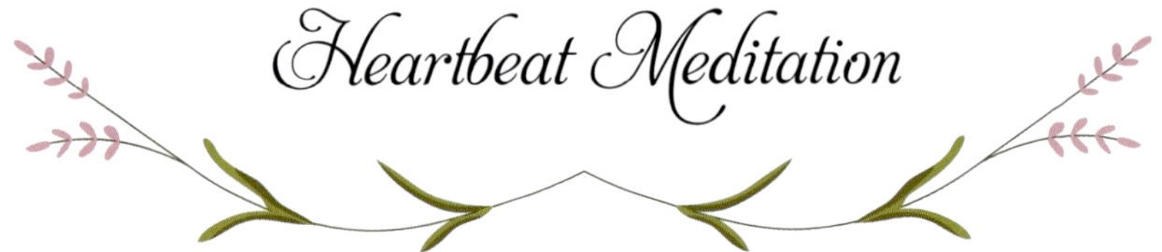

Meditating on your heartbeat brings your focus inward, and it can encourage calmness and clarity. The practice may also help increase empathy. Some people silently repeat a mantra during this meditation. The mantra is usually one or two syllables so it matches the double beat (ba-dum, ba-dum) of the heart. Kundalini yogis often use Sat Nam ("I am Truth," or "Truth is my essence"). "I am" is another choice.

Time

If you're just beginning with this meditation, start with a goal of 10 minutes. You can increase or decrease the time according to what is comfortable.

Posture

Sit in a comfortable position. Legs may be crossed or in a lotus position if you're on the floor or a cushion. If you're sitting in a chair, position yourself so your feet are flat on the floor if you can. Support yourself with cushions behind your back, under your knees, or elsewhere as needed. Keep your back comfortably straight, gaze down or eyes closed.

Remember

Your mind will wander, and that's ok. When it wanders or becomes fixed on a topic, acknowledge that it has. Then gently bring your attention back to your heartbeat.

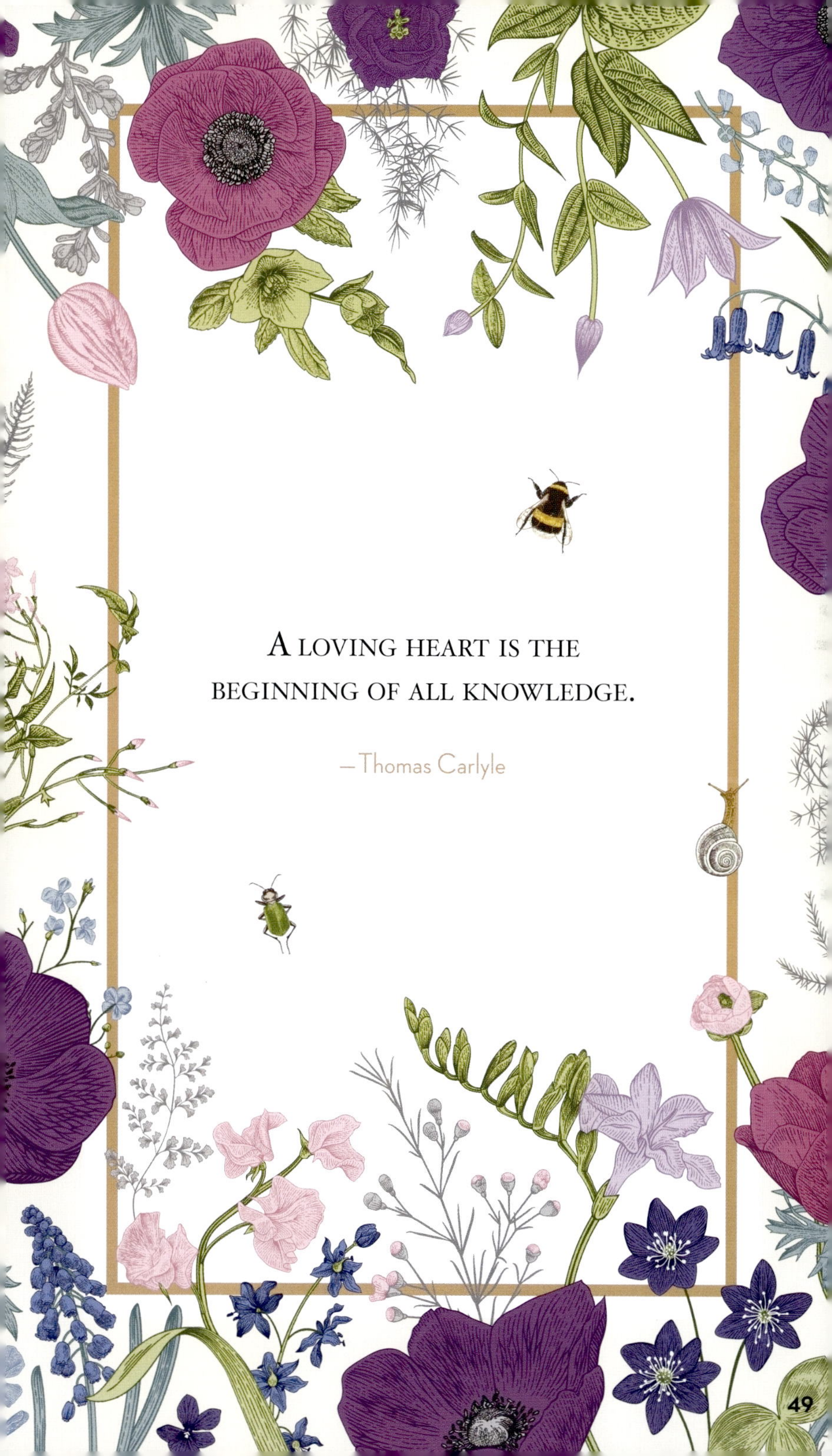

A LOVING HEART IS THE BEGINNING OF ALL KNOWLEDGE.

—Thomas Carlyle

Step 1

Breathe deeply a few times to ground yourself.

Step 2

Begin to extend your inhales and exhales to perhaps 6 or more seconds each. At the top of your inhale, pause with your breath held. Count to 3, then exhale. Adjust the lengths of your inhale, pause, and exhale if you need to make the breathing pattern comfortable.

Step 3

You should start to notice your heartbeat becoming more obvious, especially when you hold your breath. The longer you hold the breath, the more strongly you'll feel your heartbeat. If you use a mantra, begin repeating it in your mind to the rhythm of your heartbeat.

Step 4

When you're ready, place your fingers on a pulse point. It could be your wrist, throat, temple, or elsewhere. Turn your focus to that beat. Continue repeating any mantra you're using.

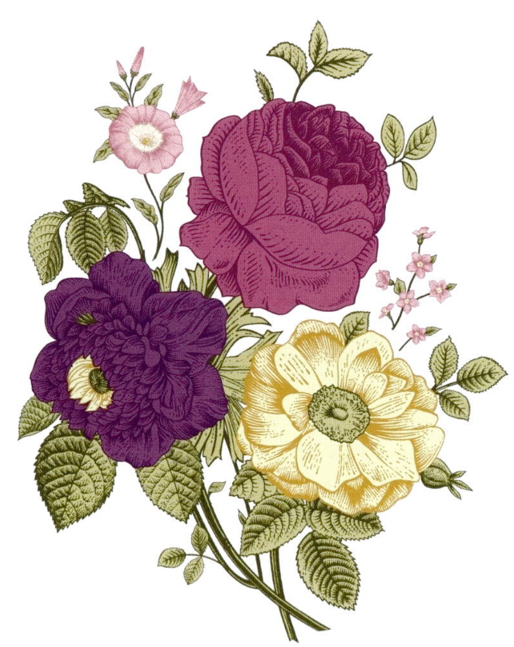

The incense of the heart may rise.

—John Pierpont

Metta Meditation

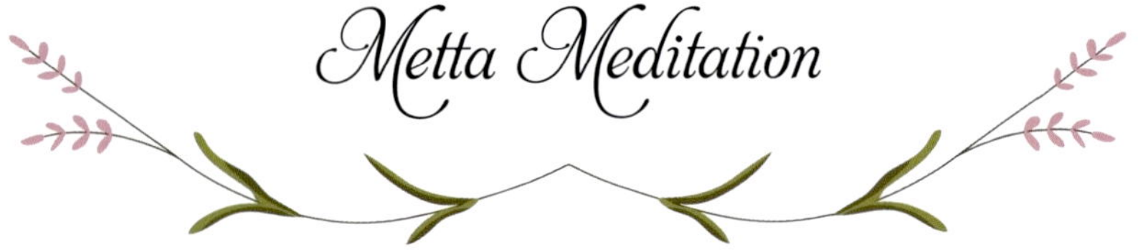

If you want to put more love and compassion into the world, Metta meditation is a wonderful way to do it. Metta is a word for a kind and friendly love in the Pali language. For this reason, English speakers often call the practice loving-kindness meditation.

Metta is a central concept in Buddhism. It is one of the four essential mental states that together can lead to enlightenment. (The other three are compassion, joy for others, and equanimity.) As such, many Buddhists include Metta meditation in their religious practice.

Time

This meditation can take as long as you need it to. Beginners may start by spending 10 or 20 minutes meditating. Those who are more practiced can spend 45 minutes or more with it. Metta meditation is done in stages, beginning with yourself and expanding outwards. If you're a beginner, take it slow. You can do the meditation in pieces, completing only the first stage or two in a session. Add stages to your practice when you're ready. Alternatively, you can complete all of the stages in one session, spending a short period on each stage and expanding that time as you become more comfortable.

Posture

Sit in a comfortable position. Legs may be crossed or in a lotus position if you're on the floor or a cushion. If you're sitting in a chair, position yourself so your feet are flat on the floor if you can. Support yourself with cushions behind your back, under your knees, or elsewhere as needed. Keep your back comfortably straight, gaze down or eyes closed.

Remember

Your mind will wander, and that's ok. When it does, acknowledge that it has, then gently bring your attention back to the light of loving-kindness and, if you are repeating a mantra, to the words and meaning of that mantra. If the practice seems mechanical or insincere at first, keep with it. Change may be happening even if you don't immediately notice it.

Metta meditation is done in stages. Visualization is a big part of it, and many people repeat mantras as well. Your mantra can be any phrase or phrases that are positive and loving, such as "May I feel happiness and peace," or "May I be safe and healthy." You can say the mantra out loud or in your head.

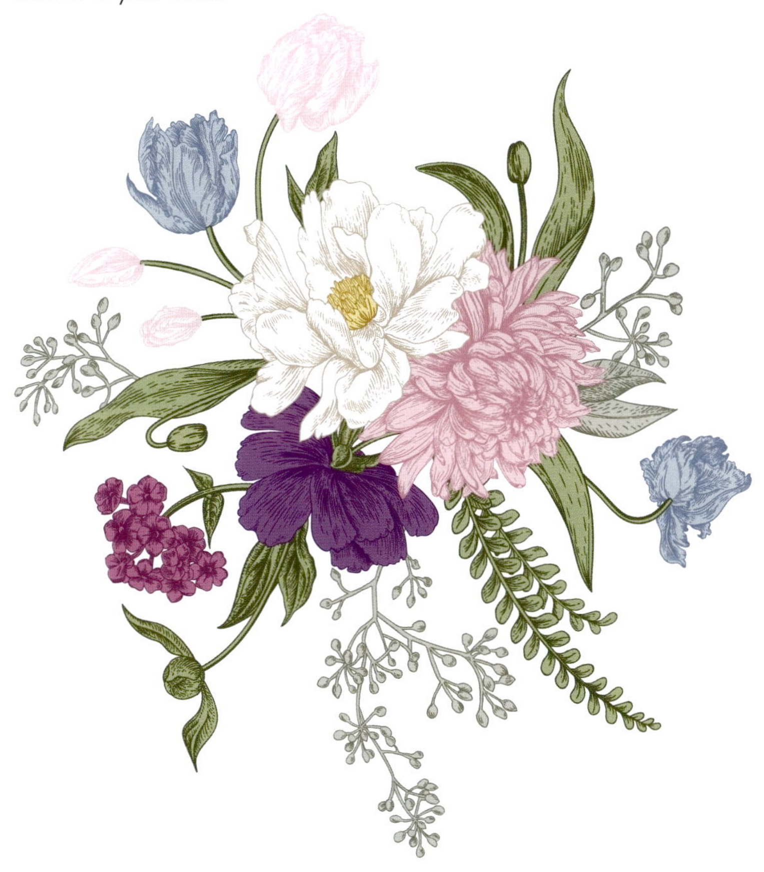

So within yourself let grow
A boundless love for all creatures.

—Gautama Buddha

Step 1

Begin with yourself. Imagine loving-kindness as a light that comes from and surrounds you. Feel the warmth of it. Repeat your mantra in the first person, as in, "May I be safe and healthy."

Step 2

When you're ready, think of a person in your life whom you like. Hold that person and all the things you love about them in your mind. Imagine your light of loving-kindness surrounding your loved one. Repeat your mantra again, turning it toward the person, as in, "May you be safe and healthy."

Step 3

Think of a person toward whom you feel neutral. This is someone you do not particularly like or dislike. Perhaps the person is an acquaintance or a stranger. In your mind's eye, see the light of loving-kindness around this person. Repeat your mantra, applying its meaning to them, too.

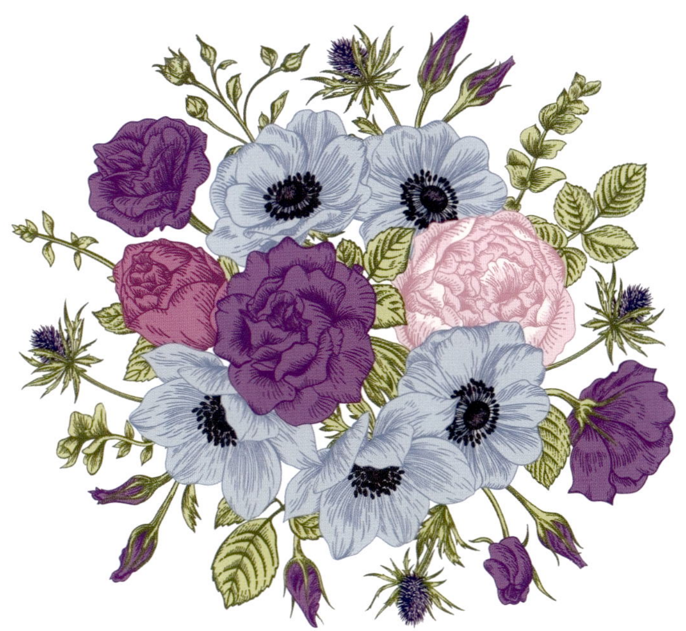

Step 4

Think of a person you do not like, or with whom you have difficulty. Be gentle with yourself if ill feelings bubble up in your mind as you think of the person. Acknowledge the feelings and let them go, reminding yourself of the person's humanity. Think of them positively. Again, surround them in the light of your loving-kindness and repeat your mantra.

Step 5

Imagine all these people—yourself, the loved one, the neutral person, and the disliked person—together in a close group. Imagine the light of loving-kindness filling and surrounding all of you at once. Repeat your mantra for the entire group, as in, "May we feel happiness and peace."

Step 6

In your mind's eye, extend that light out to include the people immediately around you. Expand it to include your neighborhood, then your town, your country, and your continent. Keep going until the light encompasses the entire world.

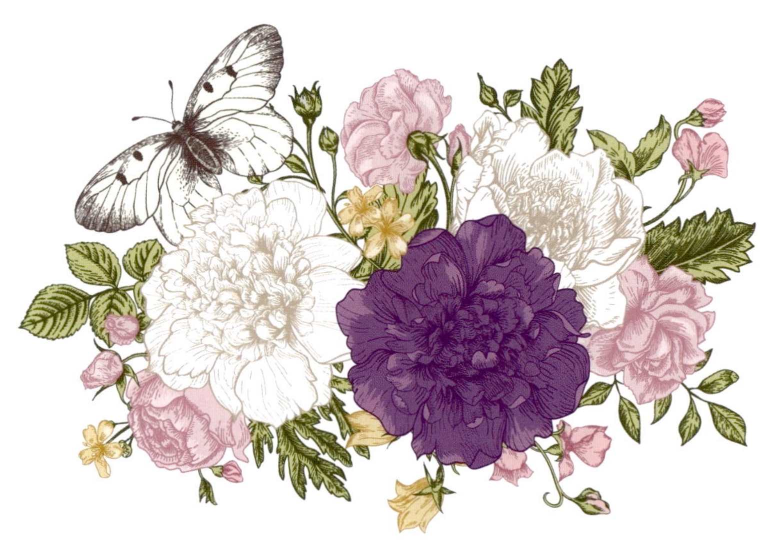

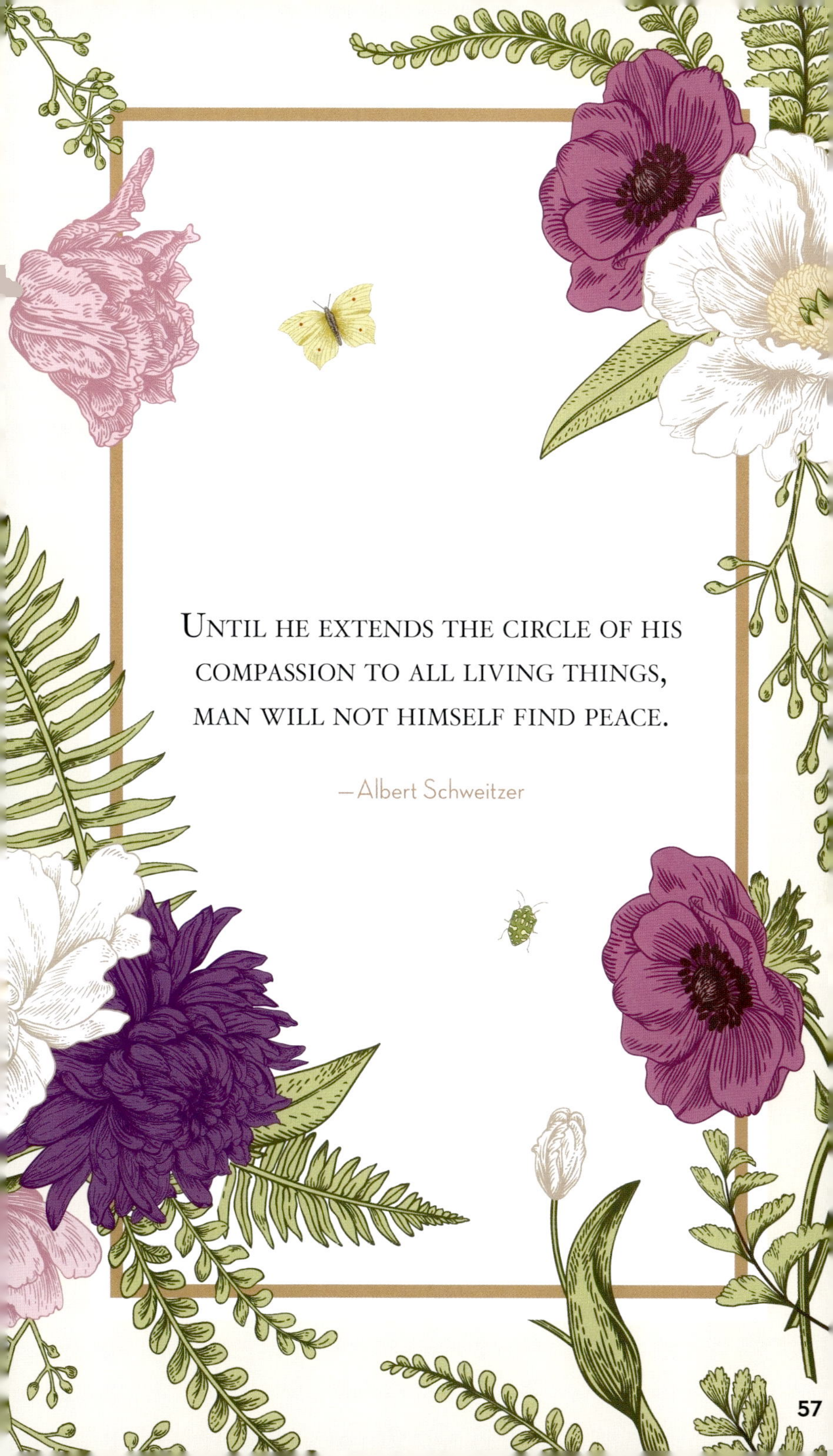

UNTIL HE EXTENDS THE CIRCLE OF HIS COMPASSION TO ALL LIVING THINGS, MAN WILL NOT HIMSELF FIND PEACE.

—Albert Schweitzer

Mindfulness Meditation

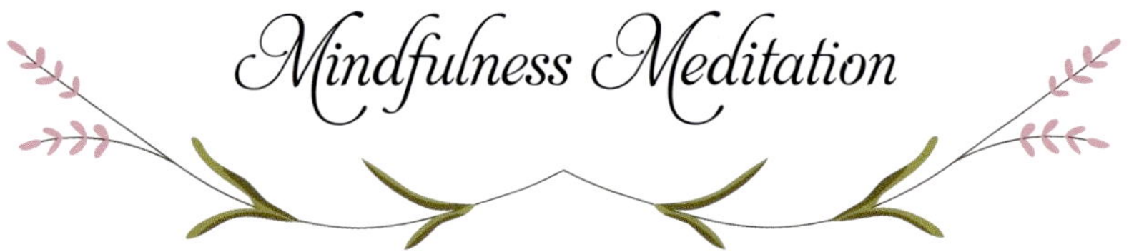

We spend a lot of time stuck in the past or the future. Whether negative (regretting something said the night before) or positive (daydreaming about an upcoming dinner date), these thoughts pull us away from the here and now. This can increase stress and wreak havoc on our ability to focus.

Mindfulness meditation is an effort to hit the brakes on runaway thoughts by focusing on one single, natural thing: the breath. The practice is less about clearing the mind, and more about becoming aware of it. This process grounds us securely in the present moment. Practitioners report calmer minds, more regenerative relaxation, and overall less stress.

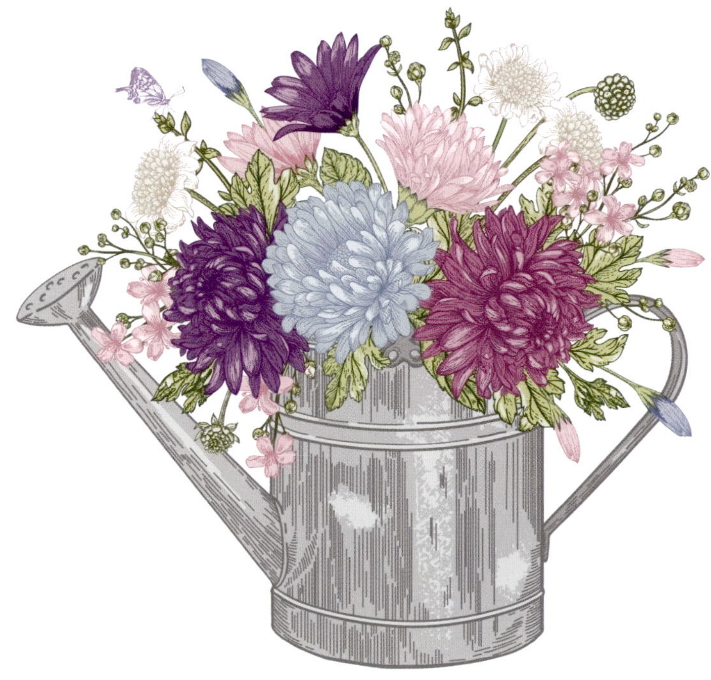

Time

It's better to practice this meditation in short sessions several times a week, rather than in one or two long sessions. With this in mind, a session may be as short as 3 to 5 minutes, especially if you're just starting out. With time and practice, you'll become more comfortable with sessions lasting 45 minutes or more.

Posture

Sit in a comfortable position. Legs may be crossed or in a lotus position if you're on the floor or a cushion. If you're sitting in a chair, position yourself so your feet are flat on the floor if you can. Support yourself with cushions behind your back, under your knees, or elsewhere as needed. Keep your back comfortably straight, gaze down or eyes closed.

Remember

Your mind will wander, and that's ok. When it wanders or becomes fixed on a topic, acknowledge that it has. Then gently bring your attention back to your breath.

Step 1

Take a few deep breaths. Breathe in through the nose and out through the mouth.

Step 2

Return to your natural breath, and gently bring your attention to it. Don't change or control your breathing, just be aware of it. Consider the physical sensation of the air moving into your body, filling your lungs, and then moving out.

Step 3

If it helps, you can count each inhale and exhale (inhale 1, exhale 2, inhale 3, and so on). Continue until you reach six, then start again from one.

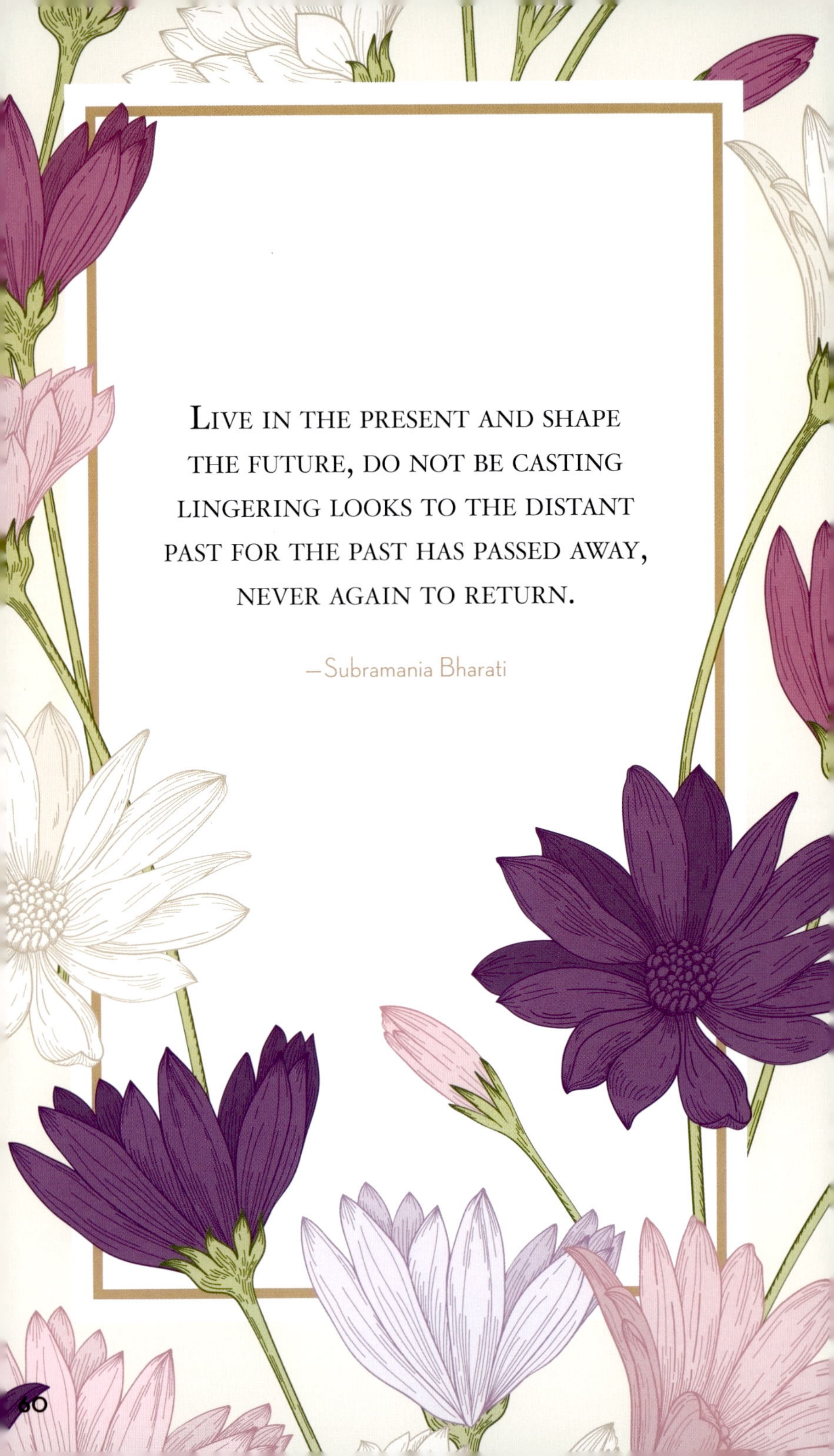

Live in the present and shape the future, do not be casting lingering looks to the distant past for the past has passed away, never again to return.

—Subramania Bharati

Noting

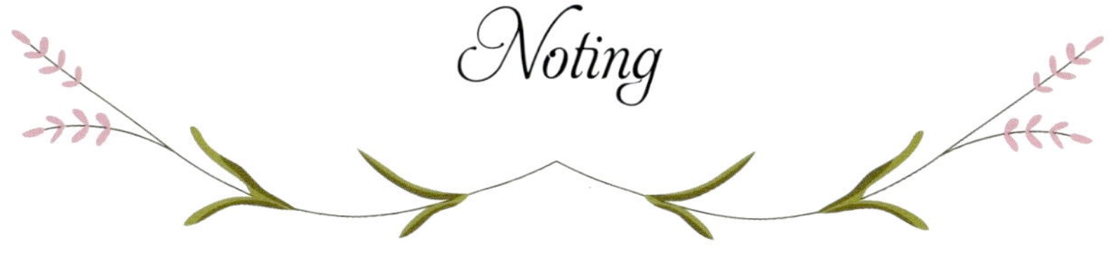

The process of noting is a tool to help you stay present in the moment. It's particularly useful for people who struggle with a wandering, preoccupied mind. In noting, you notice and label each thought, emotion, or physical sensation distracting you with a simple, single word. Every label is neutral, without judgement or any attempt to change or control.

In the short term, noting gives a wandering mind something relatively active to do, which helps you stay focused and mindful as you meditate. Noting can also help you recognize the thoughts, emotions, or physical sensations that are most heavily on your mind. In the long term, you can learn patterns in your thoughts and feelings. When the time is right, you can then respond to the patterns. This kind of awareness can also help you resist obsessive thinking or preoccupation.

There are a few different types of labeling you can use in your practice.

- Very basic, general labels, such as "this," or "here"
- More specific labels, such as "warmth," "wanting," "excitement," or "tingling"
- Labels describing the type of sensation being experienced, such as "seeing," "hearing," "feeling," or "thinking"
- Naming the parts of the breath, such as "rising" with an inhale, and "falling" with an exhale

Time

Generally speaking, you can use a noting technique when and however long you need to. It can last 20 minutes and help you enter a mindful state at the beginning of a meditation session. Or you can use the technique for a few moments, breaths, or minutes when your mind becomes particularly distracted from your meditation.

Posture

Use a posture that matches the main meditation method you're using, whether it is seated Vipassana, a prone body scan, or a body position in yoga.

Remember

If noting starts to feel mechanical, take a brief break from it. You can come back to it in a few minutes, or if you need, in a few days. There is no "right" or "wrong" label. Use whatever word comes to mind. You don't have to note everything. Note experiences that are dominating your attention. It's ok if the same label comes up over and over again. When it does, note each occurrence until the experience fades or is replaced by another thought.

Step 1

When a thought, emotion, or physical sensation starts to predominate your focus, take a moment to give it a label. Think it silently in your mind. Then move on from it.

Step 2

Your mind may calm and quieten as you meditate. Let your labels follow, becoming quieter and more nebulous. For example, you may find yourself going from "coolness," to "this," to "hmm."

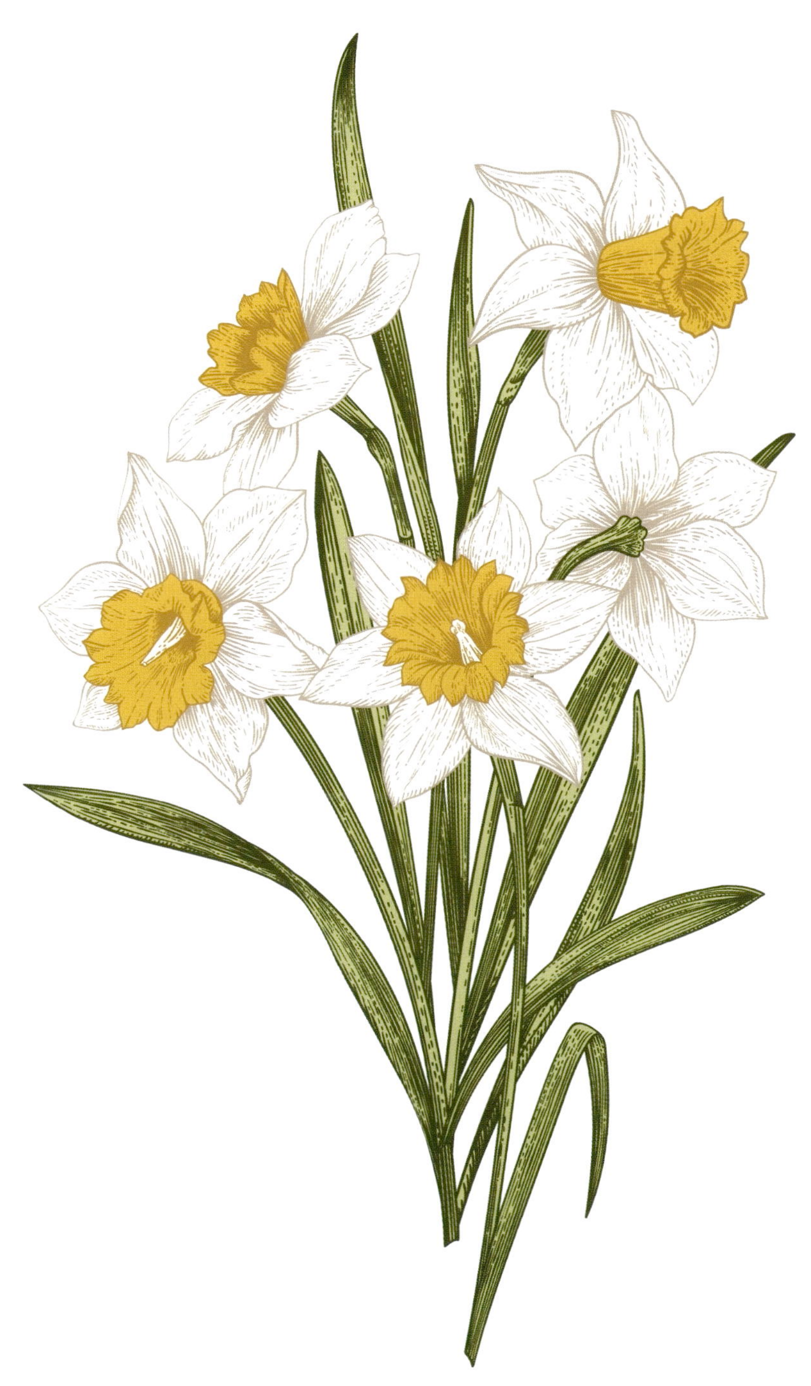

Life is not a series of gig-lamps
symmetrically arranged;
life is a luminous halo,
a semi-transparent envelope
surrounding us from the
beginning of consciousness
to the end.

—Virginia Woolf

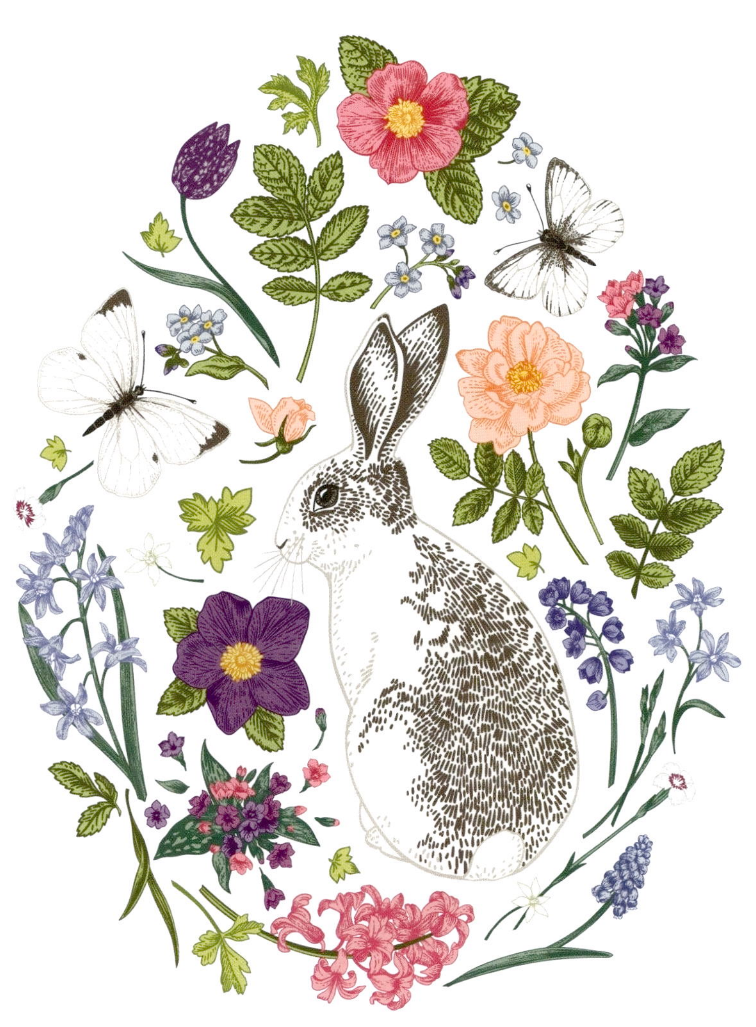

Self-reflection Meditation

While most meditations involve letting thoughts and emotions go, a more reflective method is sometimes useful. Self-reflection meditation is a conscious and deliberate effort to study and understand yourself. You can use it to regularly check in on any changes or shifts in your life or identity that have taken place. It can also be a handy tool to work through a feeling or memory that preoccupies you.

Time

Some people practice self-reflection once a week or once a month. Others practice it when the need arises. You can start with 10- or 20-minute sessions, and adjust the time as you see fit.

Posture

Sit in a comfortable position. Legs may be crossed if you're on the floor, a mat, or a cushion. If you're sitting in a chair, position yourself so your feet are flat on the floor if you can. Support yourself with cushions behind your back, under your knees, or elsewhere as needed. Keep your back comfortably straight, eyes closed.

Remember

Work to remain neutral about your thoughts and emotions. This isn't rumination! If you become distracted or find your mind wandering, bring your attention back to your intention.

Step 1

Spend 5 to 10 minutes in mindful meditation. Focus on your breath, and let thoughts come and go.

Step 2

When you're ready, call up the event, person, period of time, or other subject you've chosen to reflect on.

Step 3

Look at the details of your subject. What images, emotions, sounds, smells, or sensations does it bring with it? If you're working through a memory of an event, what were your emotions at that time? What sights, smells, and physical sensations were you experiencing?

Step 4

Focus in turn on each image, emotion, sound, smell, or physical sensation the subject conjured in Step 3. View them as a neutral outsider might. Are there patterns? Is an aspect of the subject particularly dominant? How do the emotions and circumstances surrounding that subject compare to your current state?

Step 5

One by one, let each image, emotion, sound, smell, and physical sensation go. Take time to focus on each detail, and then let it fade from your attention as you move on to the next.

Step 6

Consider the subject as a whole for a moment, with all its aspects, and then let it fade from your attention.

Step 7

Take a few minutes to come back to simple mindfulness, focusing only on your breath.

Silence more musical than any song.

—Christina Rossetti

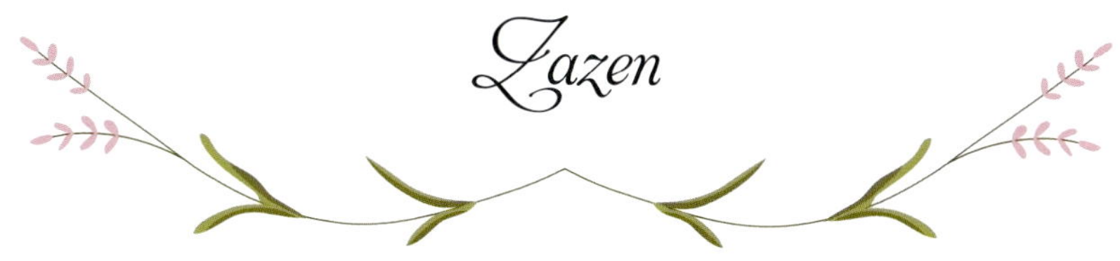

Zazen

Zazen is practiced in the Zen school of Buddhism. A core Zen belief is that anyone can achieve awakening, or enlightenment. The school also emphasizes a oneness among all living and nonliving things. Both of these concepts shape Zazen. It's a very intentional form of meditation that involves getting rid of individual identity—including likes or dislikes, desires, expectations, and goals—to exist in the present moment, as well as becoming aware of the breath, body, and mind as a single, complete unit.

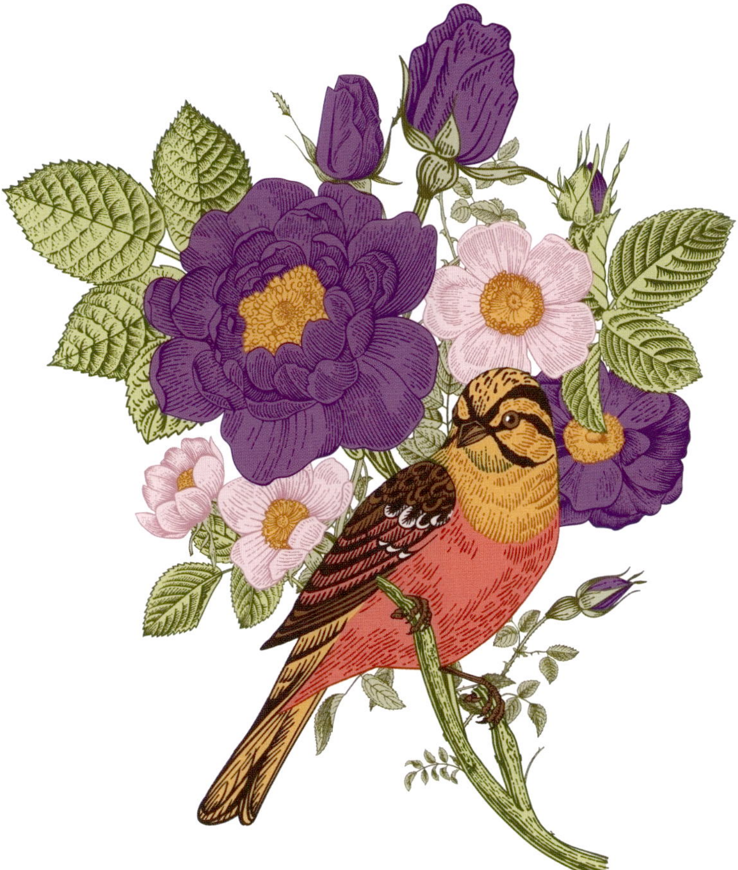

Time

Devotees often practice Zazen for 20 to 30 minutes, one or two times a day. If you're a beginner, you can work up to this kind of practice gradually, starting with 5 minutes, for example.

Posture

The body's position is an important part of Zazen practice.
Legs: You have a few options. In all poses, you can sit on a support to make the position easier to do.

- Full lotus: Sit cross-legged with each foot resting on top of the opposite thigh.
- Half lotus: One foot rests on the opposite thigh, the other foot is folded underneath the opposite leg.
- Seiza: Kneel, resting your hips on your heels. You can sit on a cushion (legs on either side) or low bench (legs folded under the bench) to make this position more comfortable.
- Chair: Sit near the edge of the chair so your back is straight and your feet rest flat on the floor. Place a cushion between your lower back and the chair back if you need some support.

Hands: Lay your hands together on your lap, palms up. Rest the fingers of one hand on top of the other, with your dominant hand on bottom (if you're right-handed, your right hand is on bottom, and vice versa for left-handers). Let the tips of your thumbs touch so your hands form an oval shape.
Spine: Keep your back comfortably erect. Tuck your chin slightly to lengthen your neck.
Eyes: Allow your gaze to rest, eyes open and unfocused, a few feet in front of you.

Remember

Your mind will wander, and that's ok. When it wanders, acknowledge that it has. Then gently bring your attention back to the breath.

Step 1

Take a moment to settle into your seated position.

Step 2

Bring your attention to your breath.

- Your breathing should be easy and comfortable, not controlled.
- Breathe through your nose, your mouth closed and relaxed.
- Rest your tongue gently against the roof of your mouth, just behind your front teeth.

Step 3 (optional)

Counting your inhales and exhales in the beginning can help you calm and focus your mind. As your mind quietens, let the counting go and just breathe. If it helps to label your thoughts and sensations in the beginning, do so, but let this go with time, too.

Step 4

Move your focus to the physical sensation of breathing, whether it's your belly moving in and out, or the air entering and leaving your lungs. If there are changes in the speed or rhythm of your breathing, note them.

Step 5

Work toward experiencing your breath as a continuous cycle. Forget any notion of parts or stages of the breath, such as inhale, pause, or exhale. It is a single, unbroken movement.

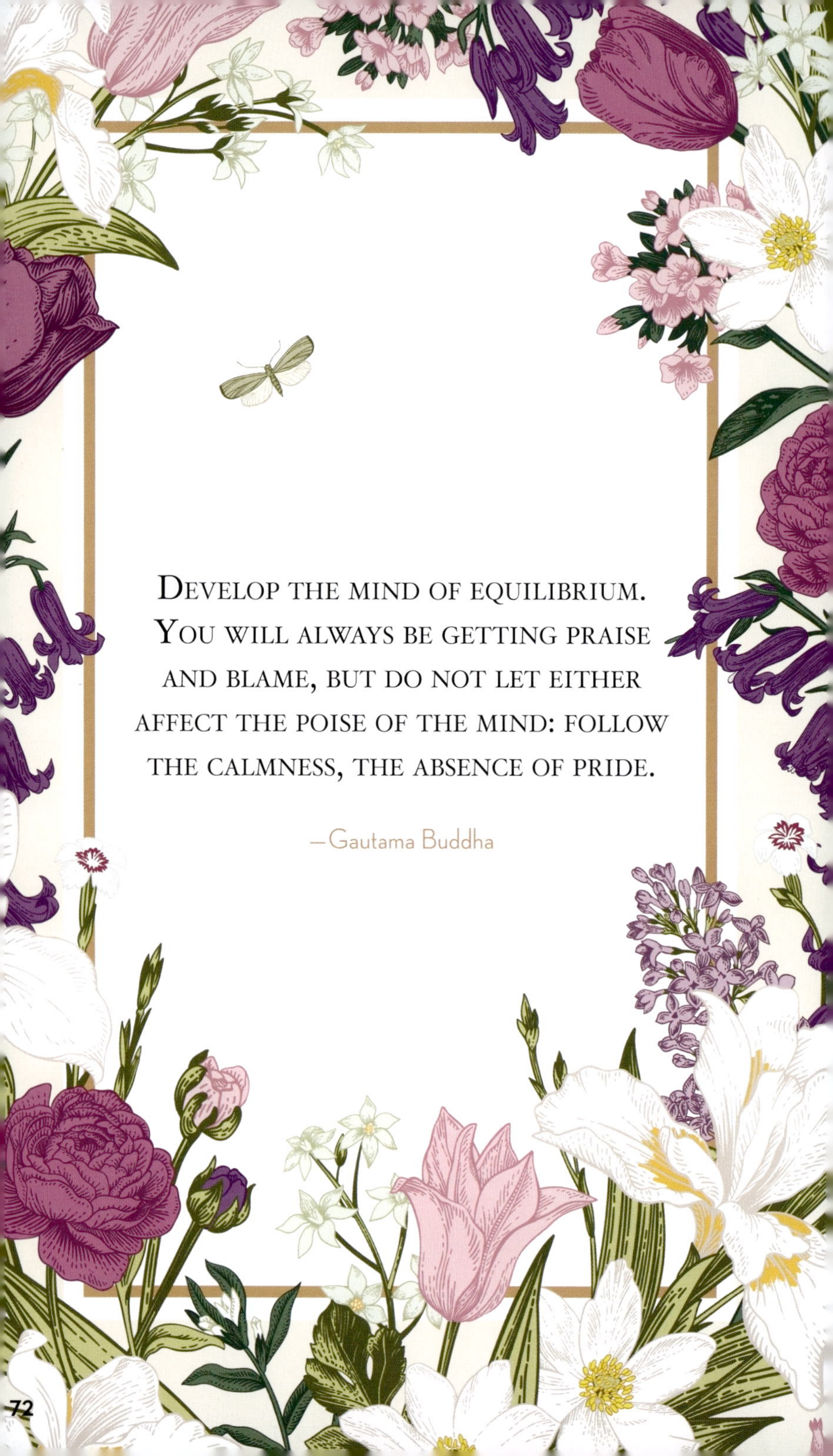

Develop the mind of equilibrium. You will always be getting praise and blame, but do not let either affect the poise of the mind: follow the calmness, the absence of pride.

—Gautama Buddha

Calming Mantras and Reflections

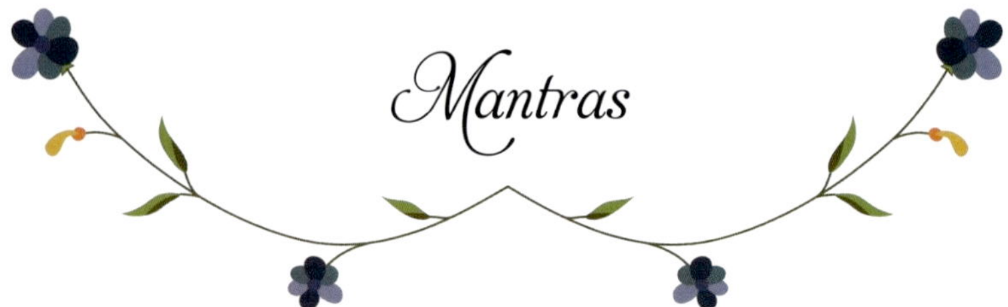

Mantras

A mantra is a repeated sound, syllable, word, or phrase that serves as a tool to cultivate focus, intention, or inspiration in the mind. It is usually spoken or thought over and over again in a steady rhythm. The word mantra is often associated specifically with Hinduism and Buddhism, though other religions also make use of repeated words, and many people have adopted mantras into non-religious meditations.

Mantras can be part of a meditation practice in a huge variety of ways. You can chant them aloud or repeat them in your head. They can be short or long, religious or secular, in any language, or in no language at all. You can add them to any part of your meditation, or just use them at stressful moments in your day. You can repeat your mantra a certain number of times, for a specific length of time, or simply until you're ready to move on. It's all up to you. All a mantra needs to do is help you stay true to the intention of your practice.

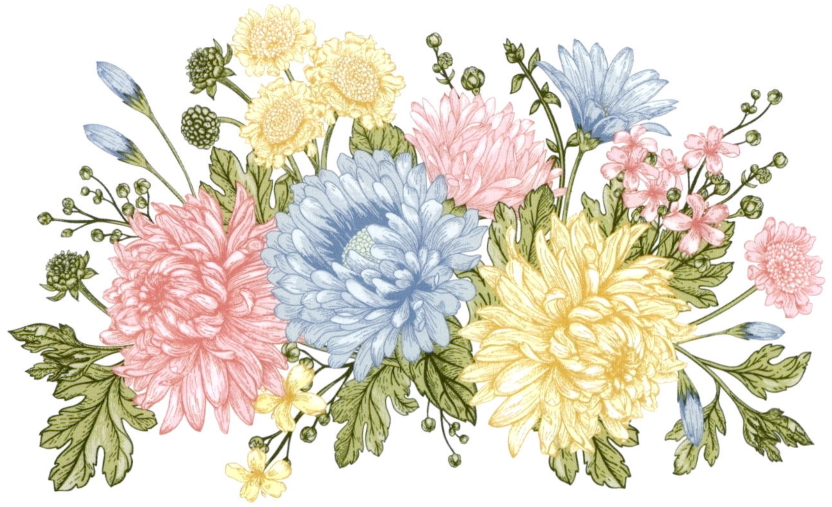

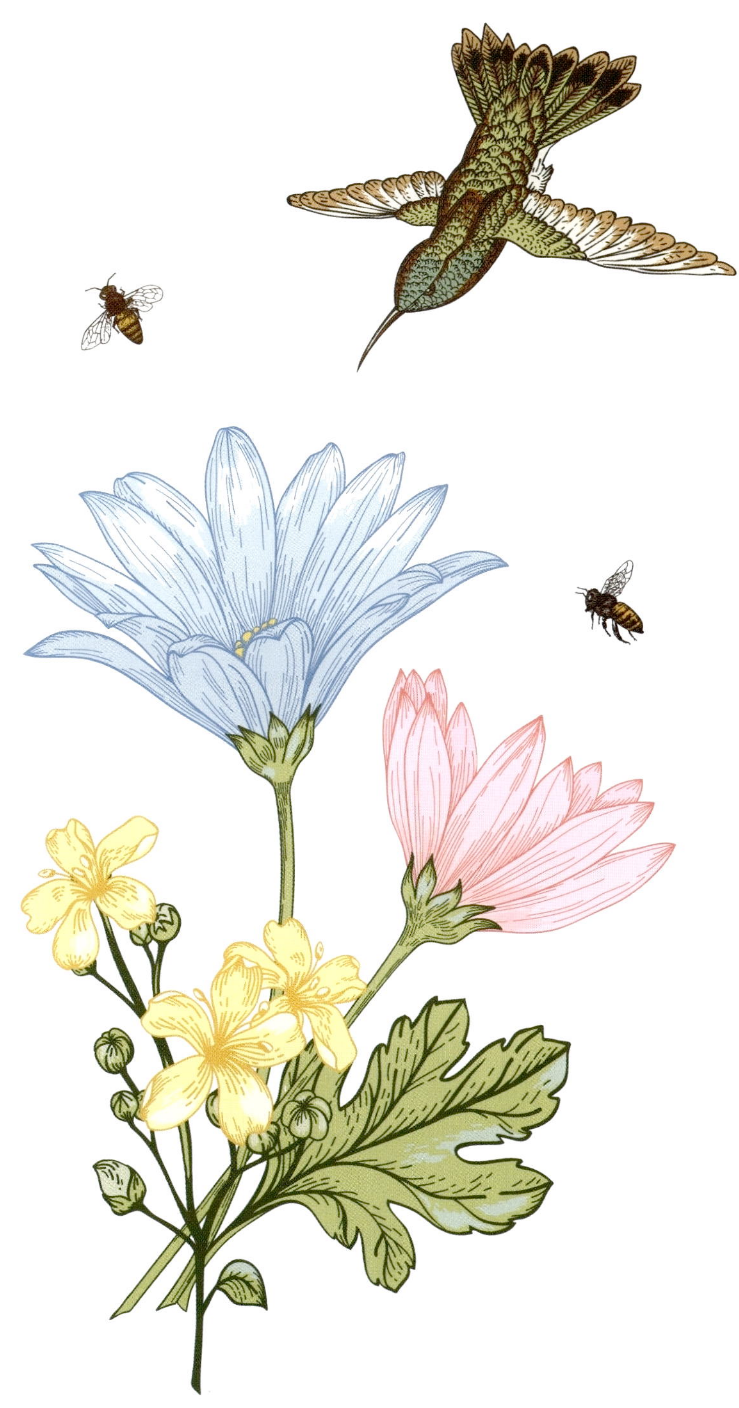

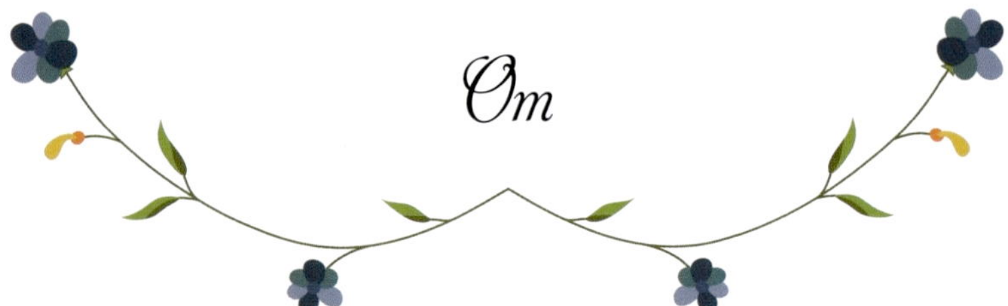

Om

You're likely familiar with Om. The syllable is synonymous with meditation, and it is sacred in Hinduism, Buddhism, and other religions. Scriptures connect it to creation and the divine, and describe it as the origin of all sounds. Many practitioners see Om as the tool that sends the spirit to enlightenment or the divine. Picture a bow, arrow, and target. The bow is Om, the arrow is the spirit, the target is the divine.

Om is pronounced with three sounds: AH-OO-MM (this is why you can sometimes find it spelled "AUM"). The three parts can represent a variety of trinities, including past, present, and future; creation, preservation, and liberation; the physical plane, mental plane, and deep-sleep state; and goodness, passion, and darkness. A fourth—and equally important—part of the syllable is the silence that comes at the end of it.

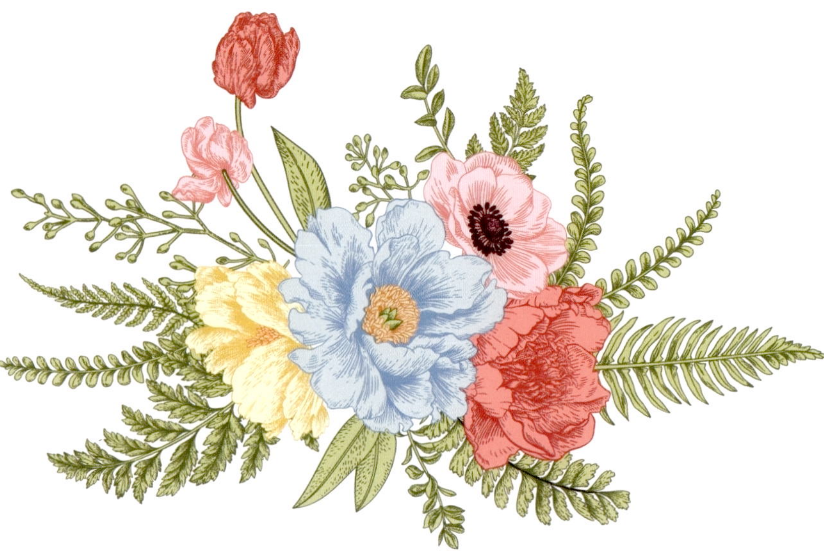

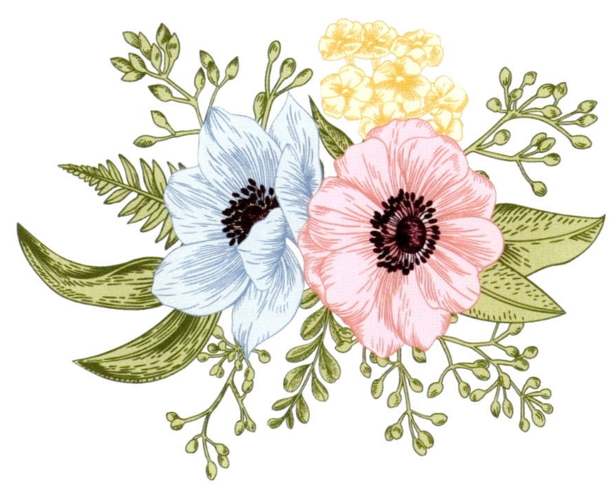

Time

Some people (yogis, for example) chant Om a few times at the beginning or end of a practice. Others chant for perhaps 45 minutes or more. Many Buddhists chant a mantra a certain number of times, keeping count on a string of beads such as a mala.

Posture

Sit in a comfortable position. Legs may be crossed or in a lotus position if you're on the floor or a cushion. If you're sitting in a chair, position yourself so your feet are flat on the floor if you can. Support yourself with cushions behind your back, under your knees, or elsewhere as needed. Keep your back comfortably straight, gaze down or eyes closed.

Remember

Your mind will wander, and that's ok. That's part of what you're working on with this meditation. When it wanders or becomes fixed on a topic, acknowledge that it has. Then gently bring your attention back to your meditation.

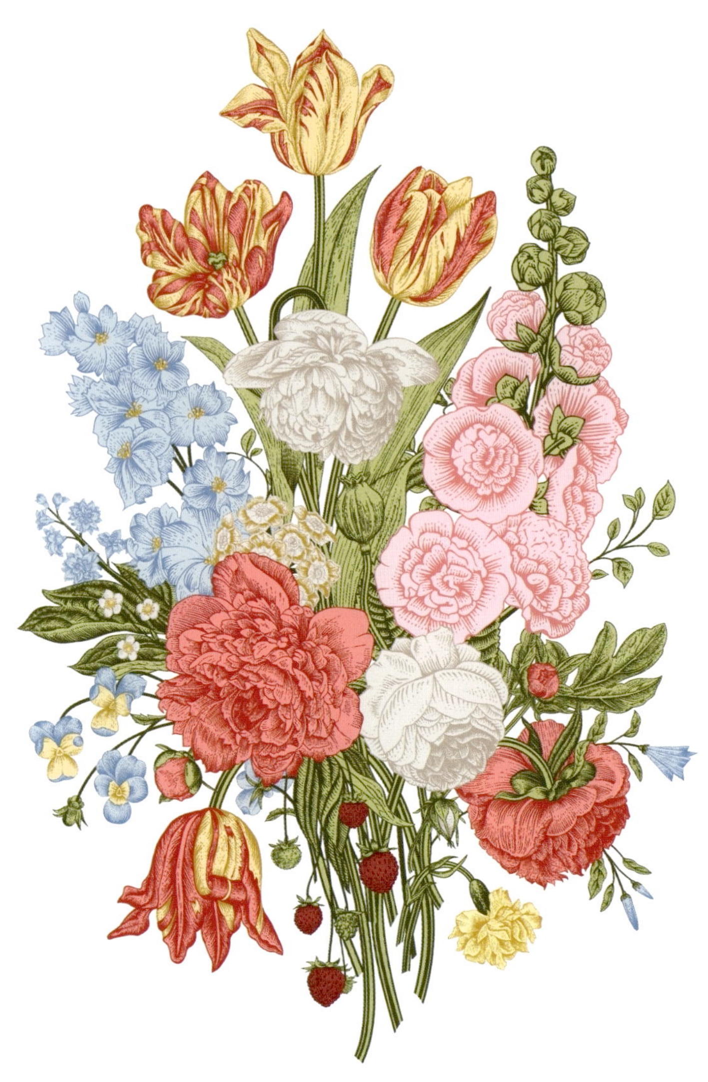

Breathe naturally. Say or think "Om" during an exhale. The length of your Om should match the time it takes to complete the exhale. Transition smoothly between each of Om's three sounds, spending a few seconds on each. You can repeat Om with every exhale, or you can take breaths in between each repetition.

I am

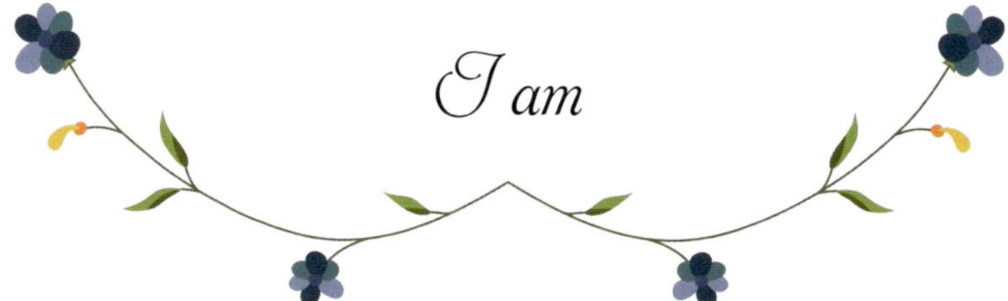

A mantra like "I am" is a very straightforward, personal method of meditation. The phrase can be said in any language, though it often resonates strongest when it is in your first language. "I am" has a particular connection to certain religions. In Sanskrit, the phrase is "So Hum," or literally "I am that/he." In Vedic philosophies, So Hum represents the connection between the individual and the universe, with "I am" being the personal and "that" the universal. In meditating, many practitioners combine this with Om, for "Om So Hum."

The mantra doesn't need to be religious. Repeating "I am" is an excellent way to include self-exploration and self-reflection in a secular meditation practice.

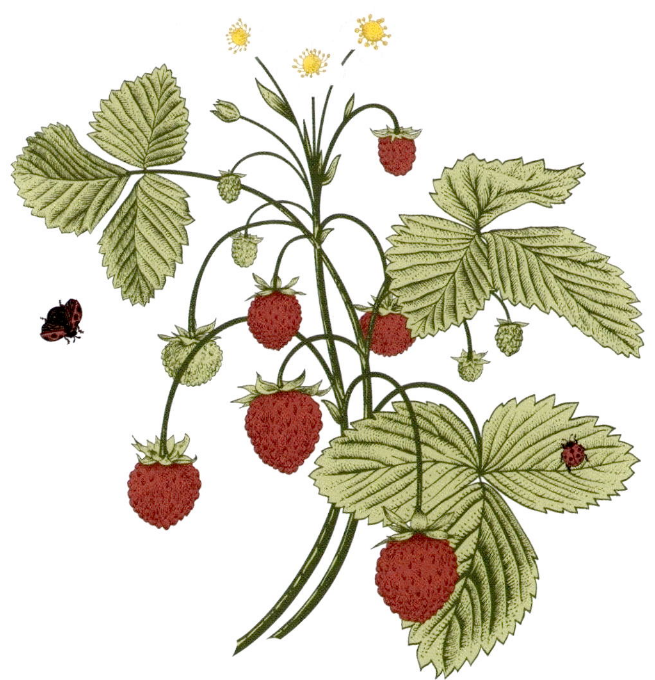

Time

A good place to start is 10 to 15 minutes. As you become more comfortable and familiar with the practice, you can increase the time to 30 minutes, 45 minutes, or more.

Posture

Sit in a comfortable position. Legs may be crossed or in a lotus position if you're on the floor or a cushion. If you're sitting in a chair, position yourself so your feet are flat on the floor if you can. Support yourself with cushions behind your back, under your knees, or elsewhere as needed. Keep your back comfortably straight, gaze down or eyes closed.

Remember

Your mind will wander, and that's ok. When it wanders or becomes fixed on a topic, acknowledge that it has. Then gently bring your attention back to the sound and meaning of the mantra.

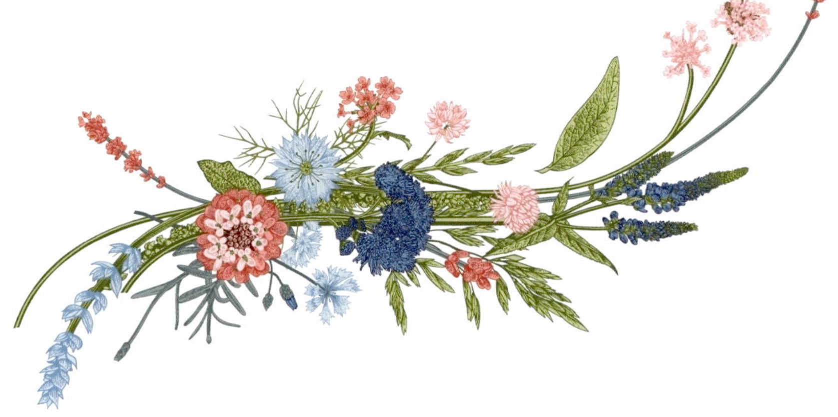

As with an Om meditation, breathe naturally. Let the rhythm of your mantra match the rhythm of your breath. For example, as you inhale, slowly go through the first part of the mantra, "I." As you exhale, go through the second part, "Am."

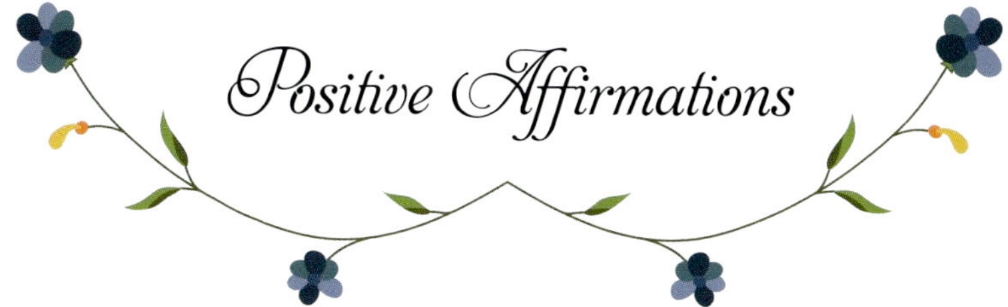

Positive Affirmations

Positive affirmations are helpful, loving thoughts. In essence, positive affirmations are sentences or phrases that describe something you love about yourself, hope for, or are working toward.

Time

You can spend 5 or 10 minutes with positive affirmations at the beginning or end of a meditation session, or you can focus on them for an entire session. You might also pull these out for a quick 30 seconds when you experience stress or just need a pick-me-up.

Posture

If you're sitting, find a comfortable position. Legs may be crossed or in a lotus position if you're on the floor or a cushion. If you're sitting in a chair, position yourself so your feet are flat on the floor if you can. Support yourself with cushions behind your back, under your knees, or elsewhere as needed. Keep your back comfortably straight, gaze down or eyes closed. If you're on the move and just taking a moment for this exercise, you can be in any posture that suits the situation.

Remember

Your mind will wander, and that's ok. When it wanders or becomes fixed on a topic, acknowledge that it has. Then gently bring your attention back to the sound and meaning of your affirmations.

Step 1

What is something you value about yourself or your life? Are you strong? Curious? Are there people around you whom you love? Do you enjoy singing, writing, shooting hoops? Turn your choice into a sentence stating that you recognize and appreciate it, such as "I appreciate that I am strong."

Step 2

What is a state of mind you wish to cultivate? Bravery? Calmness? Compassion? Use your choice in a sentence with "I am," such as "I am brave."

Step 3

How do you want to feel about yourself or the world around you, or what is something you know to be true but often lose sight of? These can be harder to pinpoint. Examples include, "I am worthy," "I love myself," and "My emotions are valid."

I TO MYSELF
AM DEARER THAN A FRIEND.

—William Shakespeare

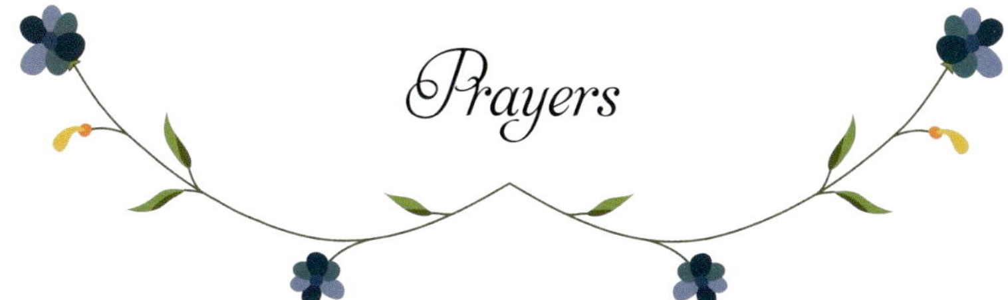

Prayers

Prayers are a form of religious meditation. Many religions have blessings, litanies, statements of praise or thanks, and other ritual words. Prayers may also be a single divine name or long quotes of scripture. Examples include Catholic rosary prayers and dhikr in Sufism.

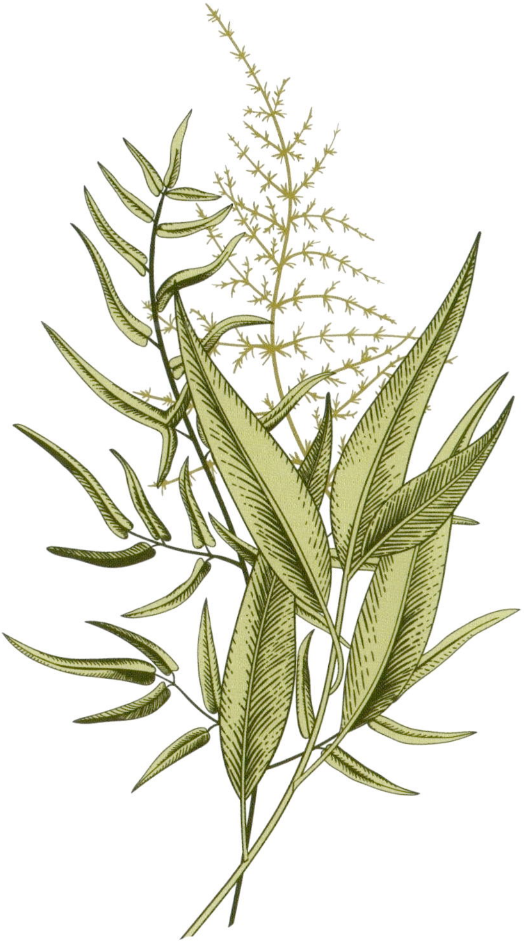

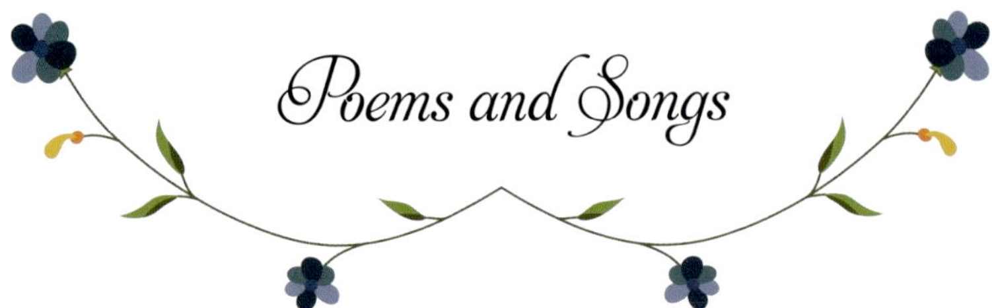

Poems and Songs

By design, poems and songs condense complex thoughts, emotions, and experiences into a series of well-chosen words. As a result, these writings are fertile ground for mantras. Whether you use a fragment of a song or the whole of an epic poem, meditating on these words can remind you of your intention, focus your mind, and reveal new layers of meaning in the words themselves.

POETRY COMES NEARER TO VITAL TRUTH THAN HISTORY.

—Ralph Waldo Emerson

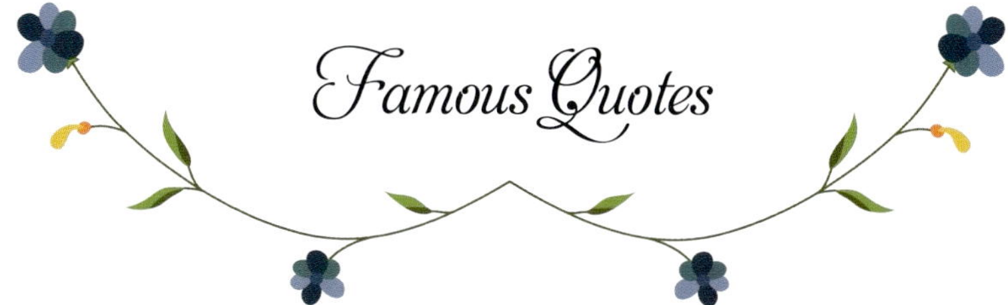

Famous Quotes

Have you ever run across a quote from a book, a speech, a film, or any other medium, that inspired or calmed you? These words can be useful as mantras as well, as you repeat them and reflect on their meaning.

THE ONLY THING WE HAVE TO FEAR IS FEAR ITSELF.

—Franklin Delano Roosevelt

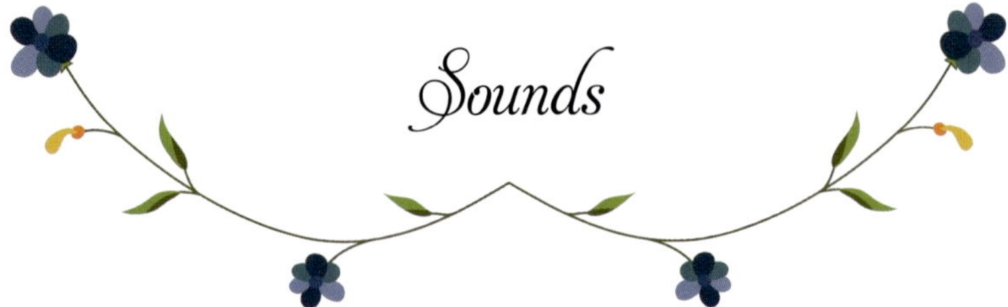

Sounds

A particular sound can help you focus or calm your mind. A basic mm or ng hum is an example. These are best done aloud so you can feel the vibration in your face, jaw, throat, or chest. It also acts as a tool to become conscious of your breathing. Repeating a melody or rhythm (simple or complex) is another method.

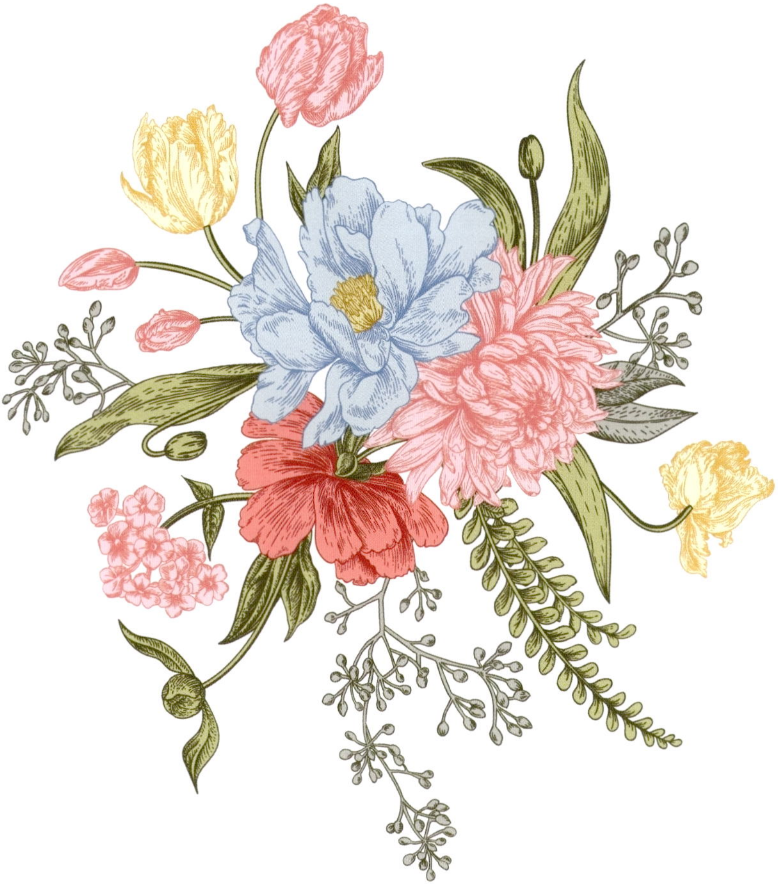

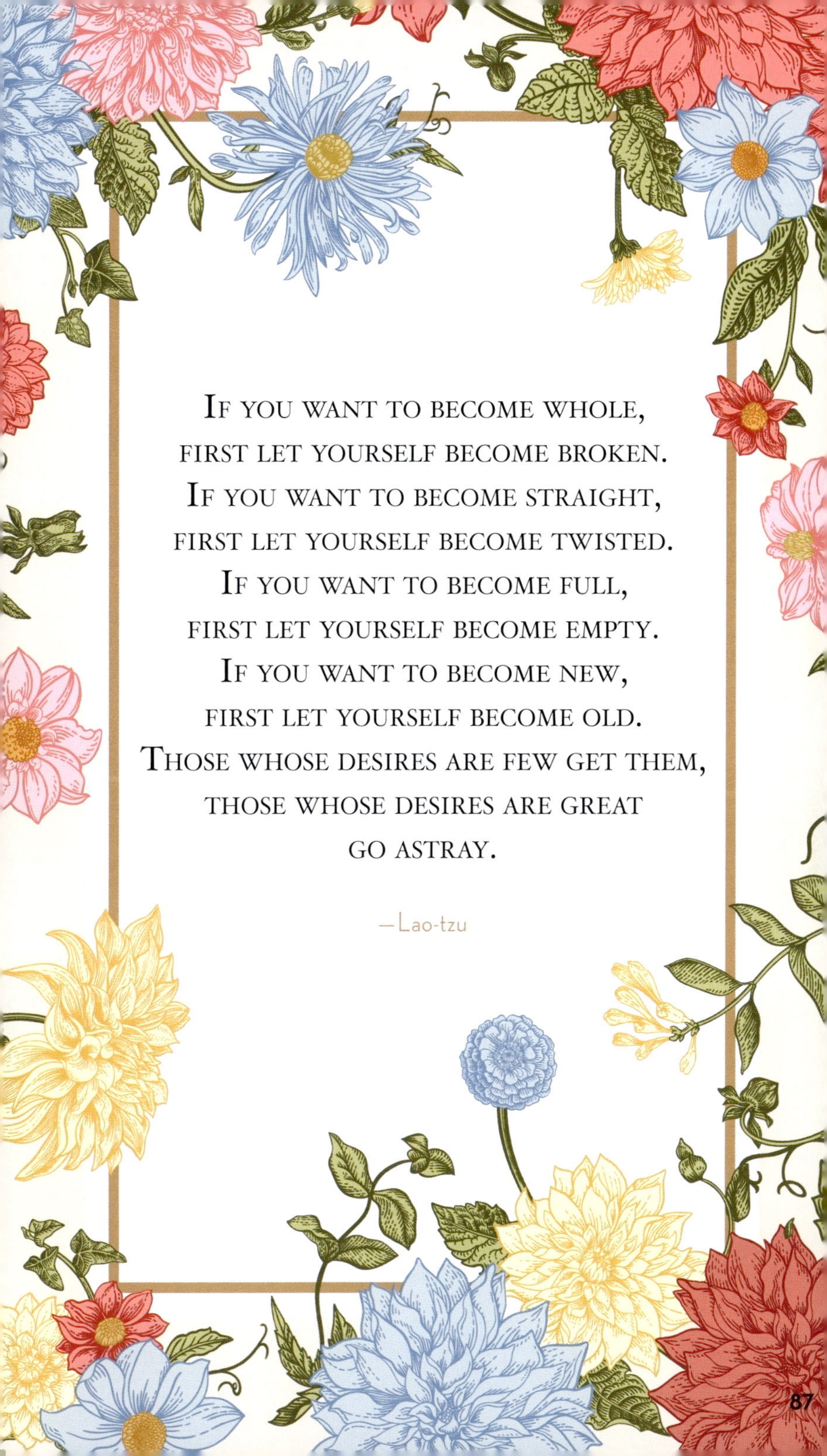

If you want to become whole,
first let yourself become broken.
If you want to become straight,
first let yourself become twisted.
If you want to become full,
first let yourself become empty.
If you want to become new,
first let yourself become old.
Those whose desires are few get them,
those whose desires are great
go astray.

—Lao-tzu

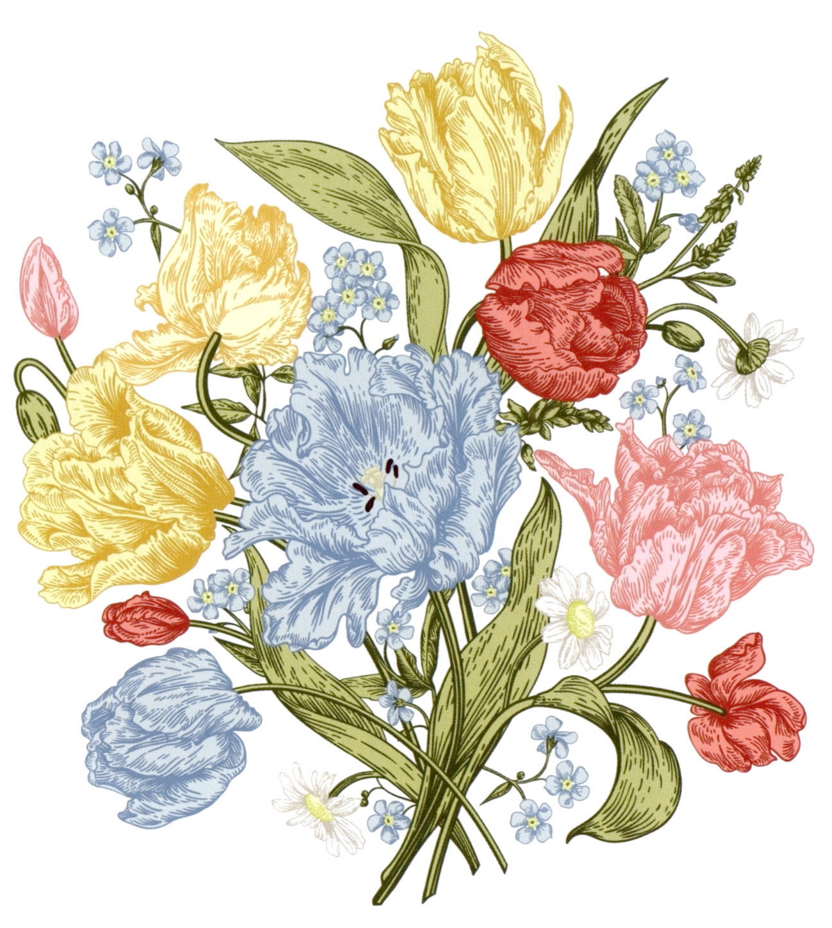

Color Reflection

Take a breath. Visualize the air as a color. The color is blue, filling you with peace. Take another breath, filling your lungs with pink, for love. Now breathe yellow, for harmony and oneness. Relax and breathe in orange, for energy and vitality. Inhale white, for union with the divine. Hold the breath for five seconds, letting the color spread to every cell, muscle, bone, and vital organ.

There is light within me. There is love throughout me. I breathe in light and release darkness from my body and my spirit. I breathe in positive energy, and release all that is negative. I invite the present into my thoughts and allow spirit to order my day. I am filled with light inward. I am expressing love outward.

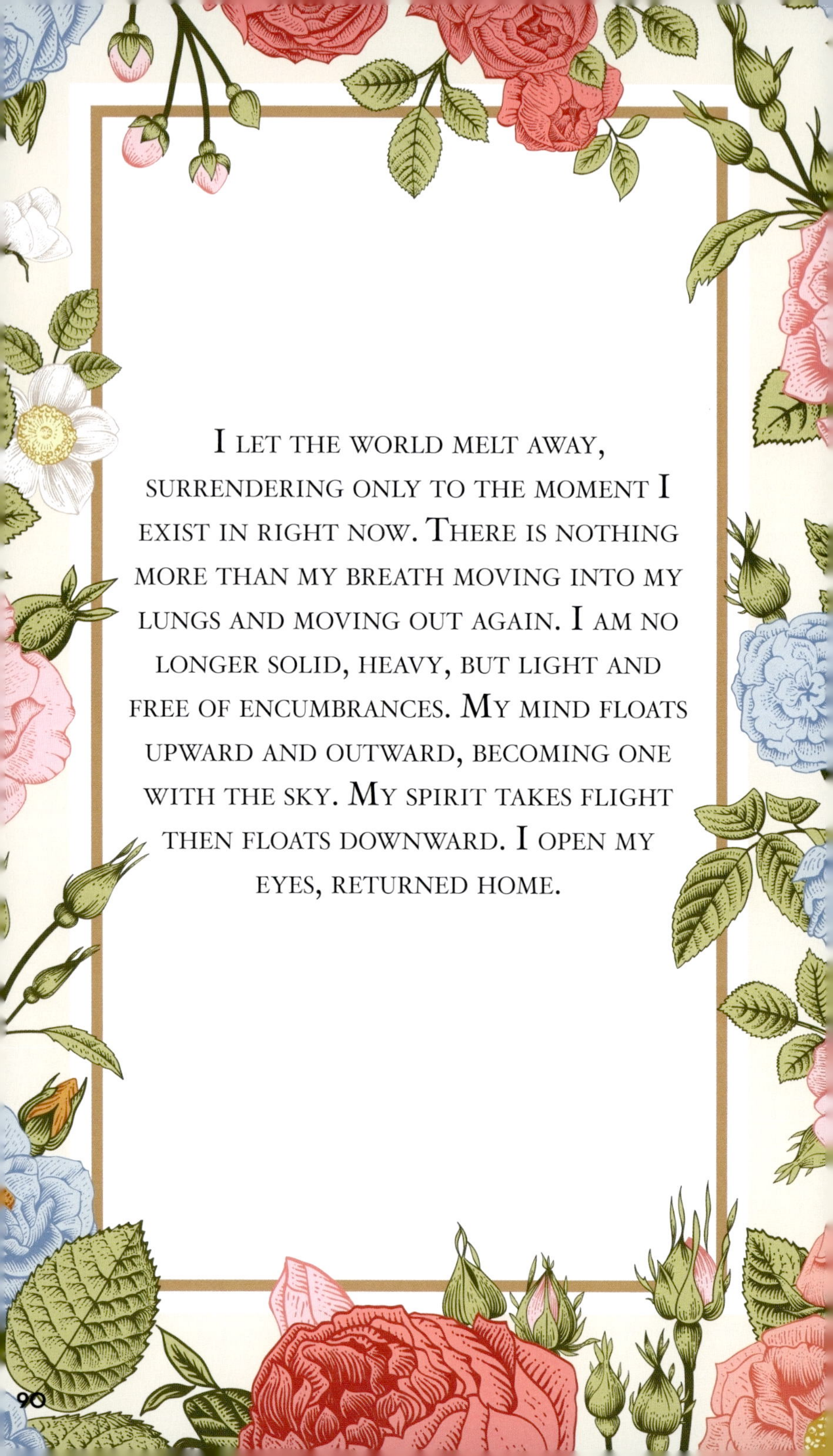

I let the world melt away, surrendering only to the moment I exist in right now. There is nothing more than my breath moving into my lungs and moving out again. I am no longer solid, heavy, but light and free of encumbrances. My mind floats upward and outward, becoming one with the sky. My spirit takes flight then floats downward. I open my eyes, returned home.

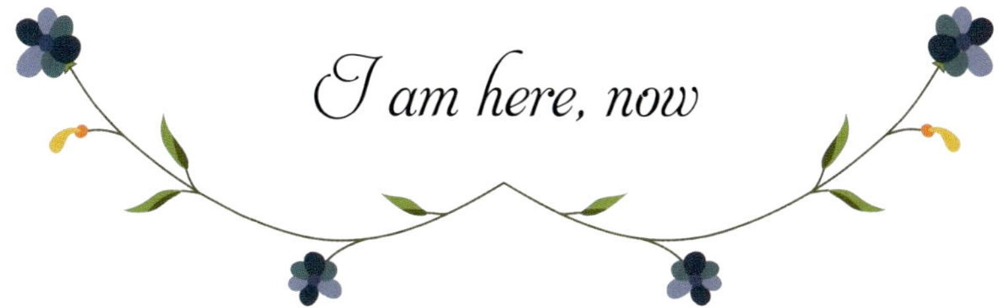

I am here, now

Close your eyes now and repeat to yourself: "I am here, now. I am here, now." Allow the chaos of the day to drift away on the ocean of your conscious awareness. "I am here, now." Let go of what weighs you down in body and in spirit. "I am here, now." Be here, now.

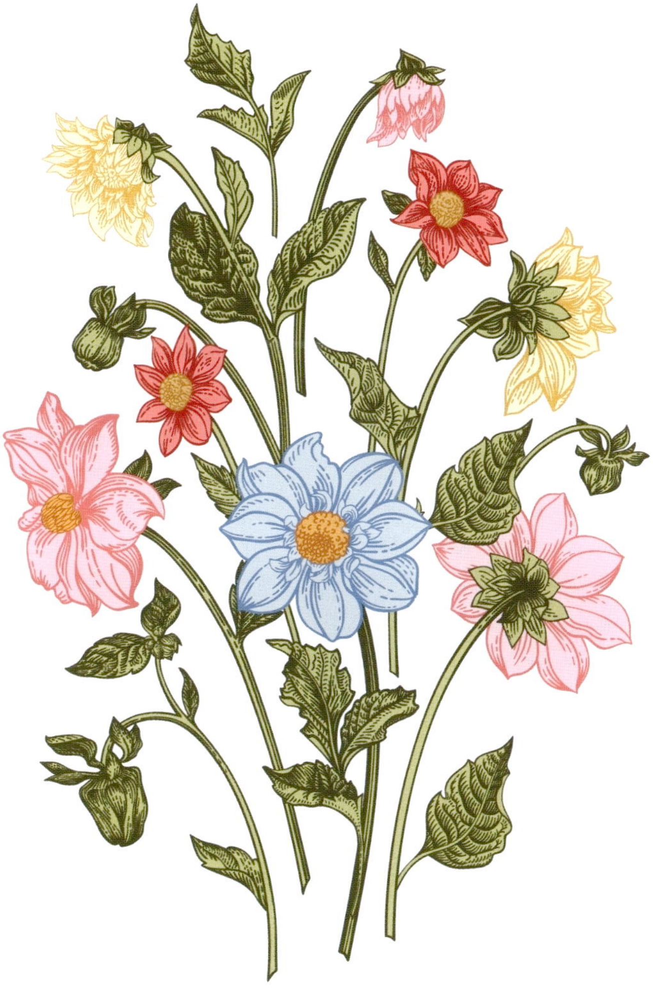

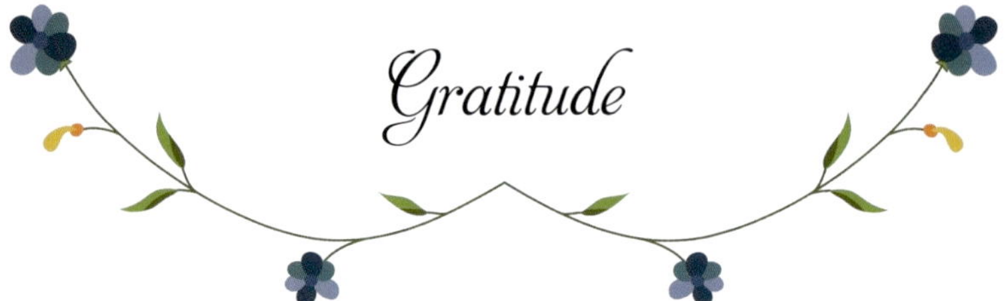

Gratitude

Upon awakening, I think of all I am grateful for. Before I sleep, I think of all I am grateful for. My mind begins and ends in a state of peace, harmony and presence, and I allow the hours between the beginning and the end to flow without resistance.

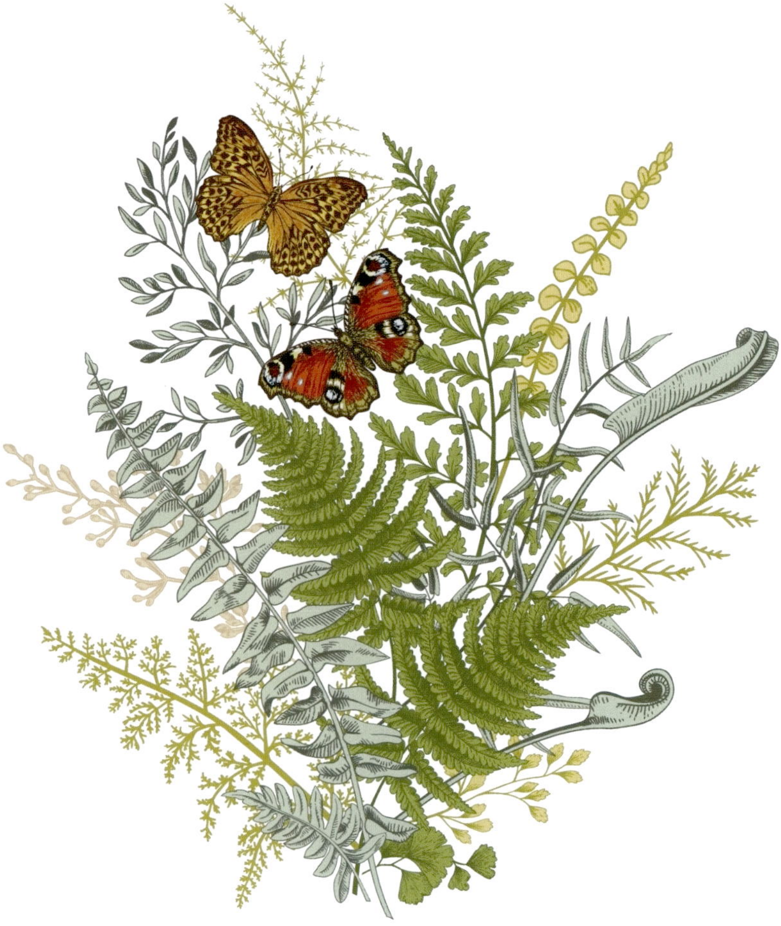

I find my quiet center and ground myself. There, I remember a time in my childhood when I felt free. I let my body absorb the feeling of freedom, of joy, playing in the grass with no cares or concerns. I am laughing, running, smelling the flowers in the garden. I melt into this memory, and I am a child again.

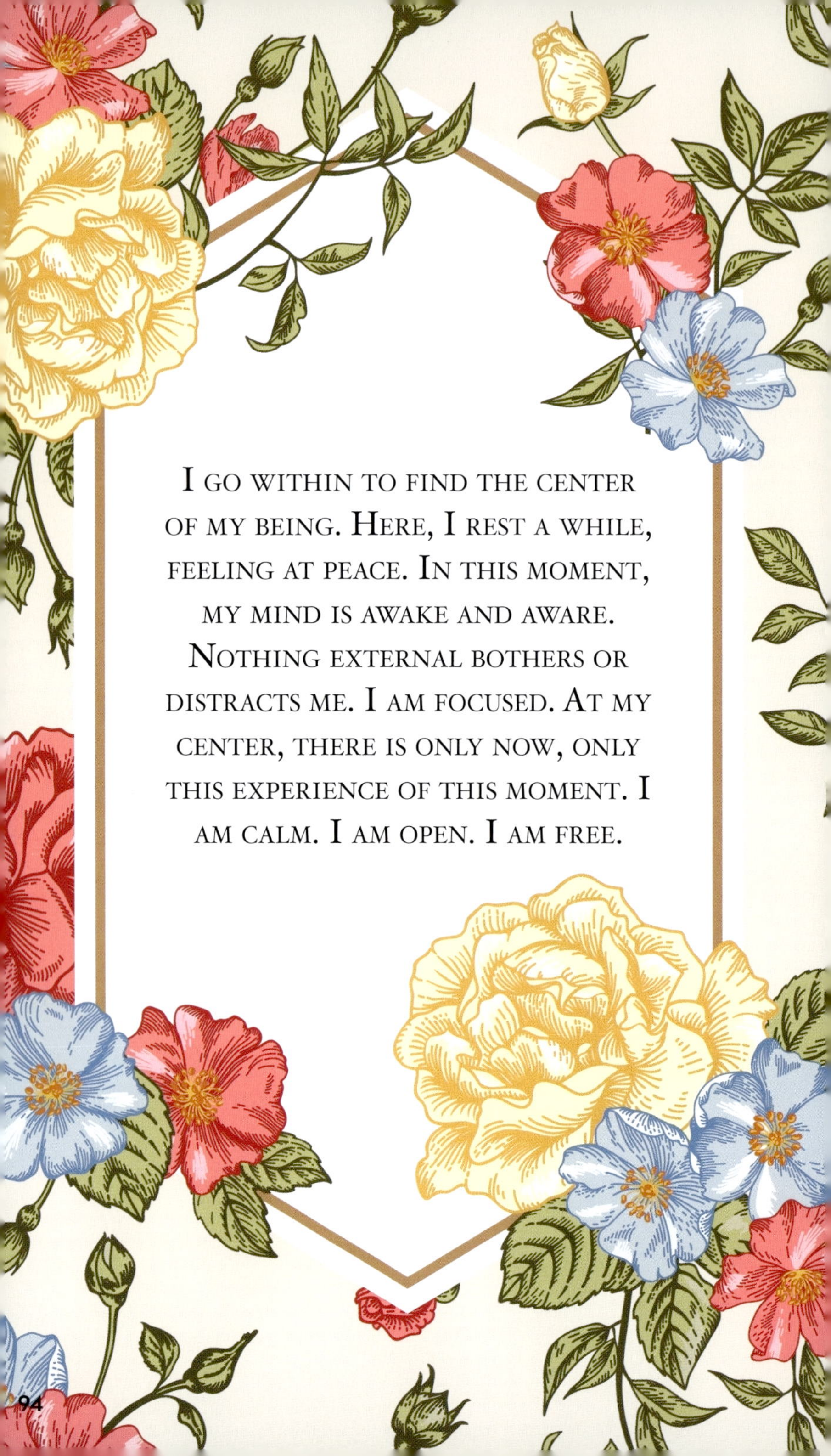

I go within to find the center of my being. Here, I rest a while, feeling at peace. In this moment, my mind is awake and aware. Nothing external bothers or distracts me. I am focused. At my center, there is only now, only this experience of this moment. I am calm. I am open. I am free.

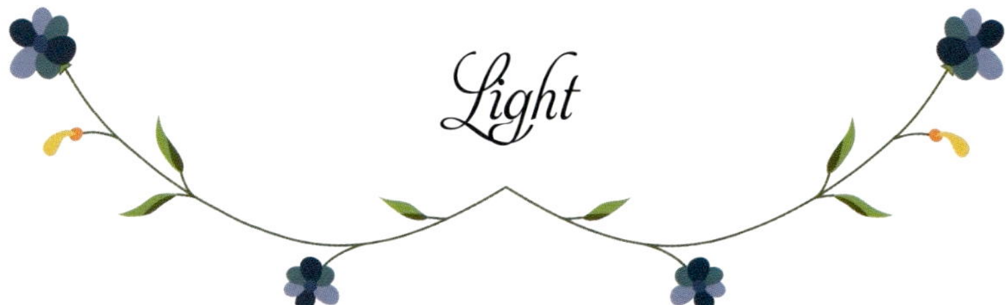

Light

My mind is like a jar of water, pouring out, emptying into the greater sea of consciousness. Now empty, I fill my mind with light. I let the light overflow and expand outward, glowing, warming. I focus on the light and let myself bask in the glow of pure love and positive energy. My mind becomes the light.

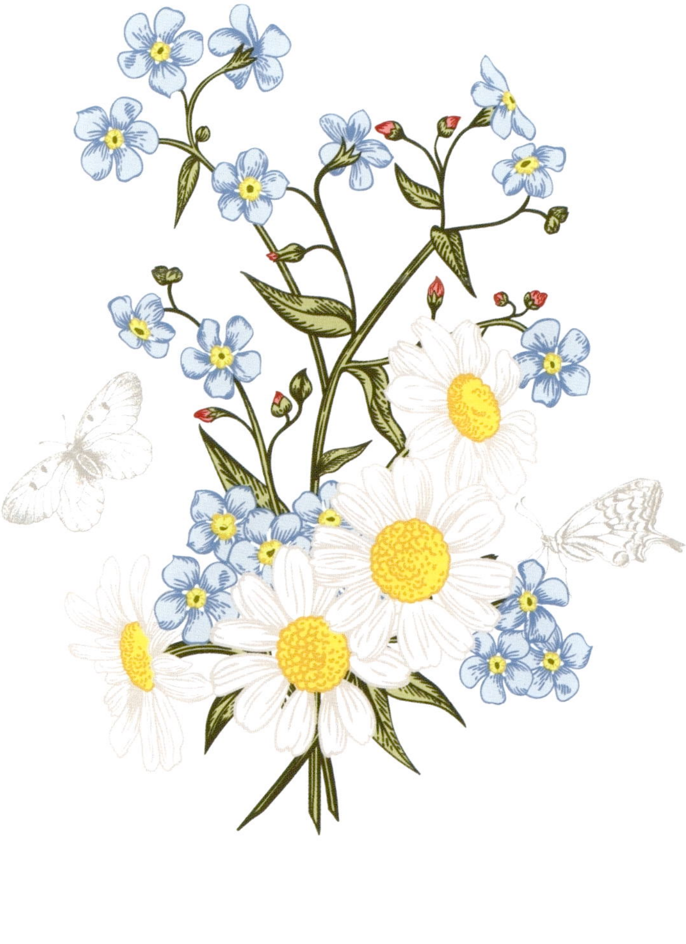

Counting backward from ten to one, let your mind become more and more quiet and calm. Breathe in with each count, holding the breath for three seconds before exhaling to the count of three. Feel your entire being relax into the pureness of the moment at hand. Breathe deeply for ten minutes: surrendering, allowing.

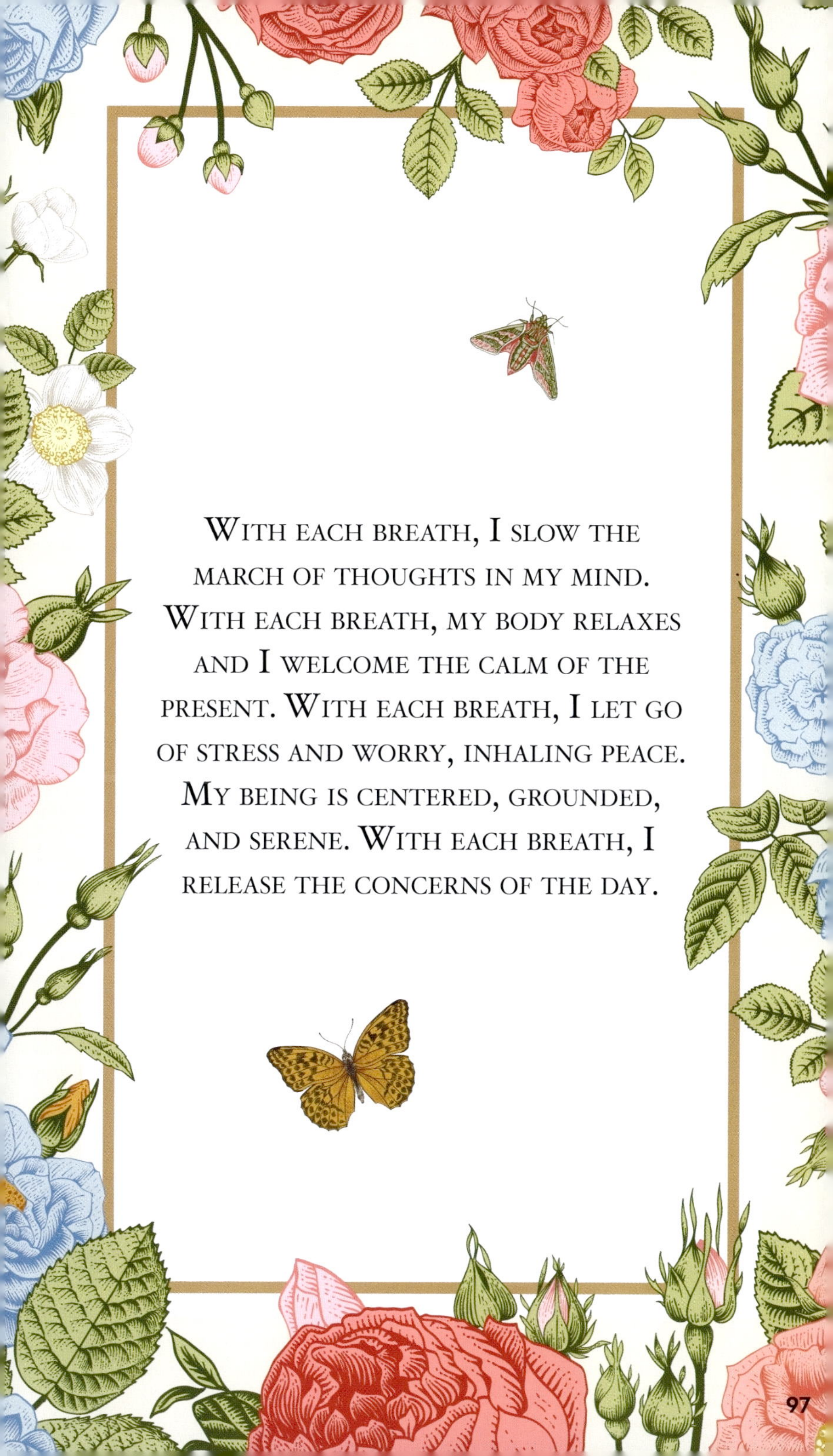

With each breath, I slow the march of thoughts in my mind. With each breath, my body relaxes and I welcome the calm of the present. With each breath, I let go of stress and worry, inhaling peace. My being is centered, grounded, and serene. With each breath, I release the concerns of the day.

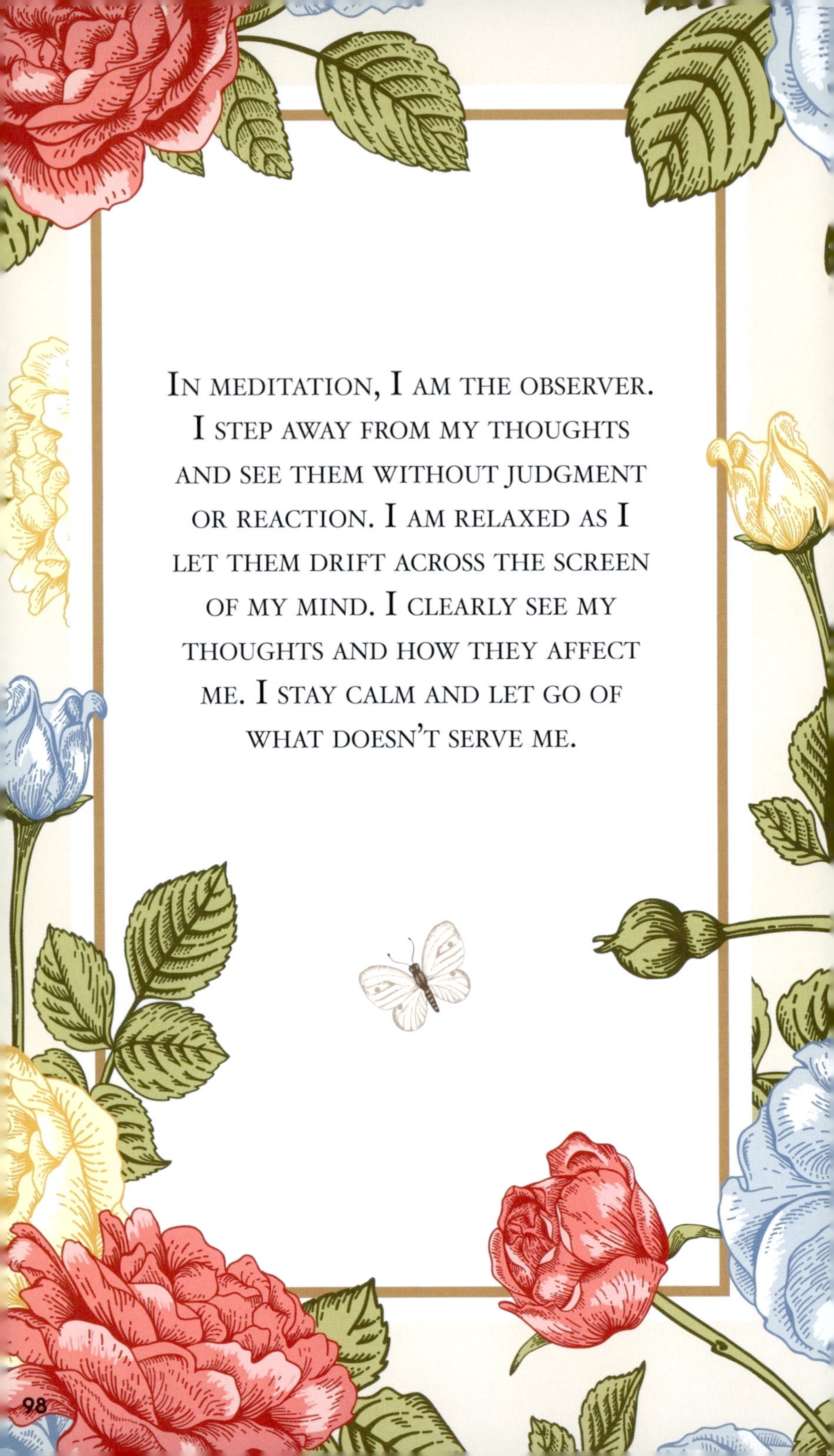

In meditation, I am the observer. I step away from my thoughts and see them without judgment or reaction. I am relaxed as I let them drift across the screen of my mind. I clearly see my thoughts and how they affect me. I stay calm and let go of what doesn't serve me.

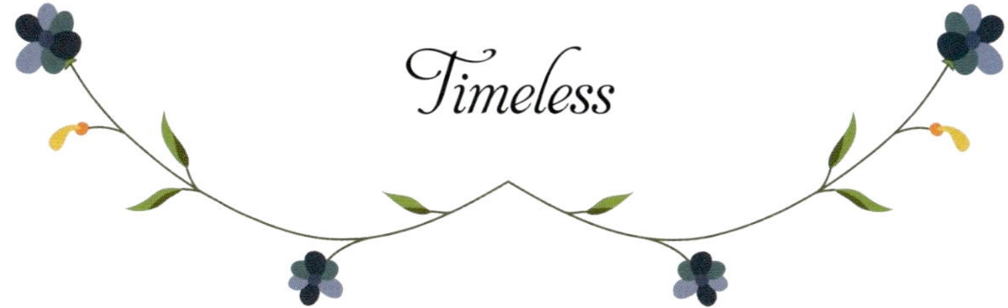

Timeless

At the center of my being there is no time, no past, present, or future. Time does not exist here, only breath, being, and awareness. I am in no hurry. I rest and relax and simply experience myself. Now I am ageless, timeless, and formless. In the center of my being, I am one with everything.

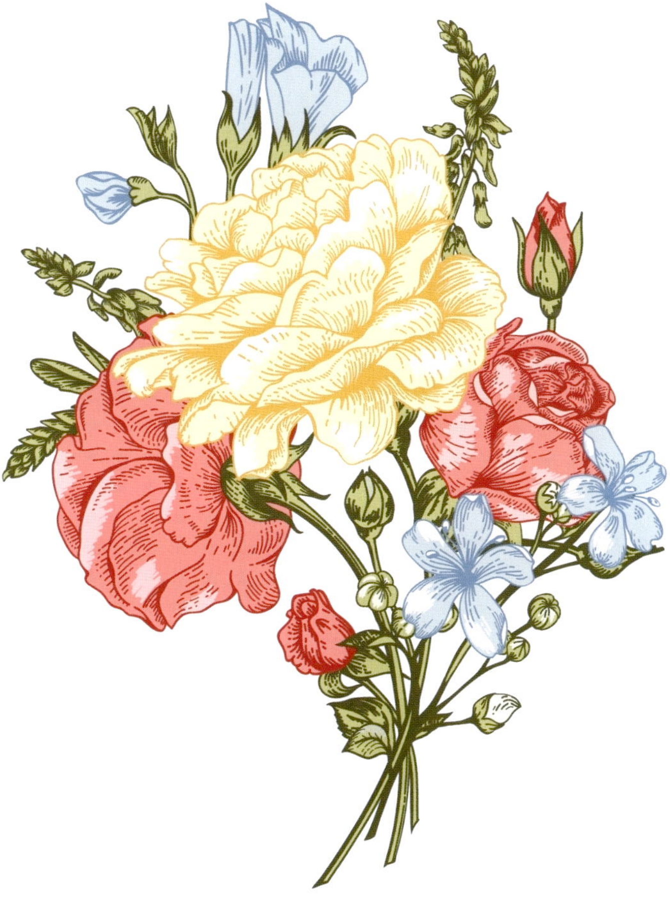

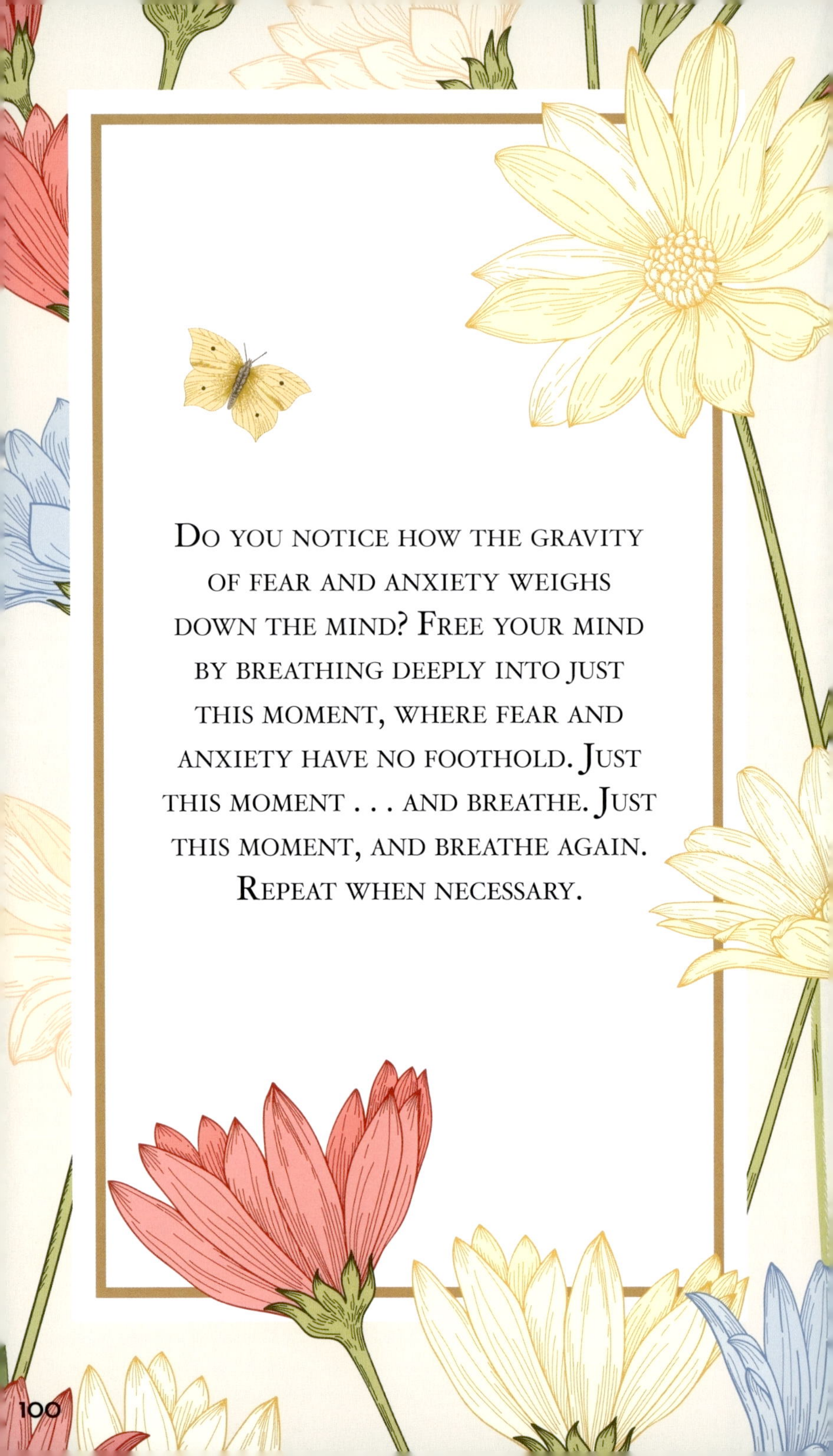

Do you notice how the gravity of fear and anxiety weighs down the mind? Free your mind by breathing deeply into just this moment, where fear and anxiety have no foothold. Just this moment . . . and breathe. Just this moment, and breathe again. Repeat when necessary.

Still the mind and let consciousness shift. Sense the oneness with all that exists. Become a part of that oneness, that wholeness. Let go of the beliefs in boundaries that separate you from that oneness. Merge with it, allowing it to fill your mind, heart, and spirit. You are connected with everything. One with all there is. Here in that oneness, all is well.
You are whole.

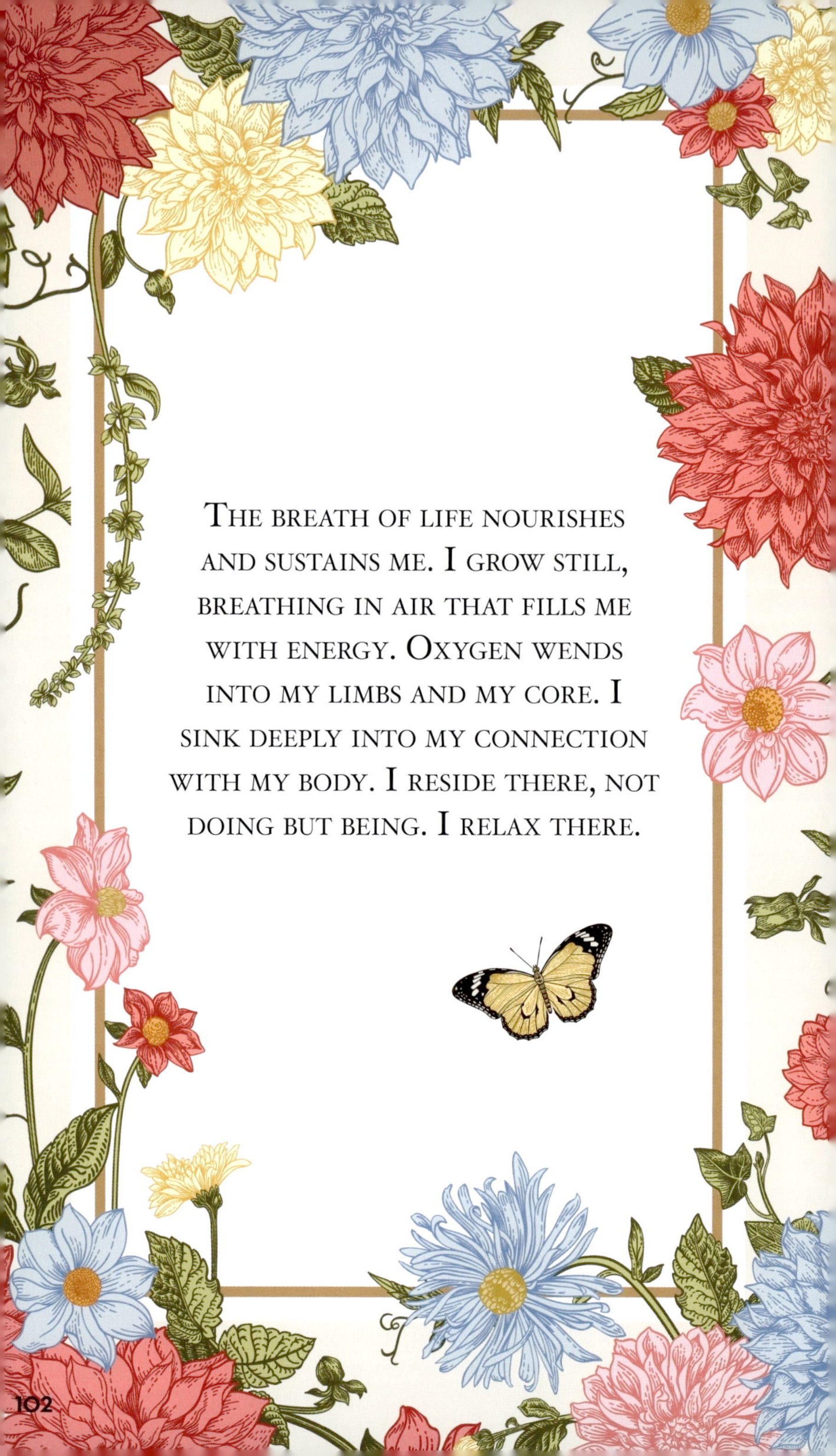

The breath of life nourishes and sustains me. I grow still, breathing in air that fills me with energy. Oxygen wends into my limbs and my core. I sink deeply into my connection with my body. I reside there, not doing but being. I relax there.

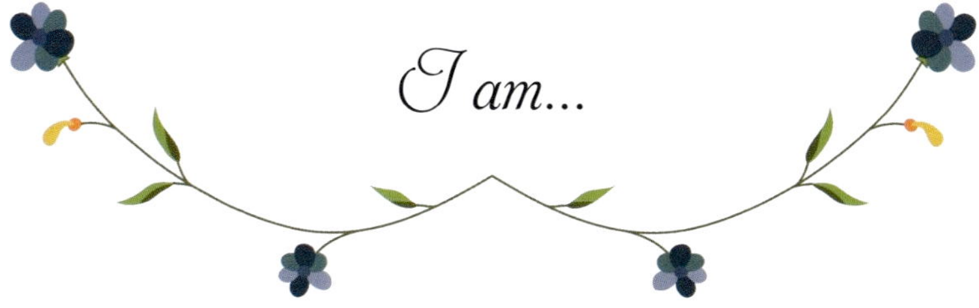

I am...

I am aware.
I am aware of my breath, giving me energy and vitality.
I am aware of my body, giving me motion and action.
I am aware of my thoughts, giving me ideas and goals.
I am aware of my spirit, giving me faith and inspiration.
I am aware of my soul, connection, and oneness.

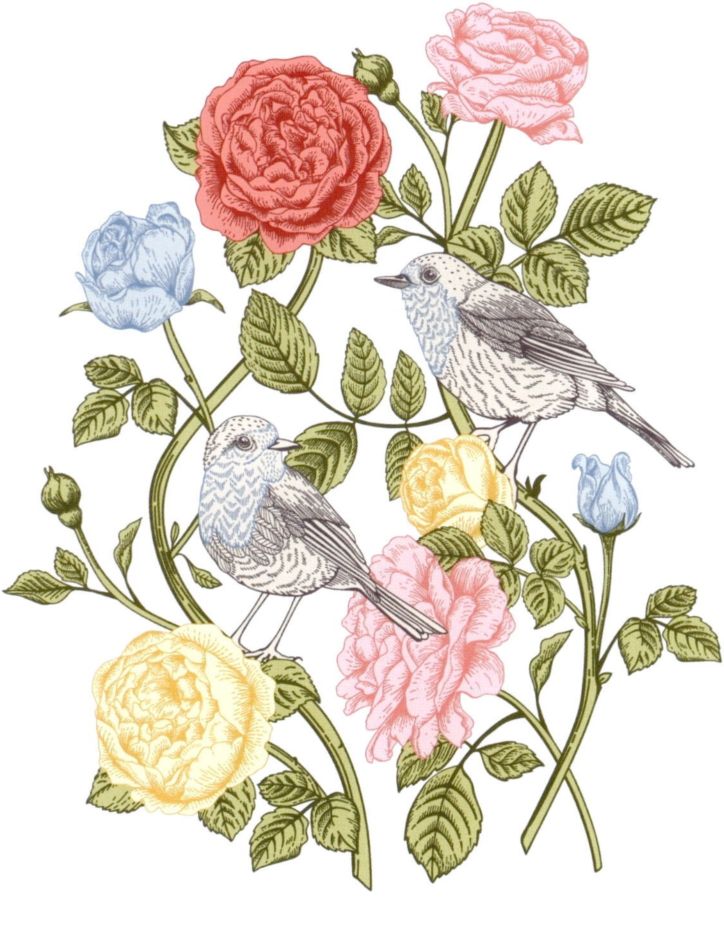

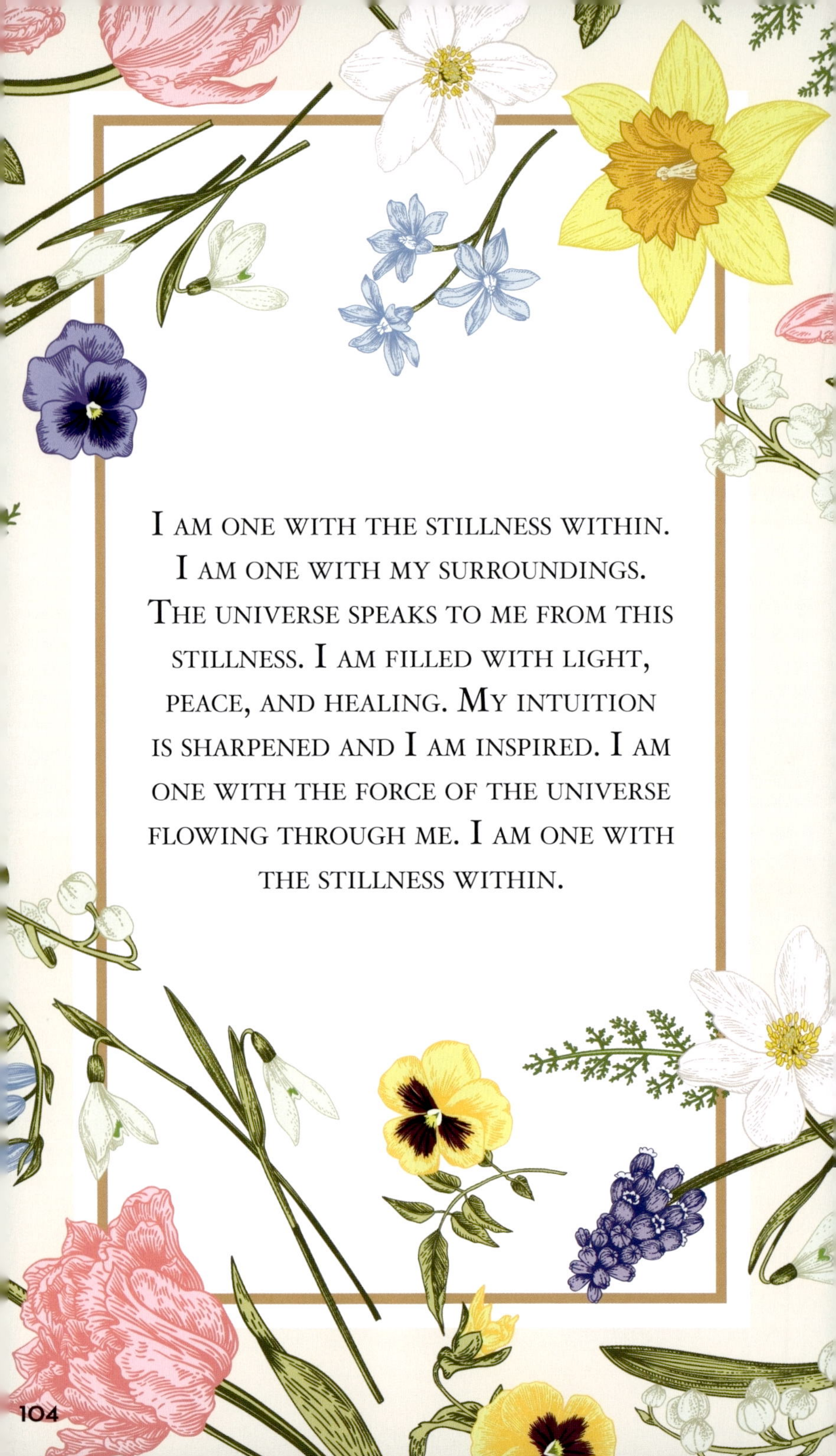

I am one with the stillness within. I am one with my surroundings. The universe speaks to me from this stillness. I am filled with light, peace, and healing. My intuition is sharpened and I am inspired. I am one with the force of the universe flowing through me. I am one with the stillness within.

Love is pure being. I turn my mind to thoughts of love, becoming present to the energies of love that express in me and through me. Love surrounds me and I am immersed in it. In the moment, there is only love, no fear. Fear cannot withstand the power of love, and I am love in its human expression. My thoughts are of the love within me, the love around me, the love I am.

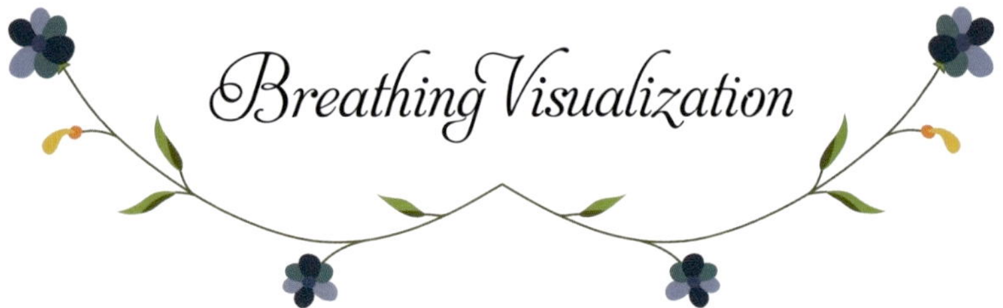

Breathing Visualization

I am formless. I am energy. I am light. I am vibration. I breathe in the energies of peace and harmony. I breathe out the energies of anger and fear. I become lighter with each breath, in and out, calming and expelling. I become free with each pass of air into my lungs, letting go of my burdens and cares. I am formless, boundless energy.

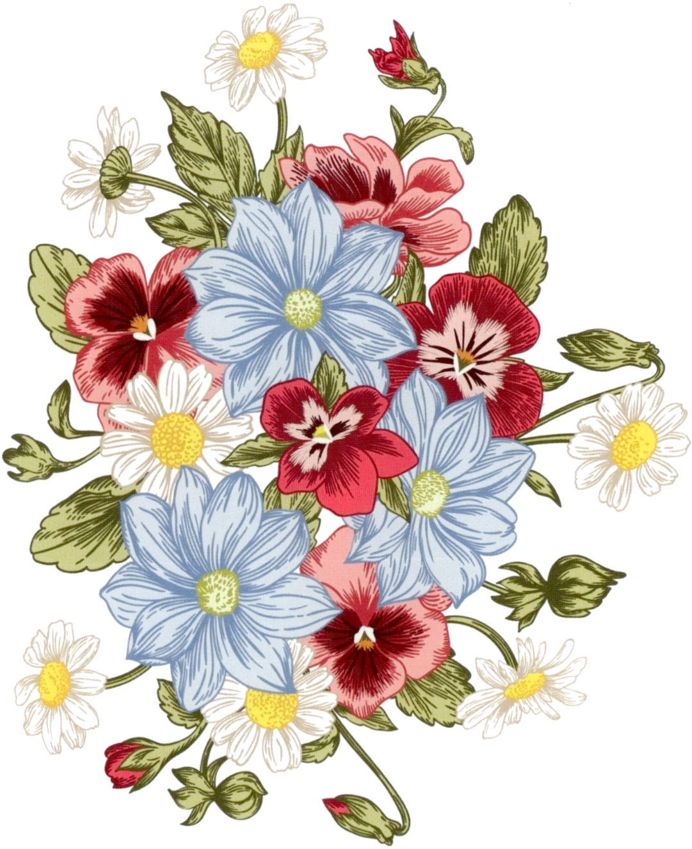

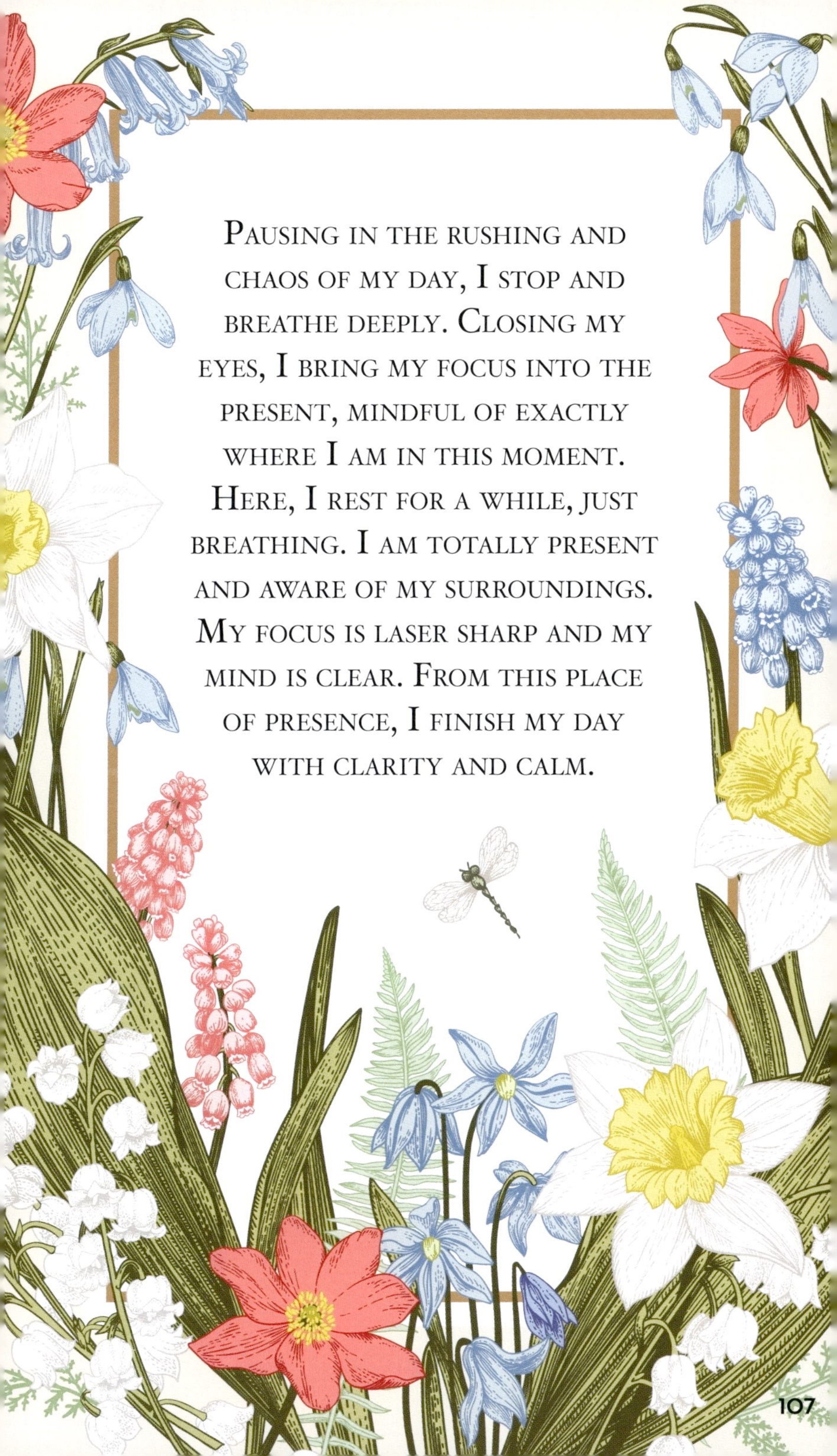

Pausing in the rushing and chaos of my day, I stop and breathe deeply. Closing my eyes, I bring my focus into the present, mindful of exactly where I am in this moment. Here, I rest for a while, just breathing. I am totally present and aware of my surroundings. My focus is laser sharp and my mind is clear. From this place of presence, I finish my day with clarity and calm.

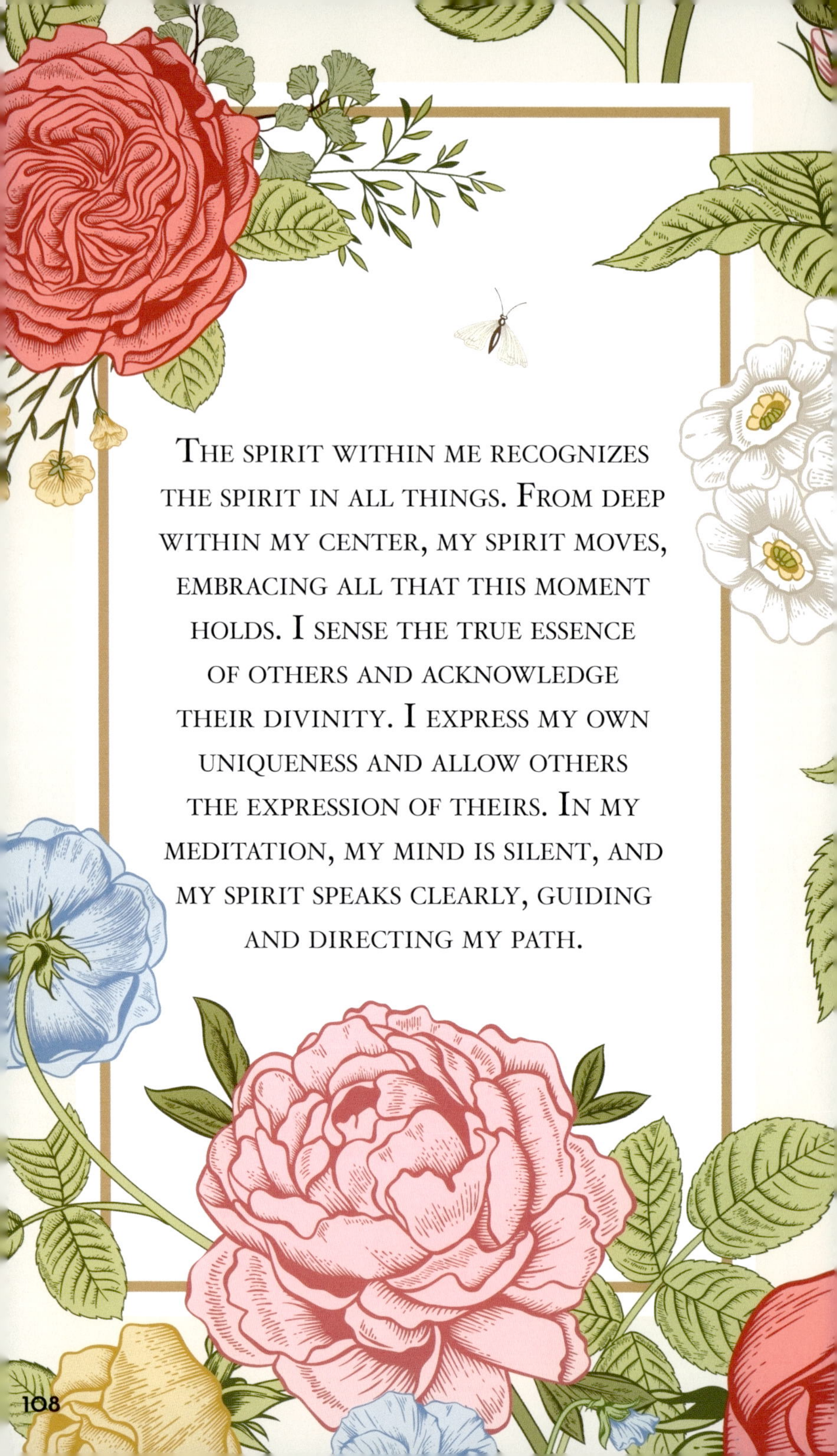

The spirit within me recognizes the spirit in all things. From deep within my center, my spirit moves, embracing all that this moment holds. I sense the true essence of others and acknowledge their divinity. I express my own uniqueness and allow others the expression of theirs. In my meditation, my mind is silent, and my spirit speaks clearly, guiding and directing my path.

I am the universe poured into one small vessel. I breathe and turn within, feeling a connection to the web of life: I am a strand in that web and a vital portion of the whole web. I release my notions of being alone, lonely, and separate. I am a piece of the whole and the whole itself. I am the universe in microcosm. I am the universe in human form.

Energy is life. During meditation, imagine you are nothing but vibrating waves of energy. Visualize your vibration rising higher. Give it a light and vivid color and a positive sensation. Experience the life energy moving through your body, lifting each cell into a vibration of healing and wholeness. Let your heart match the frequency of joy.

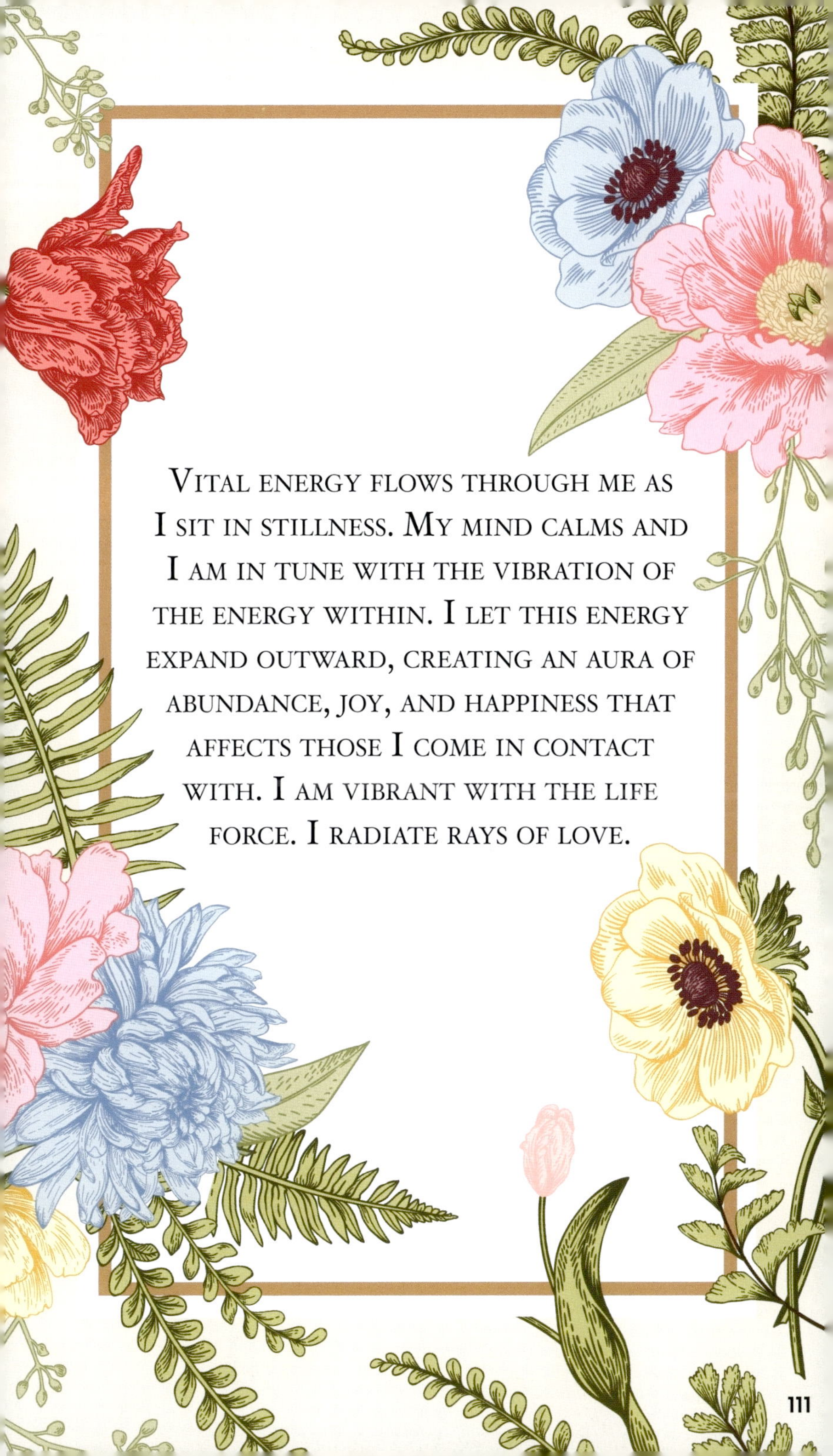

Vital energy flows through me as I sit in stillness. My mind calms and I am in tune with the vibration of the energy within. I let this energy expand outward, creating an aura of abundance, joy, and happiness that affects those I come in contact with. I am vibrant with the life force. I radiate rays of love.

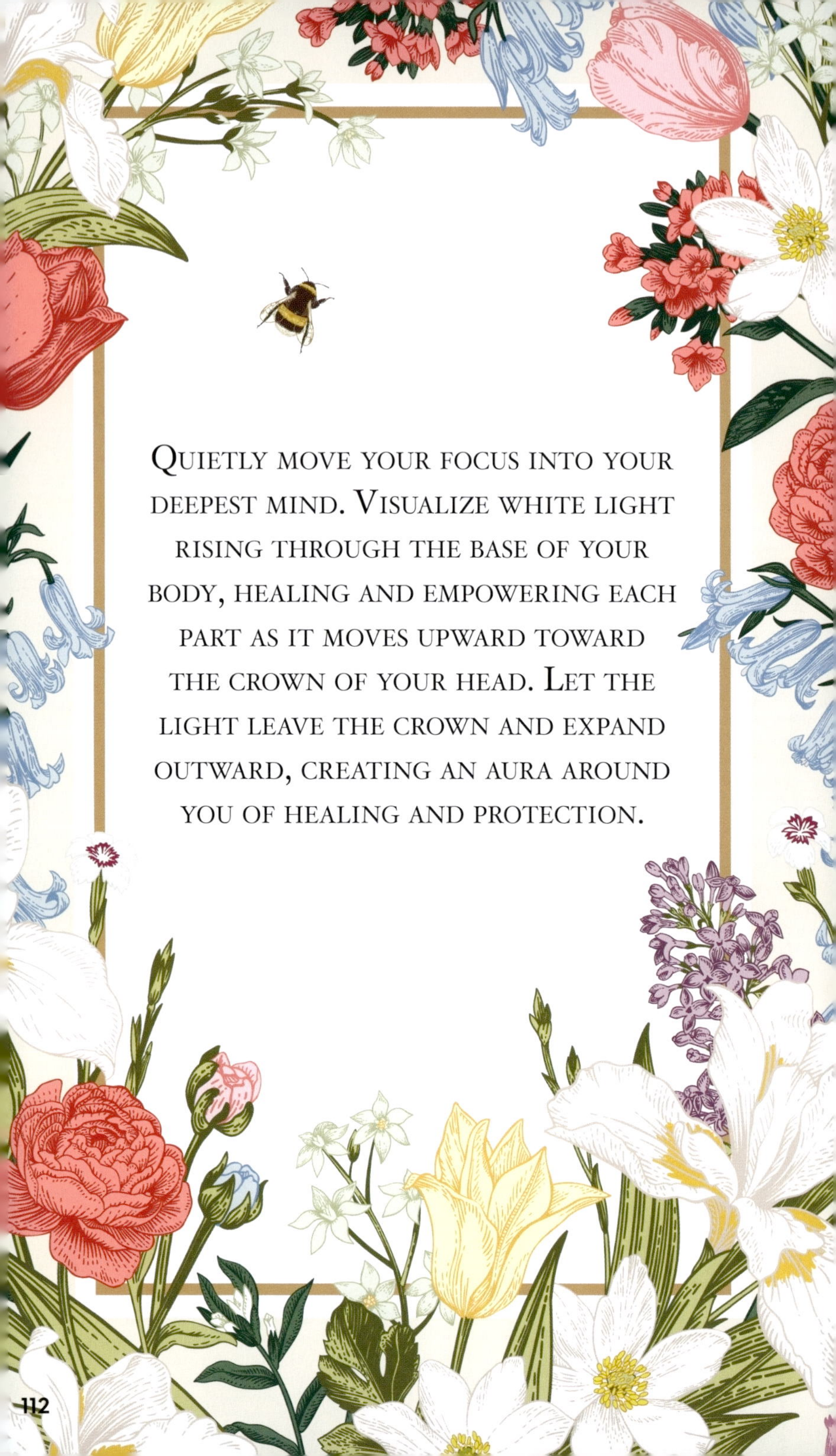

Quietly move your focus into your deepest mind. Visualize white light rising through the base of your body, healing and empowering each part as it moves upward toward the crown of your head. Let the light leave the crown and expand outward, creating an aura around you of healing and protection.

Allow the mind to drift with no end goal. Let thoughts be as they ebb and flow with no expectation. Breathe in and out, observing but not reacting. Let everything happen without necessity of control. The mind drifts. Thoughts move like waves on the sand. Breath comes and goes. Life is in this moment, here and now.

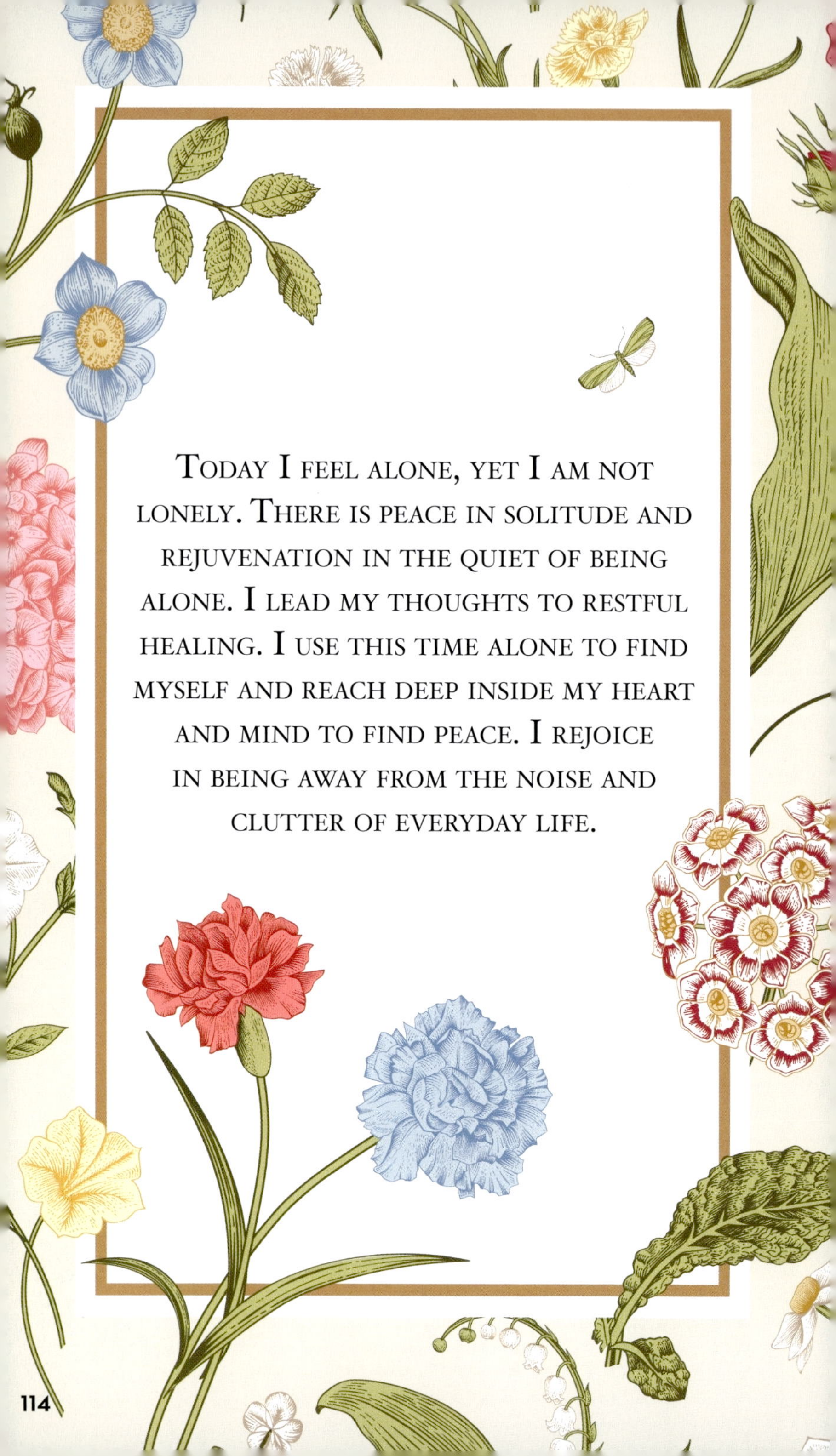

Today I feel alone, yet I am not lonely. There is peace in solitude and rejuvenation in the quiet of being alone. I lead my thoughts to restful healing. I use this time alone to find myself and reach deep inside my heart and mind to find peace. I rejoice in being away from the noise and clutter of everyday life.

As I breathe deeply, time slows down to a singular moment—the now. I relax here, sensing with a greater awareness the timelessness of experience. Spirit within knows no boundaries of time. I am spirit. I am without boundaries of time. The now I rest in is eternal, with no beginning or end. In the now, I am forever.

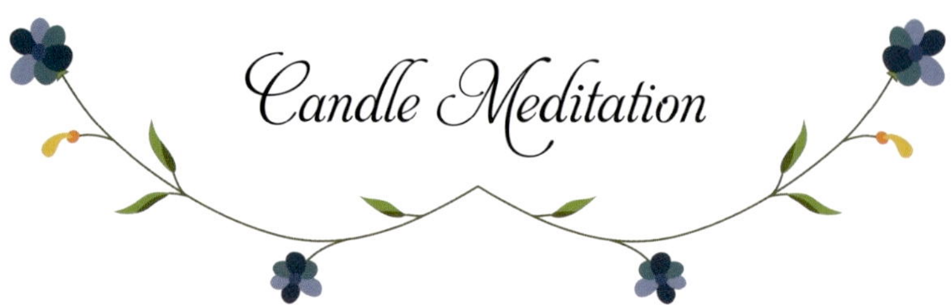

Candle Meditation

Dim the lights in a quiet room and light a candle. Watch the flame and let thoughts drift away as your mind focuses on the dance of light. Drop your shoulders and let your eyelids droop, allowing the flame to hypnotize and relax you. Breathe in through your nose and out through your mouth. Become the dancing flame as your sensation of having a body dissipates. Become the light in the darkness.

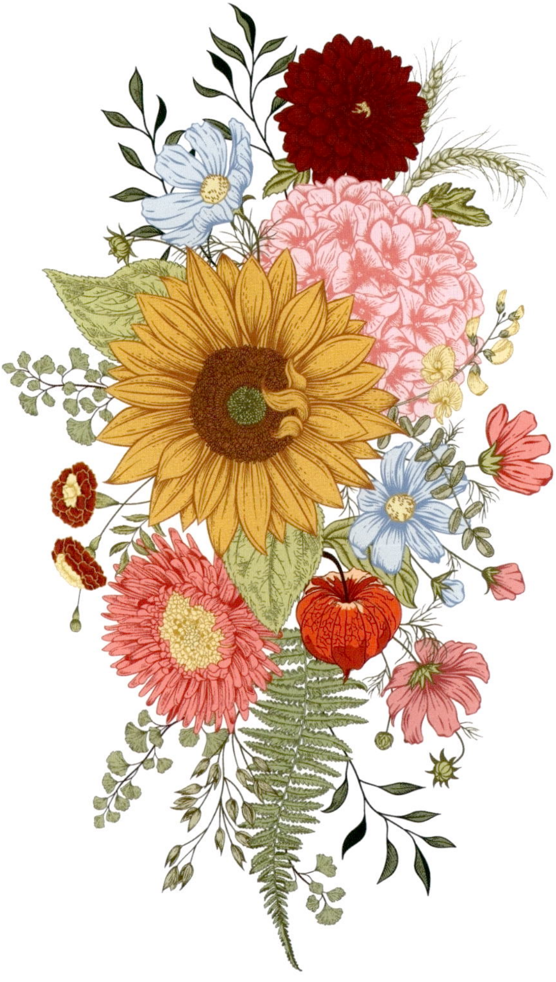

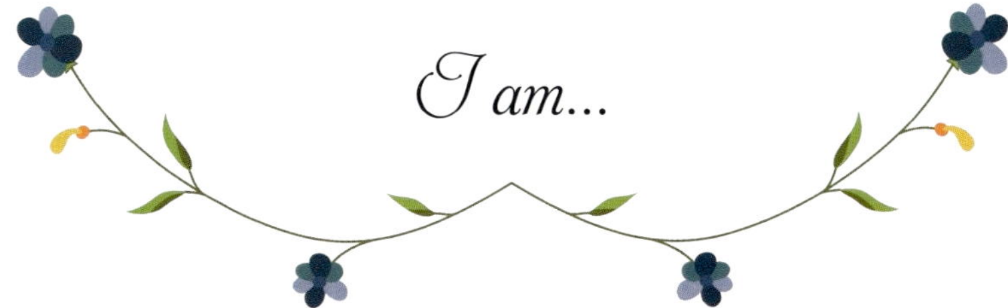

I am...

I am breath. I am energy. I am light. I am the force of life itself within my body, expressing outward into my world. I am the flow and process of life, moving in rhythm with every heartbeat. I am consciousness made manifest. With each breath, I am immersed in this vibrant, creative, and empowering energy of love.

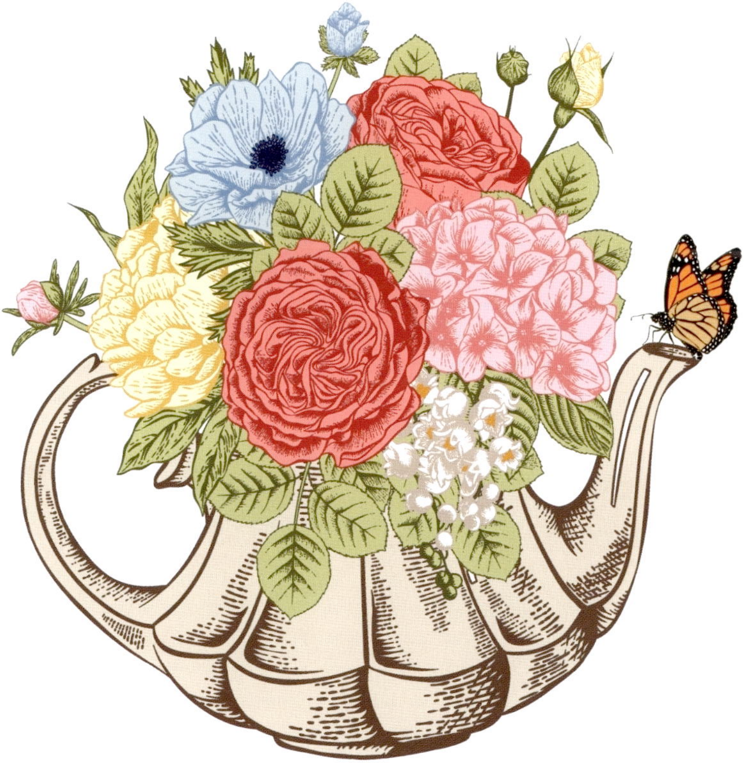

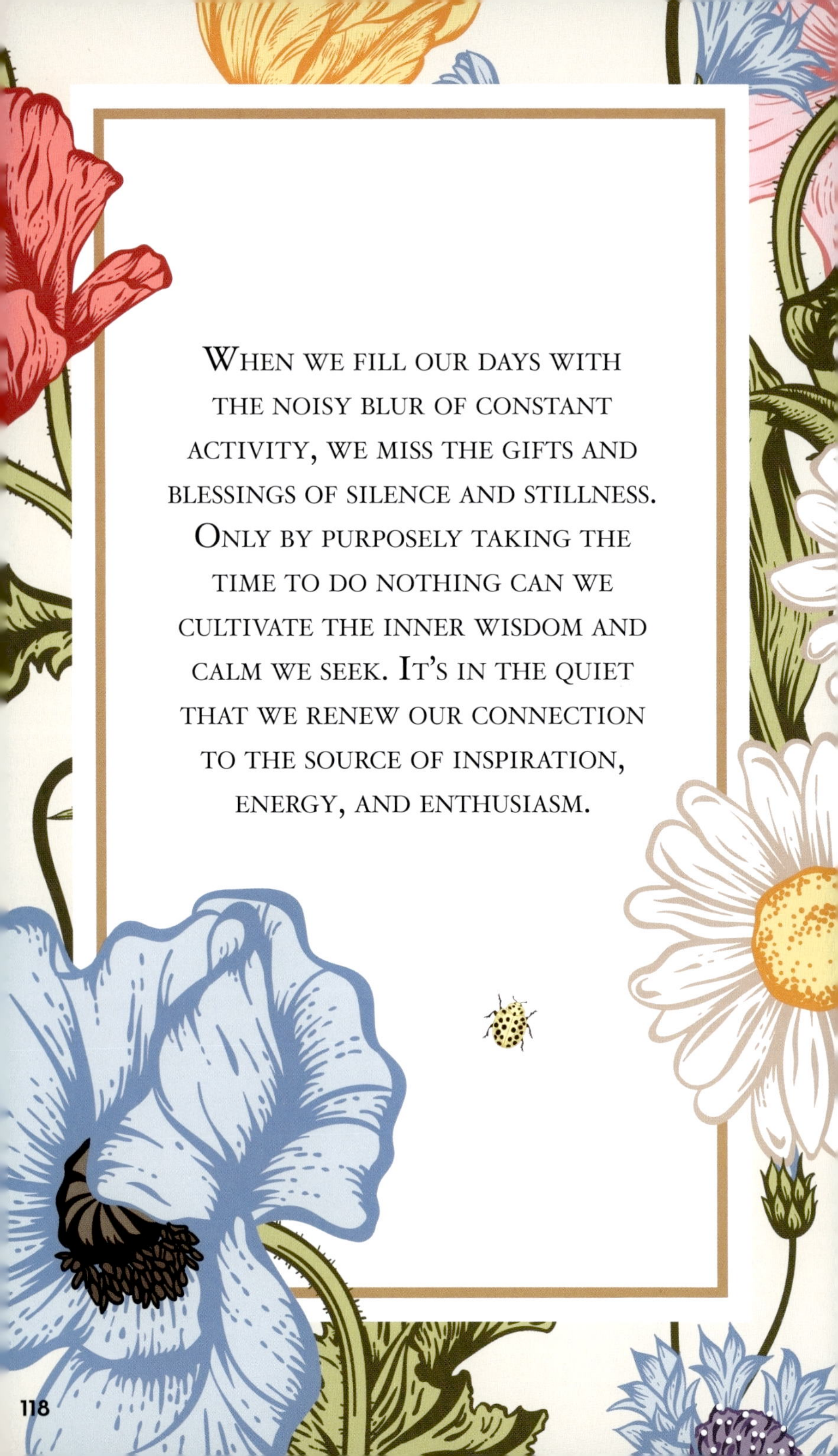

When we fill our days with the noisy blur of constant activity, we miss the gifts and blessings of silence and stillness. Only by purposely taking the time to do nothing can we cultivate the inner wisdom and calm we seek. It's in the quiet that we renew our connection to the source of inspiration, energy, and enthusiasm.

Pick up an object in the room and focus your attention on it. Feel it in your hands. Is it smooth or rough? Cool or warm? Does it have a scent? Look closely at the materials. Hold it up to the light and examine it. Focus only on this object. This exercise teaches you to see something instead of merely looking at it.

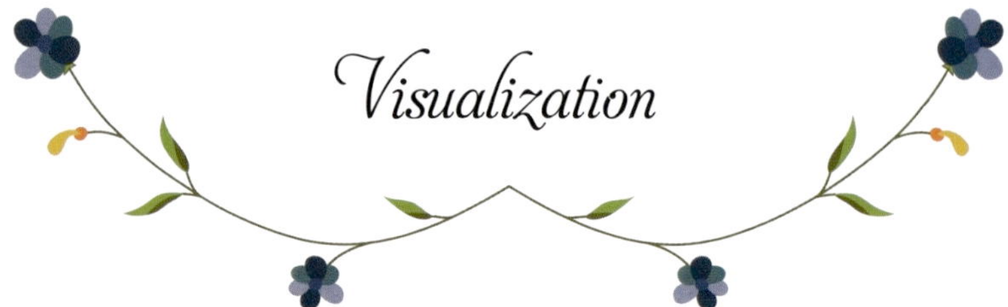

Visualization

In your mind exists a door. Visualize this door opening. Go through the door into a beautiful place vibrant with light and color. There is a wise person waiting. Sit with this person in silence, absorbing their unspoken guidance. When you feel ready, go back through the door, carrying with you the wisdom of your inner spirit.

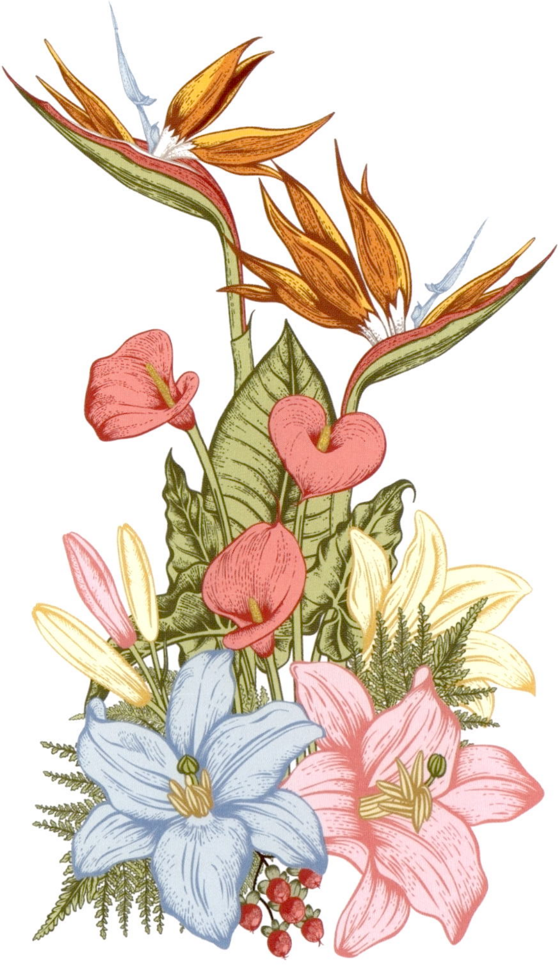

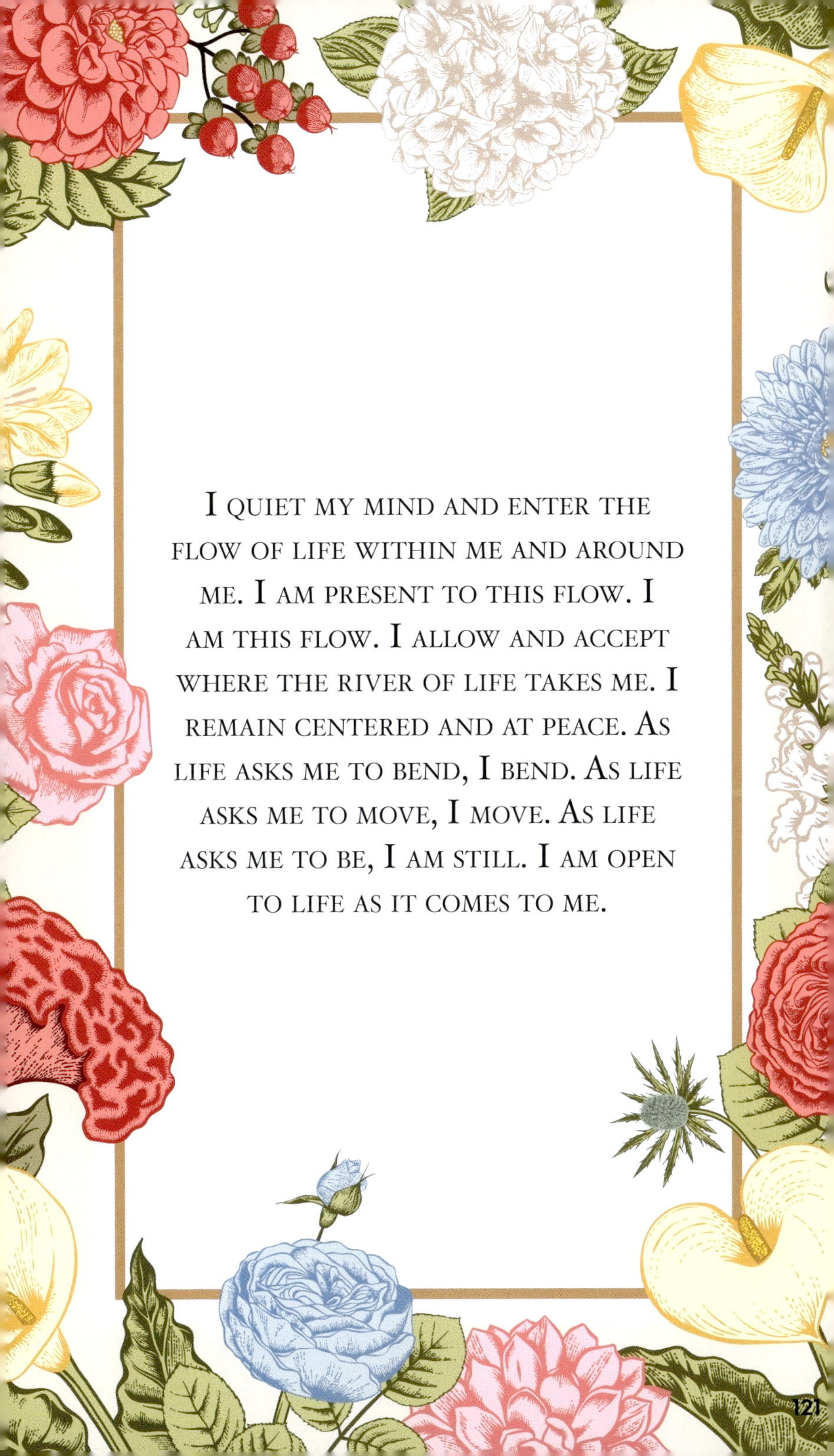

I quiet my mind and enter the flow of life within me and around me. I am present to this flow. I am this flow. I allow and accept where the river of life takes me. I remain centered and at peace. As life asks me to bend, I bend. As life asks me to move, I move. As life asks me to be, I am still. I am open to life as it comes to me.

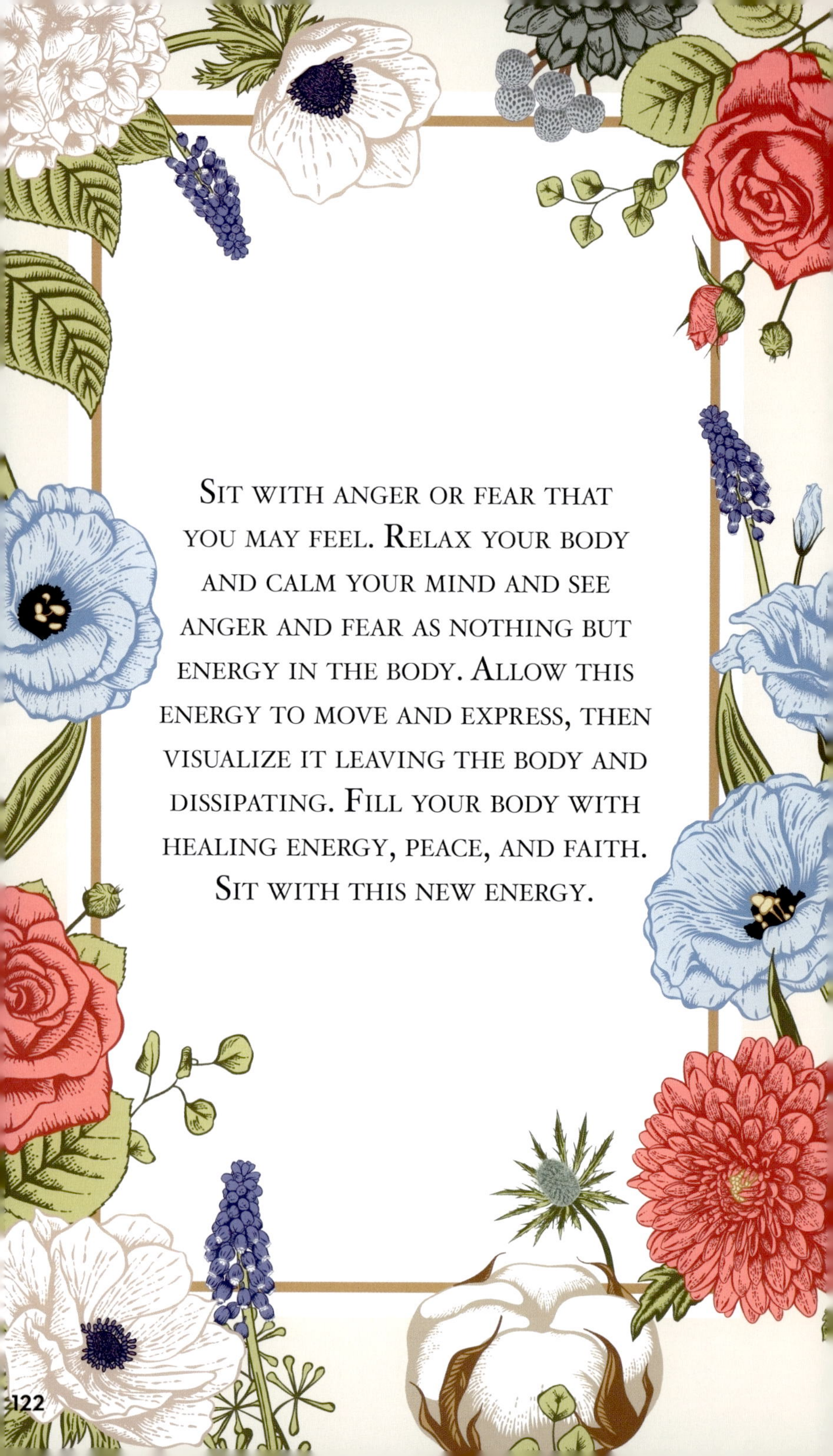

Sit with anger or fear that you may feel. Relax your body and calm your mind and see anger and fear as nothing but energy in the body. Allow this energy to move and express, then visualize it leaving the body and dissipating. Fill your body with healing energy, peace, and faith. Sit with this new energy.

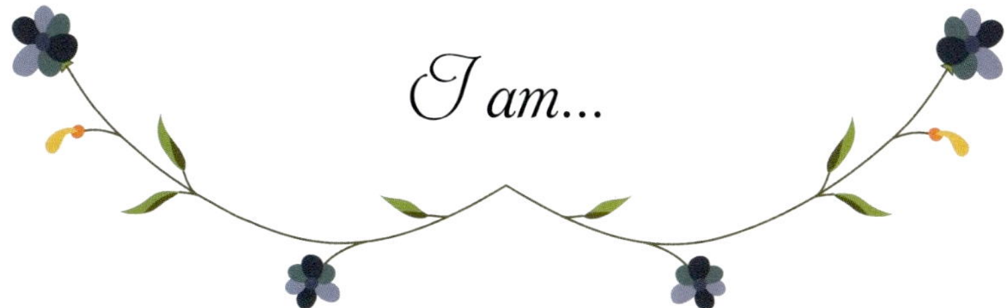

I am...

I am here. I begin breathing, inhaling and holding the breath for five beats. I am here. I exhale slowly, feeling the air move out of my lungs. I am here. I inhale again, filling my body with life-giving air. I am here. I exhale, to a count of five, letting go of stress. I am here. I breathe in, I breathe out. I am here.

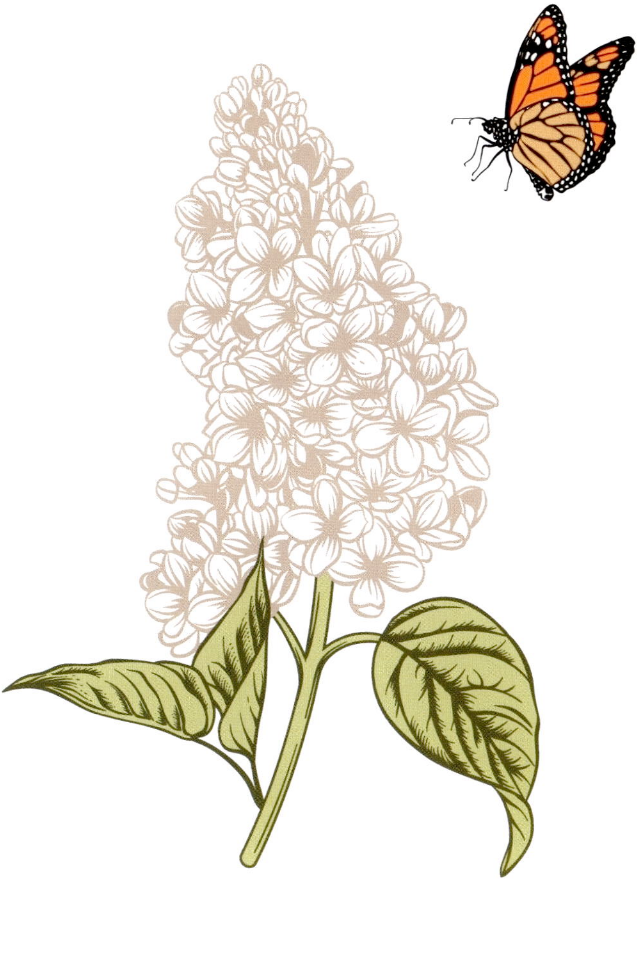

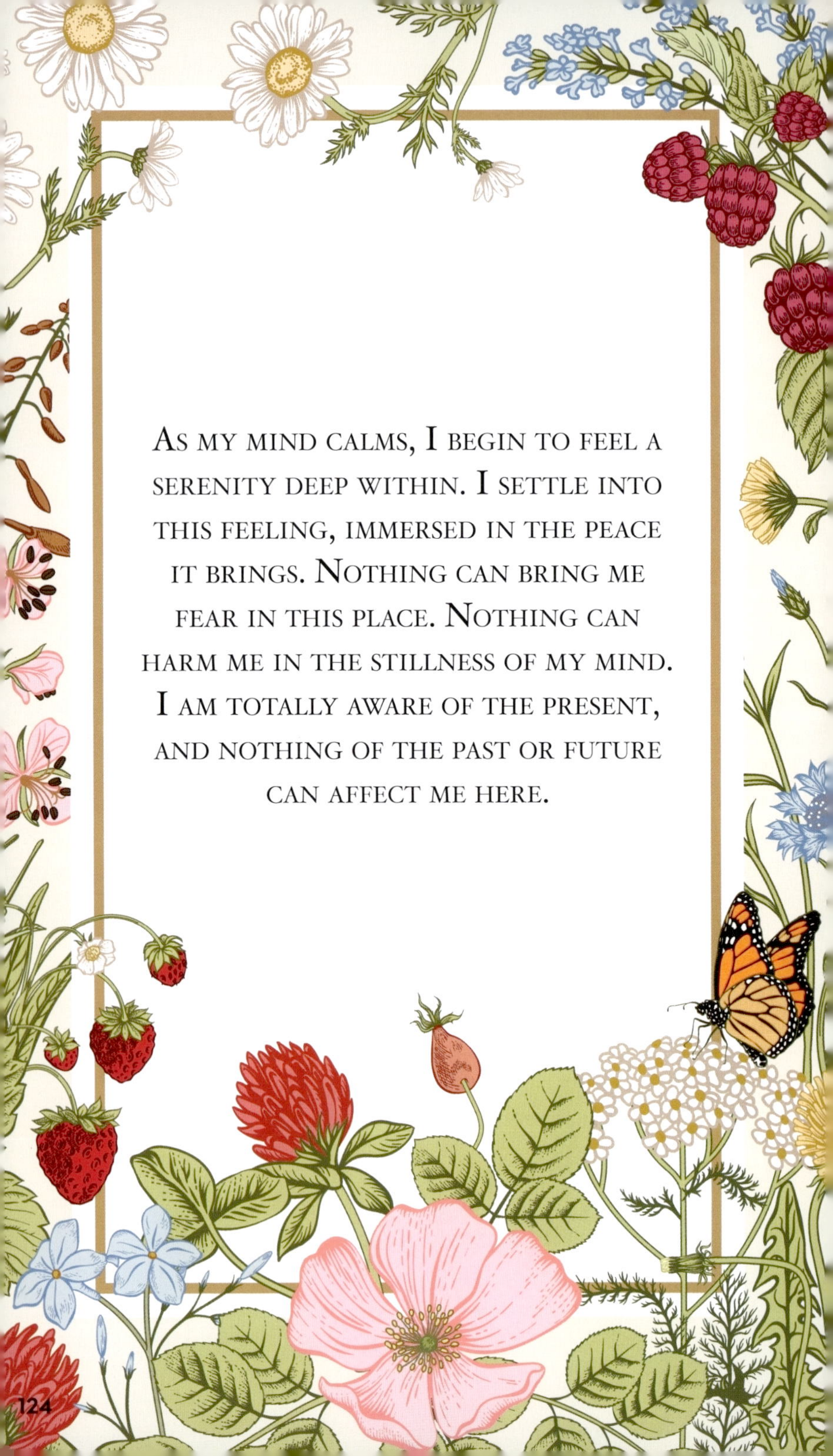

As my mind calms, I begin to feel a serenity deep within. I settle into this feeling, immersed in the peace it brings. Nothing can bring me fear in this place. Nothing can harm me in the stillness of my mind. I am totally aware of the present, and nothing of the past or future can affect me here.

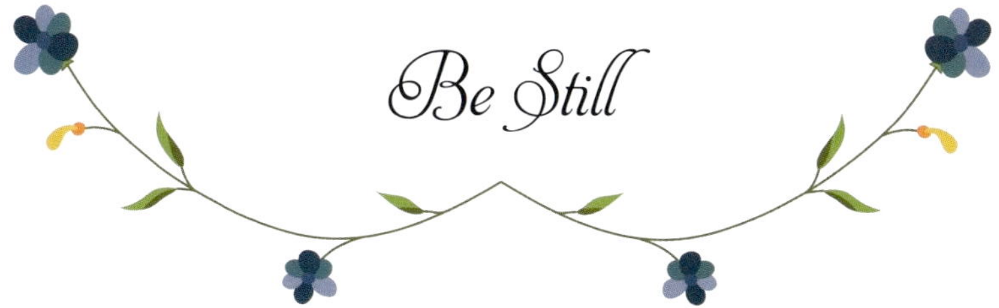

Be Still

Be still and listen to the whisper of your intuition within. Let it speak to you with the guidance and wisdom you seek. Relax the body, rest the intellect, and quiet the mind—allow your heart to have its voice. Be still in this loving and safe place, and know that you are precious, unique, and important.

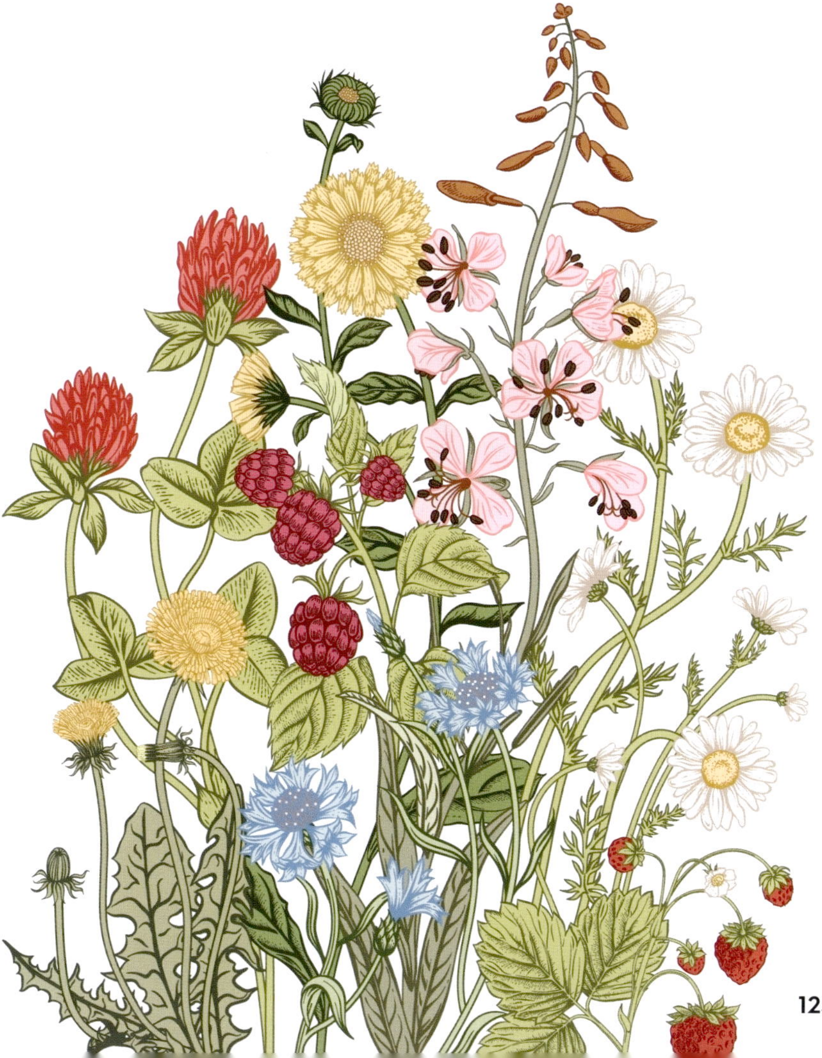

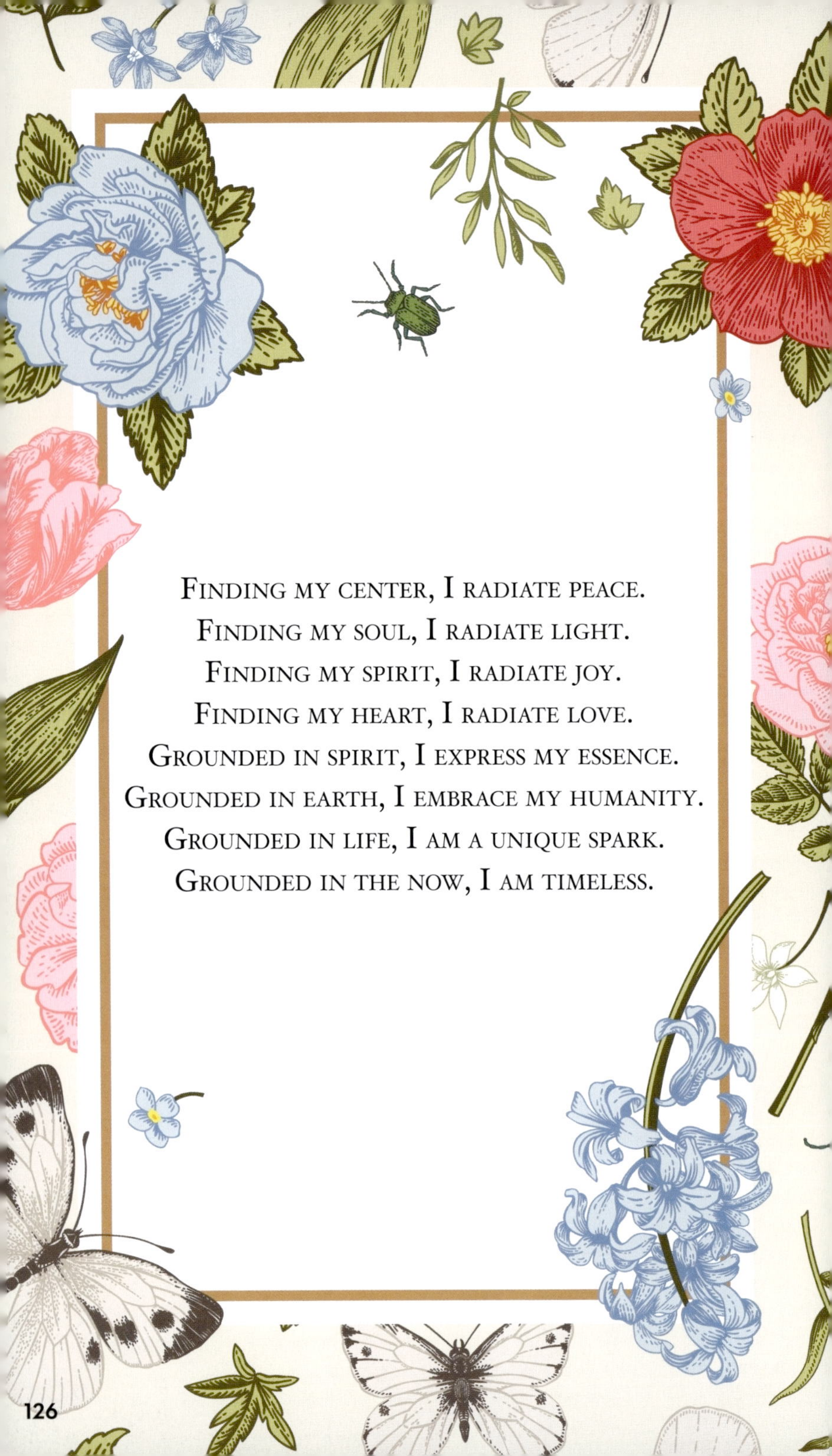

Finding my center, I radiate peace.
Finding my soul, I radiate light.
Finding my spirit, I radiate joy.
Finding my heart, I radiate love.
Grounded in spirit, I express my essence.
Grounded in earth, I embrace my humanity.
Grounded in life, I am a unique spark.
Grounded in the now, I am timeless.

Light is energy. I breathe in light and energize my body, mind, and spirit. The light washes over every part of me that is tired, rejuvenating and refreshing it with pure and joyful enthusiasm. I envision the light surrounding my body like an aura of good vibrations. My mind is clear and focused. I am ready.

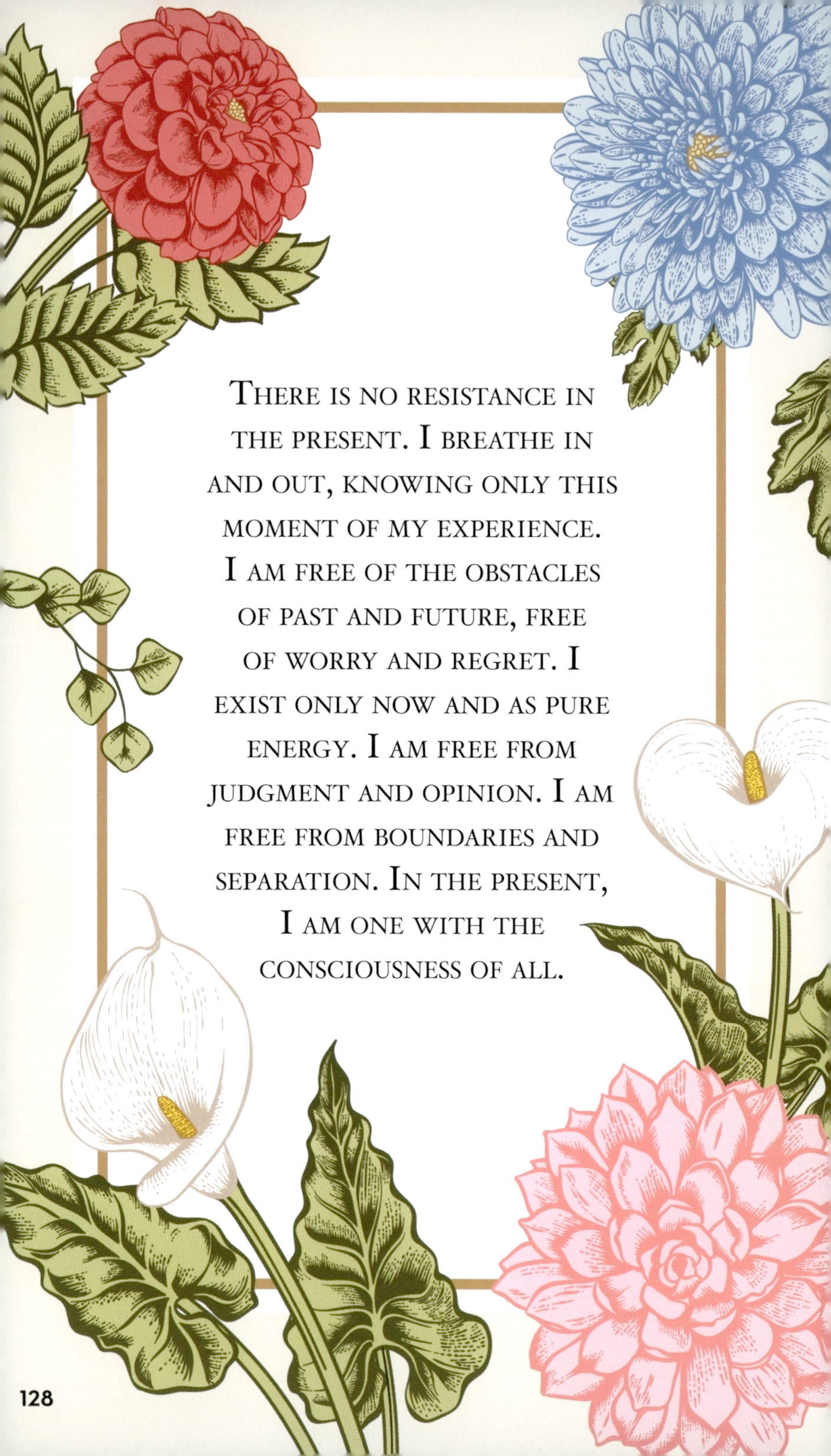

There is no resistance in the present. I breathe in and out, knowing only this moment of my experience. I am free of the obstacles of past and future, free of worry and regret. I exist only now and as pure energy. I am free from judgment and opinion. I am free from boundaries and separation. In the present, I am one with the consciousness of all.

I watch thoughts drift by like debris on ocean waves. In the stillness of my spirit, I am the observer. I don't hold onto things or let go of things. I let them float past. I feel no need to own or demand. I have no goals or motivations. In the stillness of my spirit, I am everything and anything I need already. I am complete and whole and free.

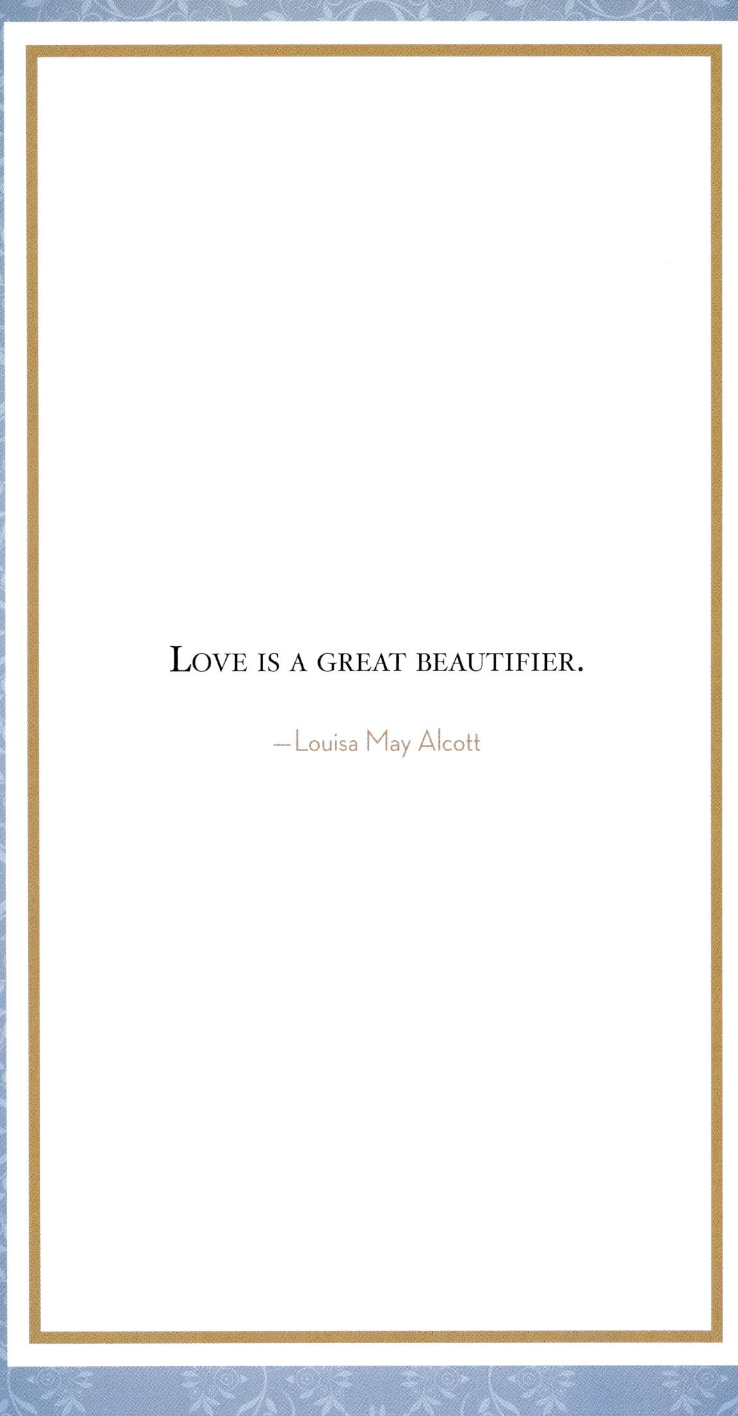

LOVE IS A GREAT BEAUTIFIER.

—Louisa May Alcott

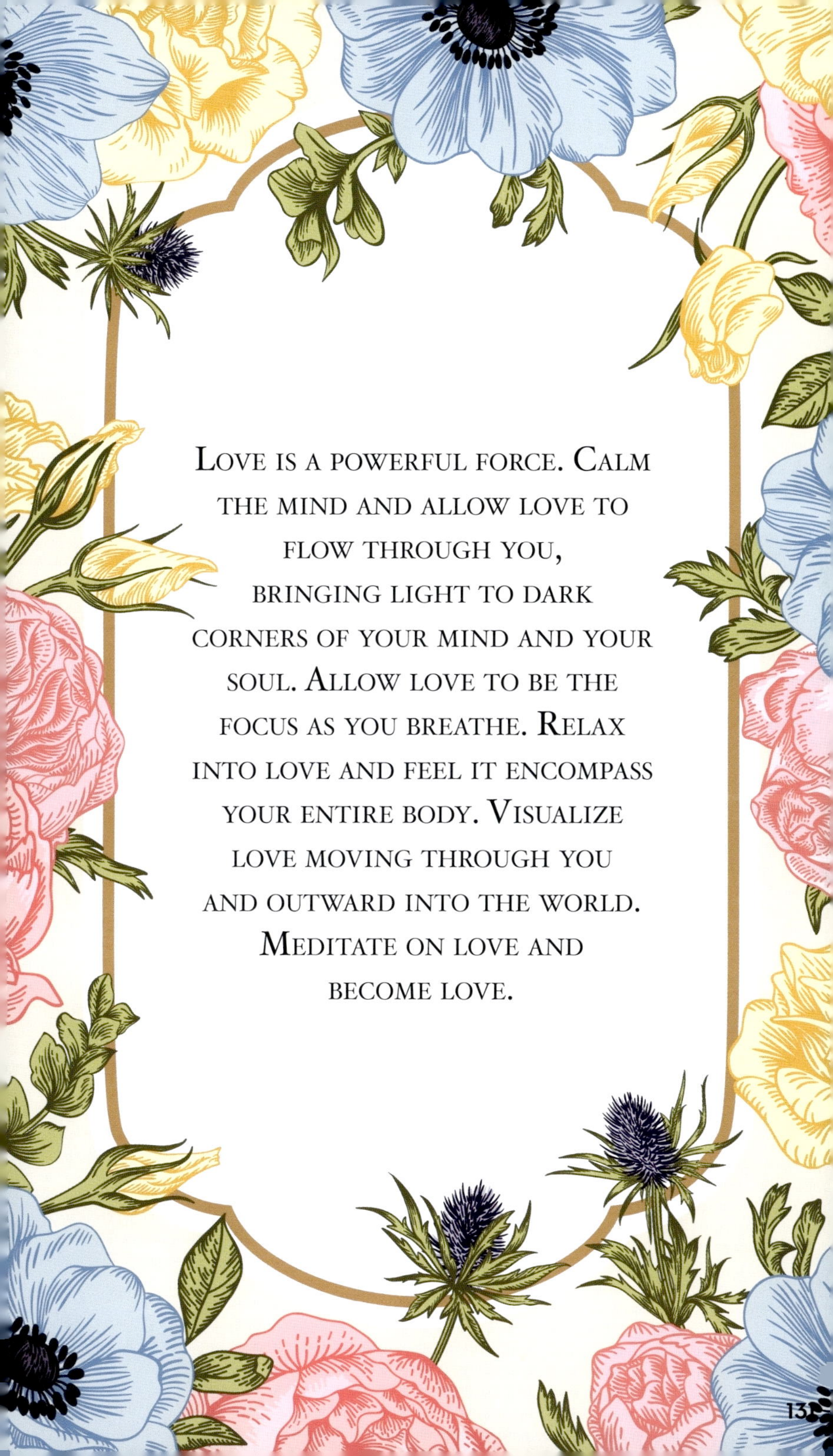

Love is a powerful force. Calm the mind and allow love to flow through you, bringing light to dark corners of your mind and your soul. Allow love to be the focus as you breathe. Relax into love and feel it encompass your entire body. Visualize love moving through you and outward into the world. Meditate on love and become love.

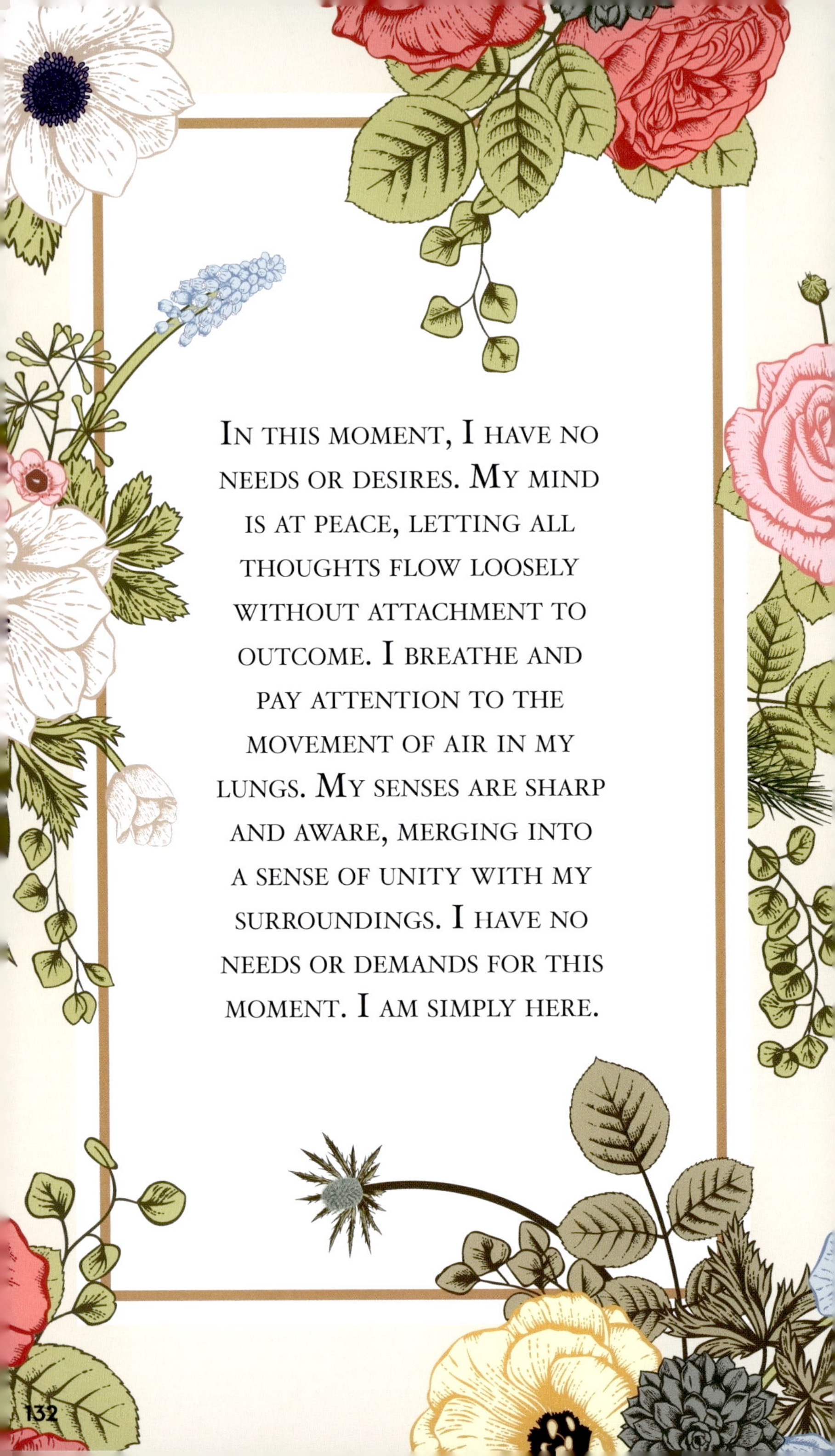

In this moment, I have no needs or desires. My mind is at peace, letting all thoughts flow loosely without attachment to outcome. I breathe and pay attention to the movement of air in my lungs. My senses are sharp and aware, merging into a sense of unity with my surroundings. I have no needs or demands for this moment. I am simply here.

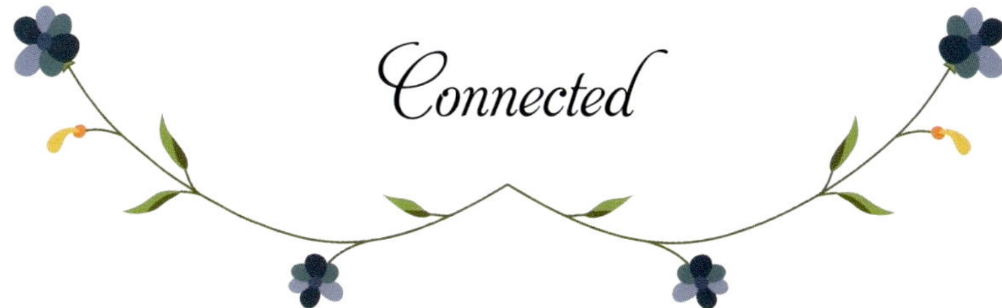

Connected

You are not alone. Breathe into the connection with life around you. Feel your ego and boundaries melt away as union with all of nature fills you with peace. Stay in this peace, fully present, aware of yourself but a part of the greater whole. With each breath, you are merging into that energy. You are not alone.

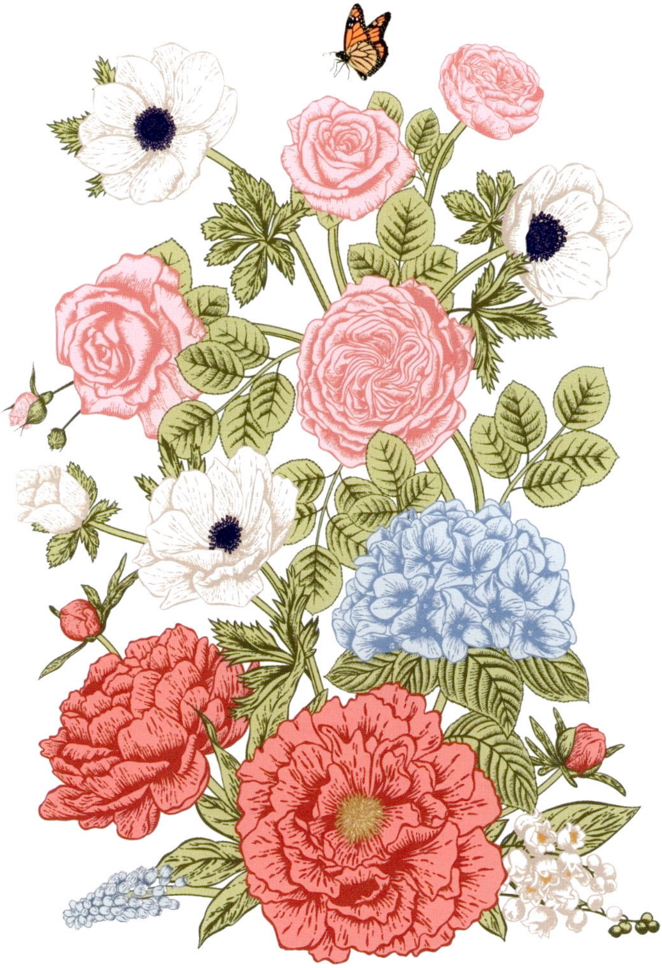

I am living my life—
my life is not living me. I
turn within to the stillness
and feel the source of life stirring
up, desiring expression through
me. I am aware and mindful of my
connection to this source,
and I let it move without
restriction. I am living mindfully,
authentically, and joyfully.

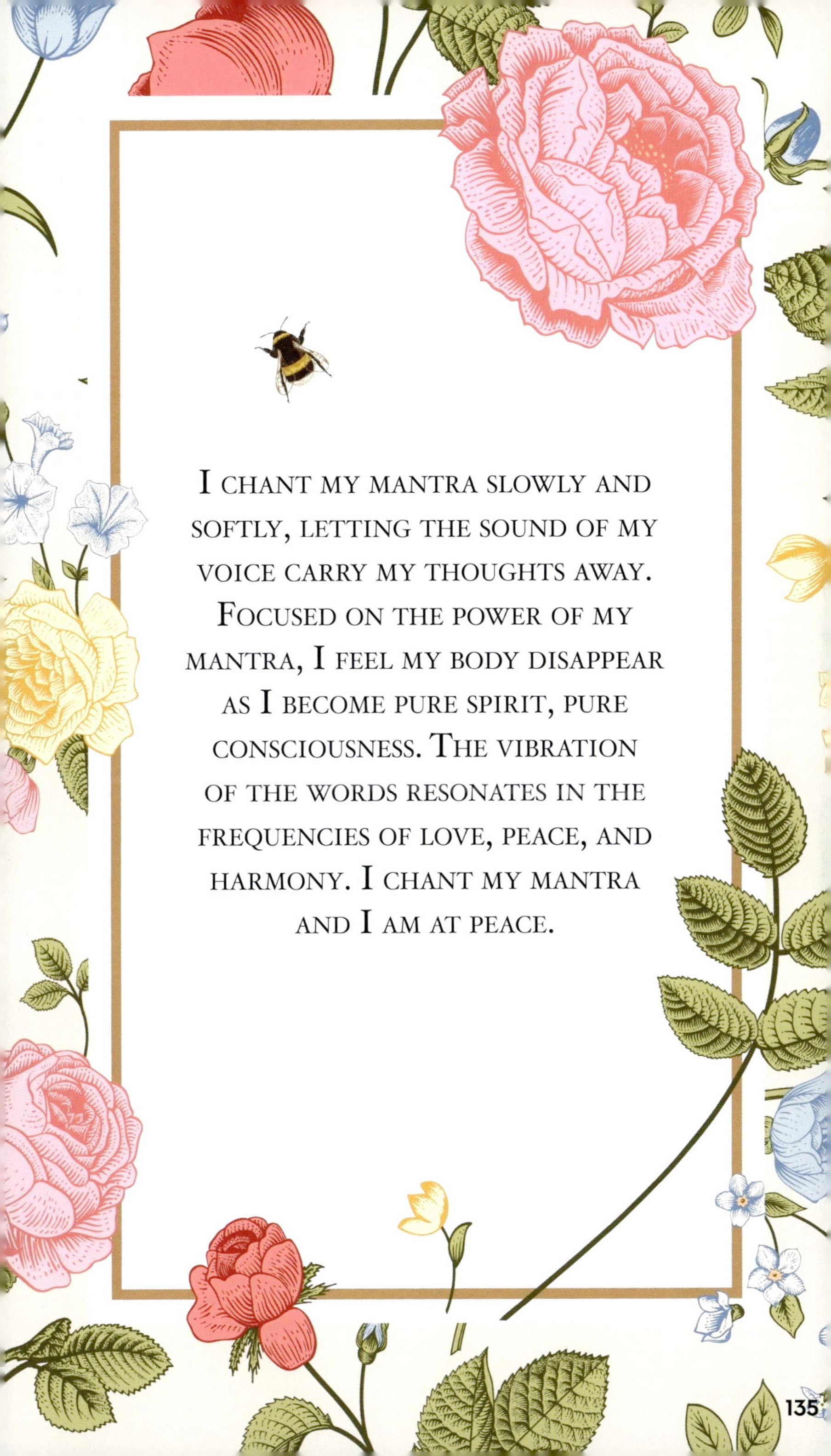

I chant my mantra slowly and softly, letting the sound of my voice carry my thoughts away. Focused on the power of my mantra, I feel my body disappear as I become pure spirit, pure consciousness. The vibration of the words resonates in the frequencies of love, peace, and harmony. I chant my mantra and I am at peace.

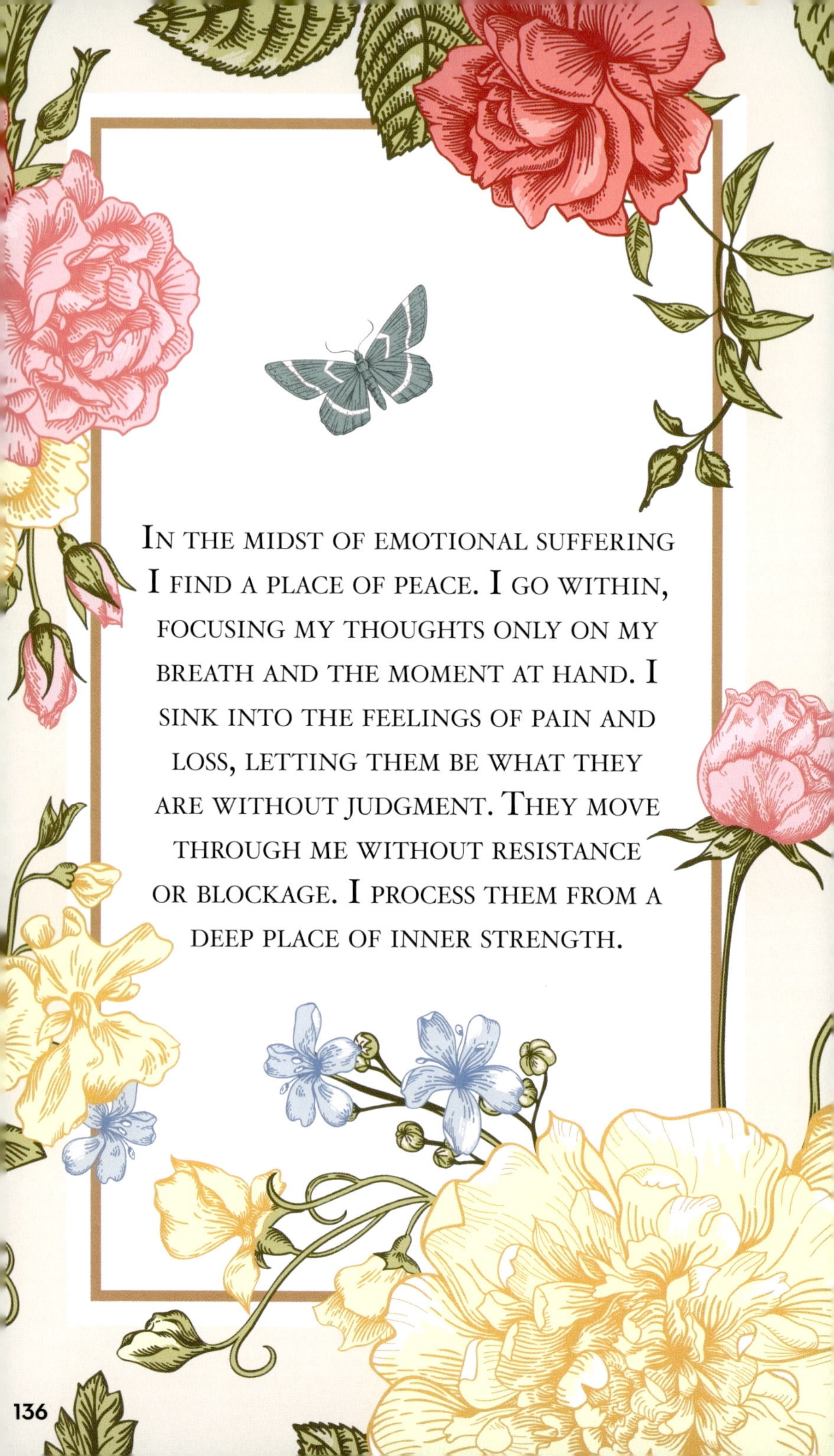

In the midst of emotional suffering I find a place of peace. I go within, focusing my thoughts only on my breath and the moment at hand. I sink into the feelings of pain and loss, letting them be what they are without judgment. They move through me without resistance or blockage. I process them from a deep place of inner strength.

Slow the pace of your life and your thoughts. Life is not a race. Sit quietly for a few moments, paying attention to what your mind is doing. Free it from worry, fear, and to-do lists, and let it wander where it wants to go. Sense the deeper mind beneath, and go there. Here, there is peace and beauty. Here, there are no lists or clocks. Dwell here for a while.

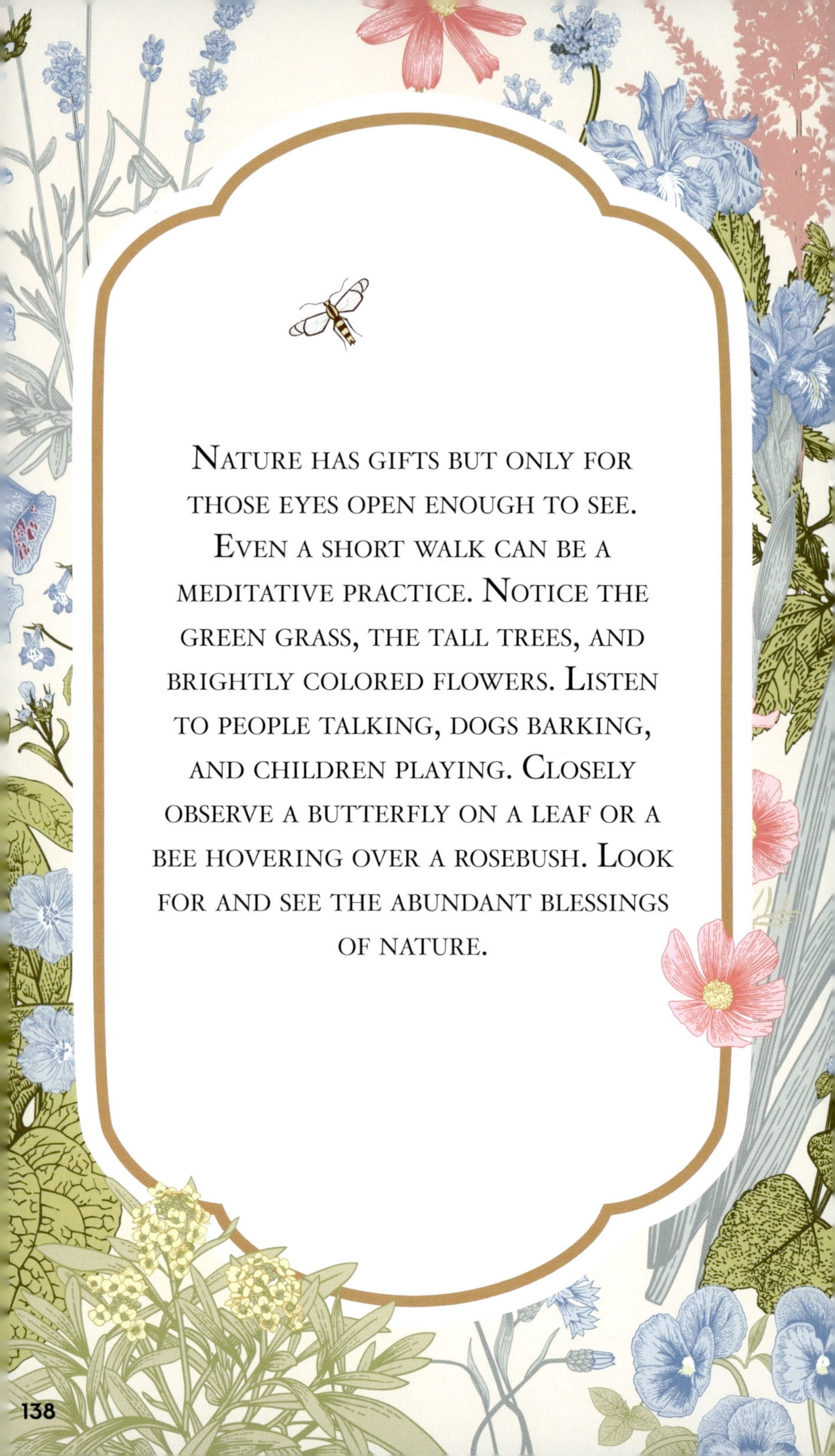

Nature has gifts but only for those eyes open enough to see. Even a short walk can be a meditative practice. Notice the green grass, the tall trees, and brightly colored flowers. Listen to people talking, dogs barking, and children playing. Closely observe a butterfly on a leaf or a bee hovering over a rosebush. Look for and see the abundant blessings of nature.

There's a place of renewal and happiness within you. All you need to do to reach it is withdraw your attention from the outside world and focus on the strength and the energy inside yourself. A calm spirit pours water on the hottest fire.

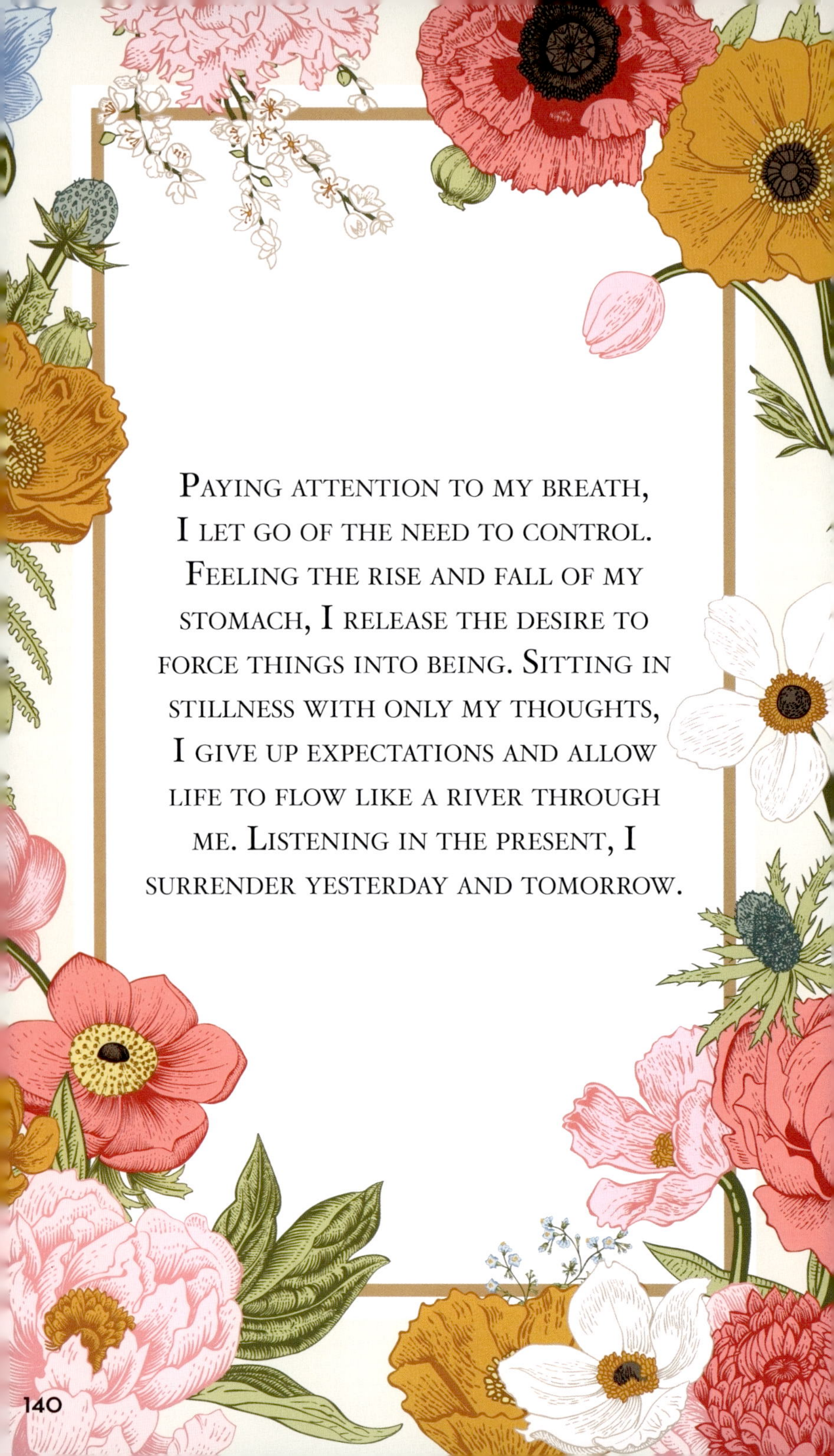

Paying attention to my breath, I let go of the need to control. Feeling the rise and fall of my stomach, I release the desire to force things into being. Sitting in stillness with only my thoughts, I give up expectations and allow life to flow like a river through me. Listening in the present, I surrender yesterday and tomorrow.

I sit quietly and let my stress go, visualizing it washing away from my body. I breathe, listening to the sound of air entering and exiting my lungs, bringing oxygen to my blood and brain. I continue to let go of worry, fear, doubt, and regret. In the present, I simply breathe and hold onto nothing.

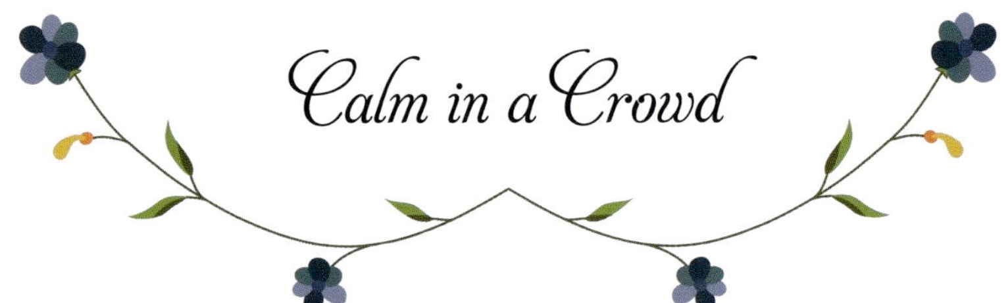

Calm in a Crowd

Sit in a crowded place. Look around and absorb every aspect of your environment. See how people rush about. Listen to their chatter. Allow sounds to move through you. You are the observer. Breathe deeply, noticing any smells or sensations. Let them move through you. Be in the chaos, but be still.

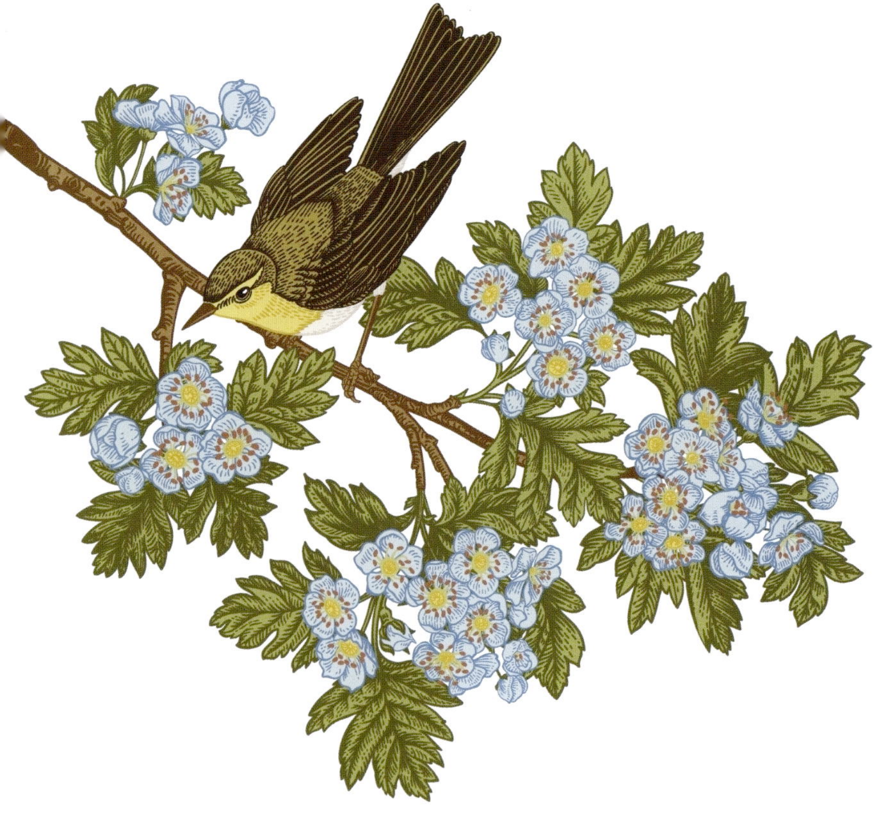

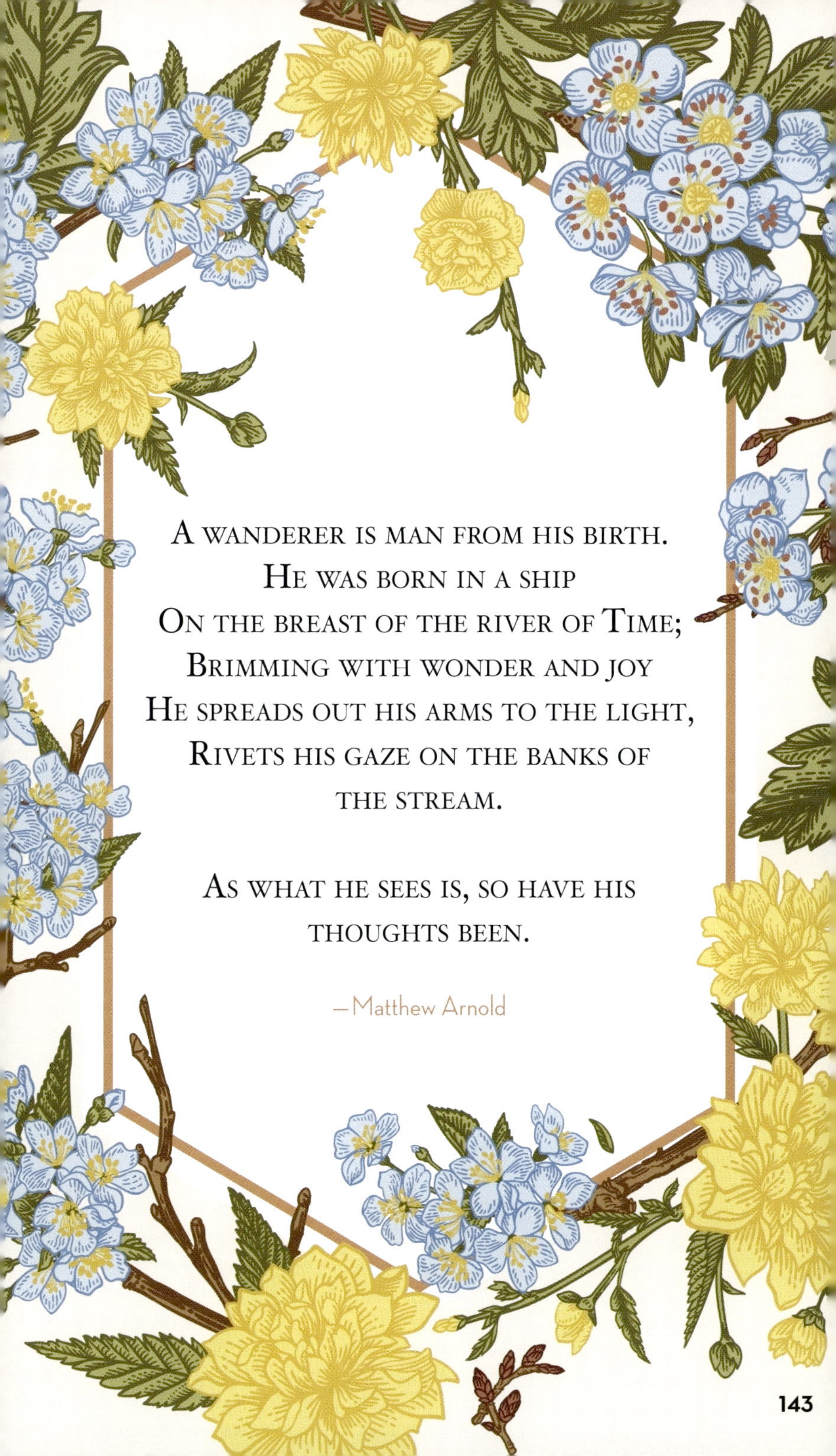

A wanderer is man from his birth.
He was born in a ship
On the breast of the river of Time;
Brimming with wonder and joy
He spreads out his arms to the light,
Rivets his gaze on the banks of
the stream.

As what he sees is, so have his
thoughts been.

—Matthew Arnold

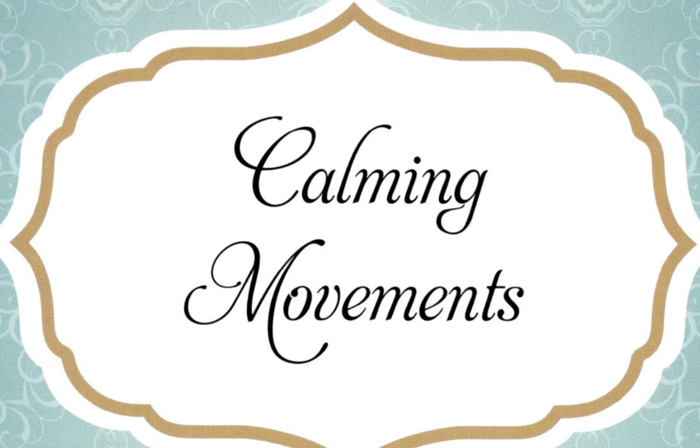
Calming
Movements

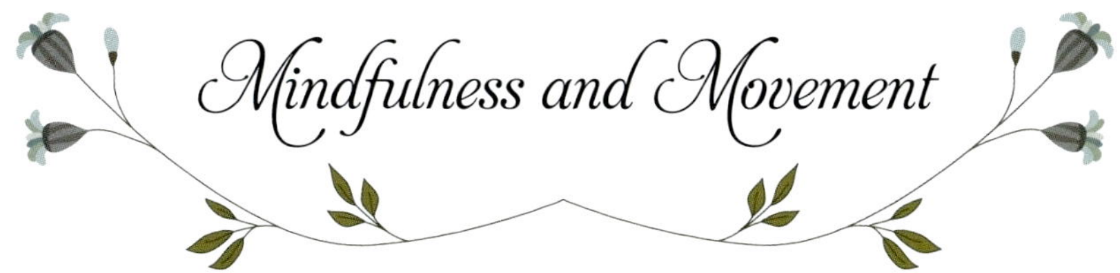

Mindfulness and Movement

Being mindful means different things to different people. Some focus on silence and a strong sense of present-moment awareness. Others chant a mantra to keep the mind from wandering to thoughts of the past or future. Others still use music, art, or movement to reach a meditative state. None are right; none are wrong. Whatever works to bring about a connection with the present is all that is necessary to be mindful and awake to the possibilities of life.

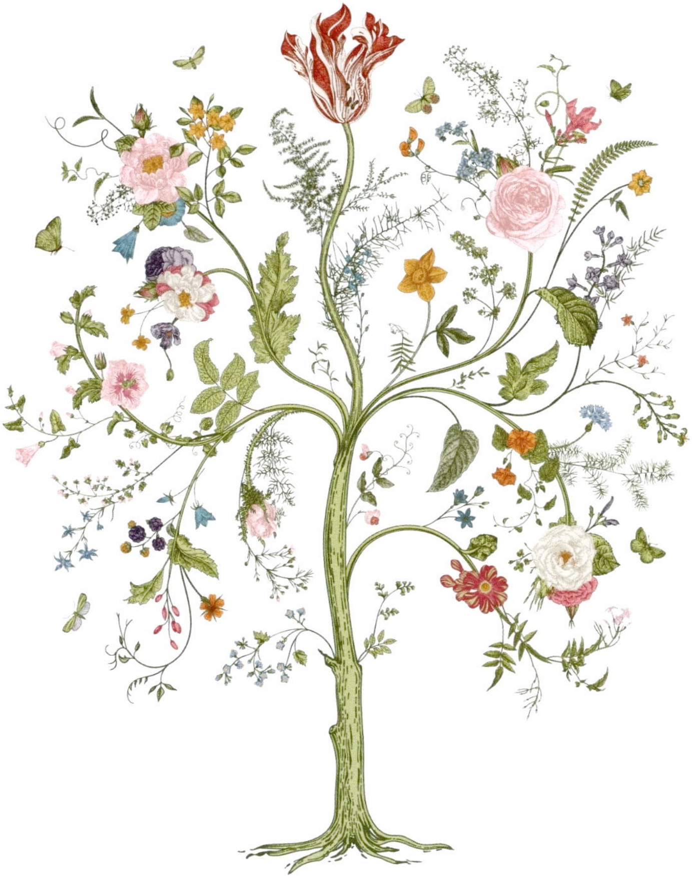

How rarely we check in with our bodies. Our minds are filled with distractions, yet our bodies are always speaking to us, through pain, soreness, or stiffness. By tuning in to what is happening to us physically, we can hear the guidance our bodies offer. Are we working too hard? Moving too fast through our days? Not slowing down enough to enjoy the moments? Listen...the body speaks a wisdom all its own.

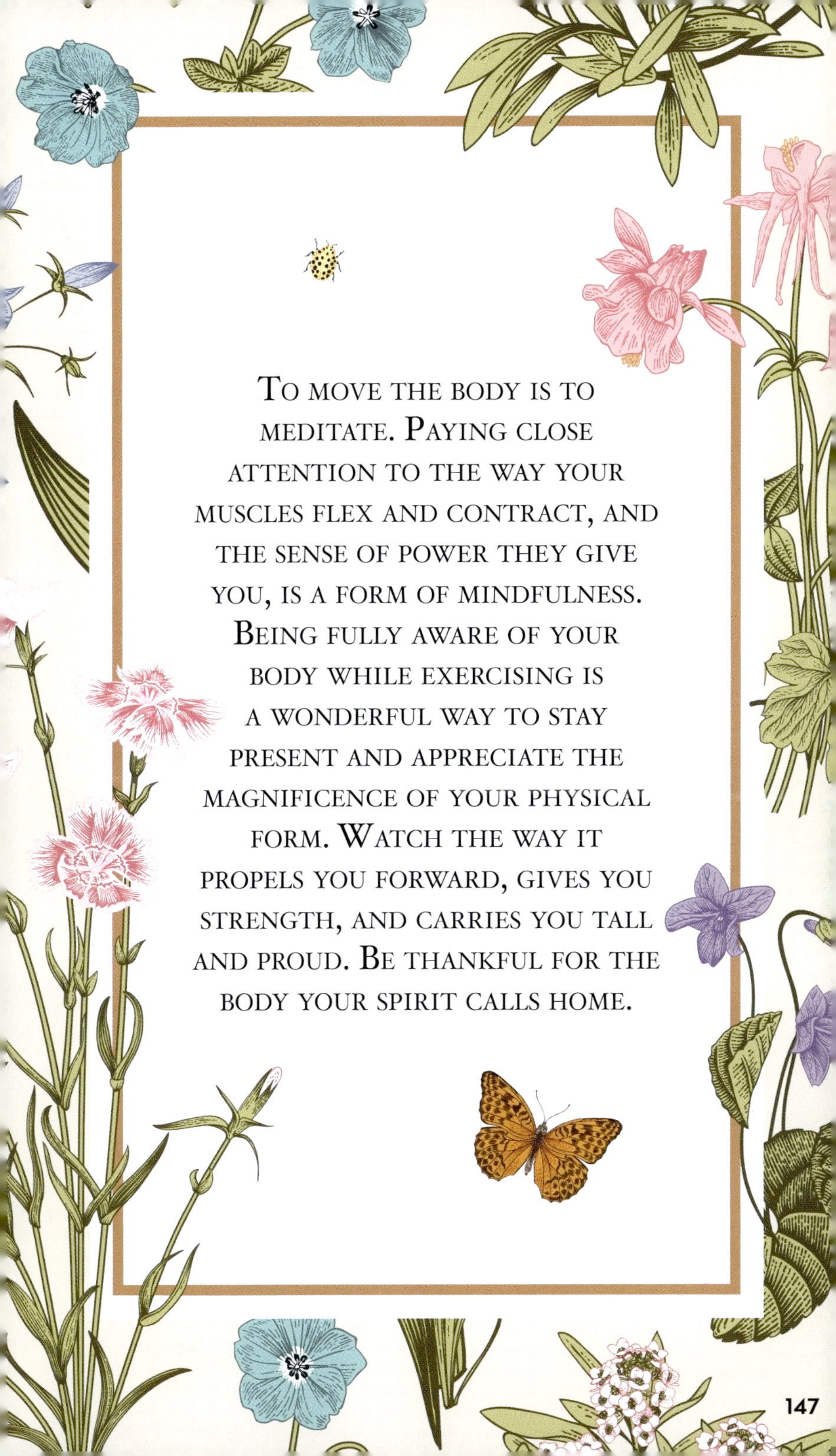

To move the body is to meditate. Paying close attention to the way your muscles flex and contract, and the sense of power they give you, is a form of mindfulness. Being fully aware of your body while exercising is a wonderful way to stay present and appreciate the magnificence of your physical form. Watch the way it propels you forward, gives you strength, and carries you tall and proud. Be thankful for the body your spirit calls home.

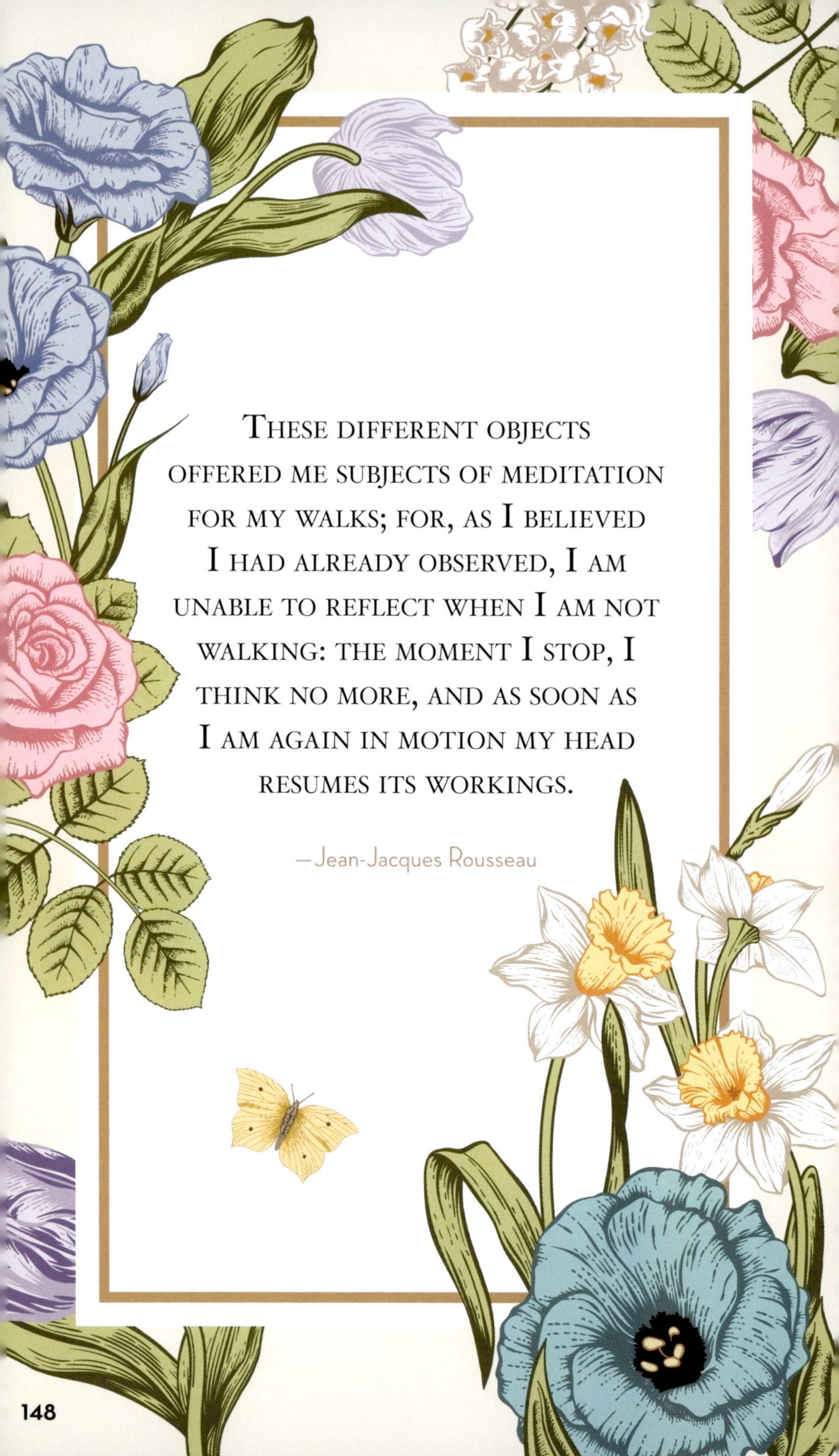

THESE DIFFERENT OBJECTS OFFERED ME SUBJECTS OF MEDITATION FOR MY WALKS; FOR, AS I BELIEVED I HAD ALREADY OBSERVED, I AM UNABLE TO REFLECT WHEN I AM NOT WALKING: THE MOMENT I STOP, I THINK NO MORE, AND AS SOON AS I AM AGAIN IN MOTION MY HEAD RESUMES ITS WORKINGS.

—Jean-Jacques Rousseau

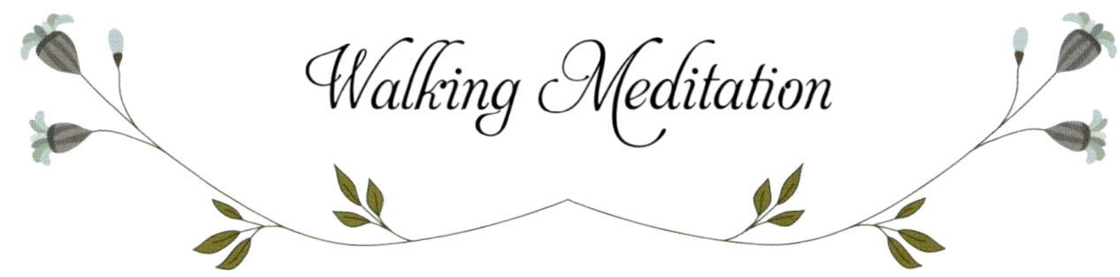

Walking Meditation

Not all meditation is about sitting still. Walking meditation involves bringing deliberate mindfulness to each step you take. Like other mindfulness exercises, walking meditation can help you cultivate a clearer mind and reduce some of your stress.

Time

If you're practicing this meditation for the first time, you can keep a session relatively short. Try a five-minute session. See how you feel and adjust from there. Experienced practitioners may meditate for 45 minutes or more.

Posture

Keep your back comfortably straight. You neck should be long, and your gaze relaxed and down. Your hands can hang loosely at your sides, or you can gently clasp your hands in front of or behind you.

Pace

You'll walk much more slowly as you meditate than you do when you're just walking to a destination. Walk slow enough that you can give each stage of each step the attention it deserves. Keep a steady, even rhythm.

Remember

You mind will wander, and that's ok. If you have trouble bringing it back to a meditative focus, there are a couple of things to try:

- Pause in your walking and address the distraction. Why is it demanding your attention? Is it a tumultuous thought, a beautiful sight, or a loud sound? Stop for as long as you need. When you're able to bring your attention back to walking, continue on.
- It may help to increase or decrease your pace slightly.

Step 1
Find a spot inside or outside where you can walk 10 to 15 paces safely and with few distractions.

Step 2
Take your first step: Raise the heel of one foot. Lift the foot off the ground. Move the foot forward, feeling your body shift its weight as it does so. Drop the foot gently to the ground, heel first. Press the sole of the foot into the ground.

Step 3
Repeat the process with the other foot. Continue step-by-step, focusing on each sensation as it arises, each muscle as it flexes and relaxes.

Step 4
When you've gone 10 to 15 steps, turn around and return to your starting spot. Then turn and start again.

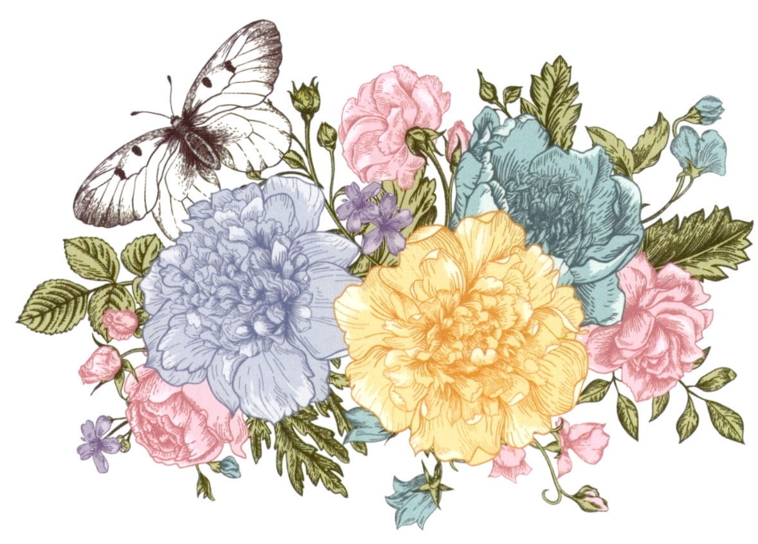

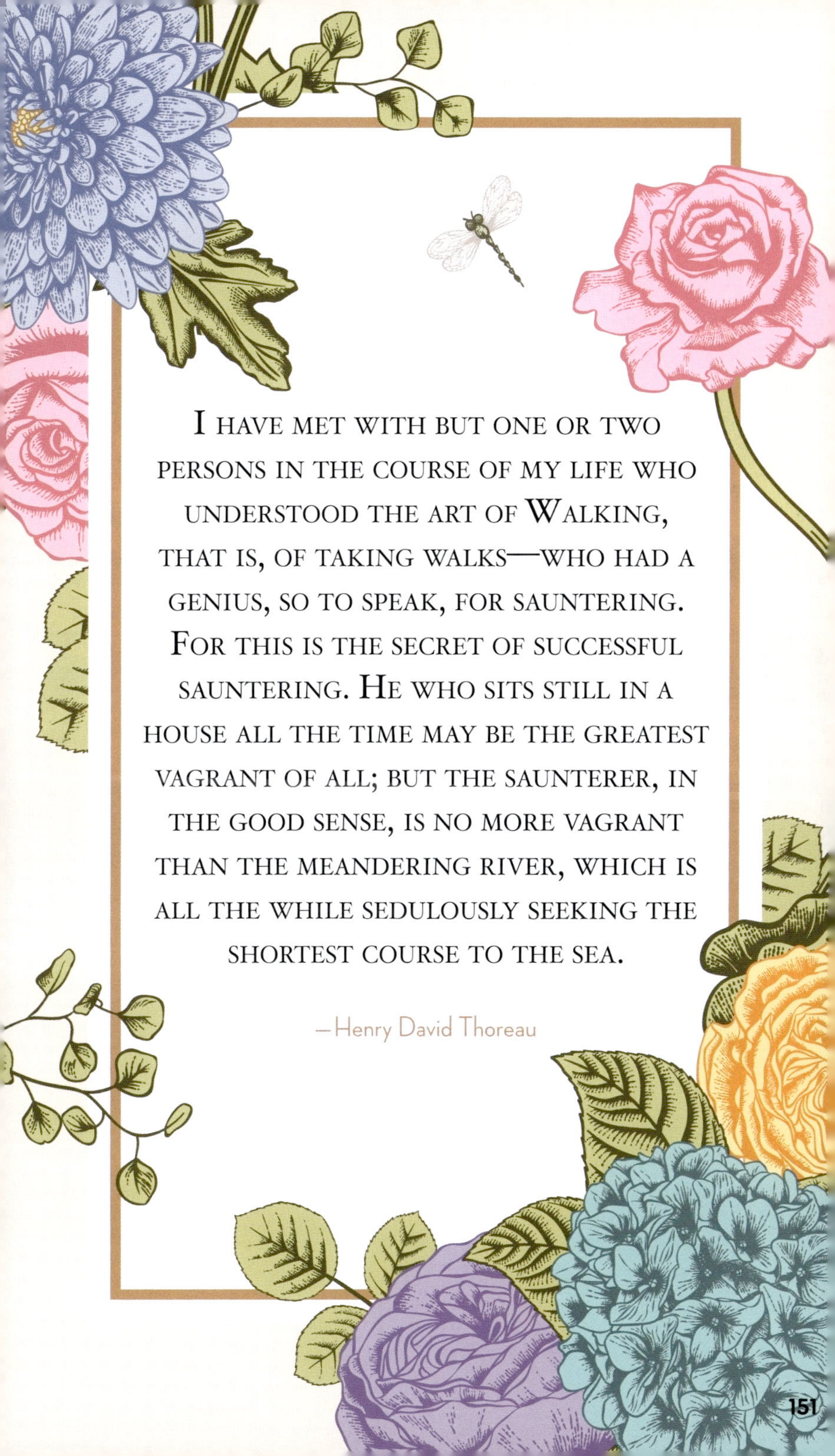

I have met with but one or two persons in the course of my life who understood the art of Walking, that is, of taking walks—who had a genius, so to speak, for sauntering. For this is the secret of successful sauntering. He who sits still in a house all the time may be the greatest vagrant of all; but the saunterer, in the good sense, is no more vagrant than the meandering river, which is all the while sedulously seeking the shortest course to the sea.

—Henry David Thoreau

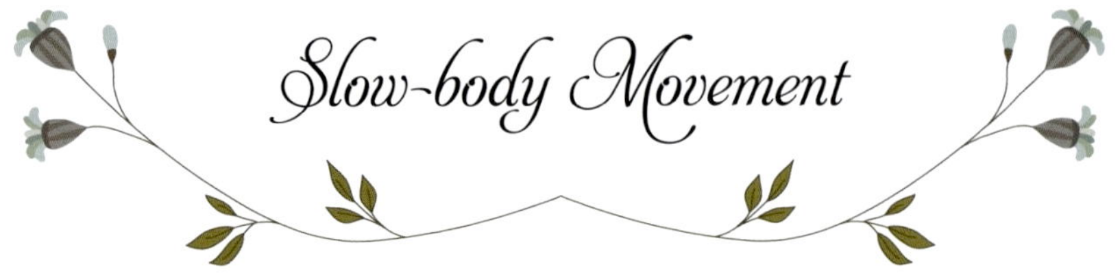

Slow-body Movement

You can bring laser-sharp focus to a single part of your body as you slowly move that part around. This is a kind of mindful meditation. The trick is to move slowly, so slowly that you have time to note all of the muscles, bones, and tendons that make the movement possible. You can also experience the pull of gravity, the temperature, and the movement of the air around your body in a new way. Sometimes this meditation is just about the movement. At other times, it involves a gradual stretch. You can apply slow-body movement to any part of the body. The ones described here are just a few examples to get you started.

Hands

Step 1

Come to a seated position, either on the floor with your legs crossed, or on a chair with your feet flat on the floor. Keep your back comfortably erect. You can also adjust this meditation to do it lying down.

Step 2

Rest your hands, palms down, on your knees.

Step 3

Bring your focus to your hands. What sensations are you experiencing in your hands?

Step 4

Raise your hands very slowly and steadily until they hover at about chest height. Keep your attention on your hands and arms as they lift. Let them feel heavy as gravity pulls on them. Consider each muscle, tendon, and bone that supports this movement.

Step 5
Slowly rotate your hands so the palms face each other.

Step 6
Move the hands together until the palms touch.

Step 7
Reverse the movements. Move your hands slowly apart, rotate your palms to face down, and bring your hands down to gently rest on your knees.

Arms

Step 1
Come to a standing position with your back comfortably erect. Let your arms hang loosely at your sides. You can also adjust this meditation to do it lying down.

Step 2
Bring your attention to your left arm, first focusing on the fingertips, then moving up to your shoulder. What sensations are you experiencing there?

Step 3
Keeping your shoulders down, lift your elbow with your hand following behind. Continue moving until your arm is pointing straight up. Focus on the feeling of this movement as you do so.

Step 4
Stretch your arm up even farther—pulling from your back, to your shoulder, up through your fingers—as though you're trying to grab an apple in a tree. You can come to your toes to reach higher.

Step 5
Reverse the movement. Come back to flat feet, if you were on your toes. Bring your arm down slowly, leading with the elbow, the hand following behind, until the arm again hangs loosely at your side.

Step 6

Repeat the movement with your right arm.

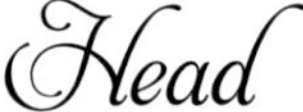

Head

Step 1

Come to a seated position, either on the floor with your legs crossed, or on a chair with your feet flat on the floor. Keep your back comfortably erect. You can also adjust this meditation to do it lying down.

Step 2

Bring your attention to your head and neck. If it helps, shift your head around a little. Feel the heaviness of the head as it balances on your neck.

Step 3

Keeping your shoulders still, move your head slowly forward until you're looking straight down.

Step 4

Gradually turn your head so it faces left.

Step 5

Lift your head so it sits up straight on your neck, your face looking left.

Step 6

Turn your head to face forward.

Step 7

Move your head forward until you're looking straight down, and repeat the process, this time looking to the right.

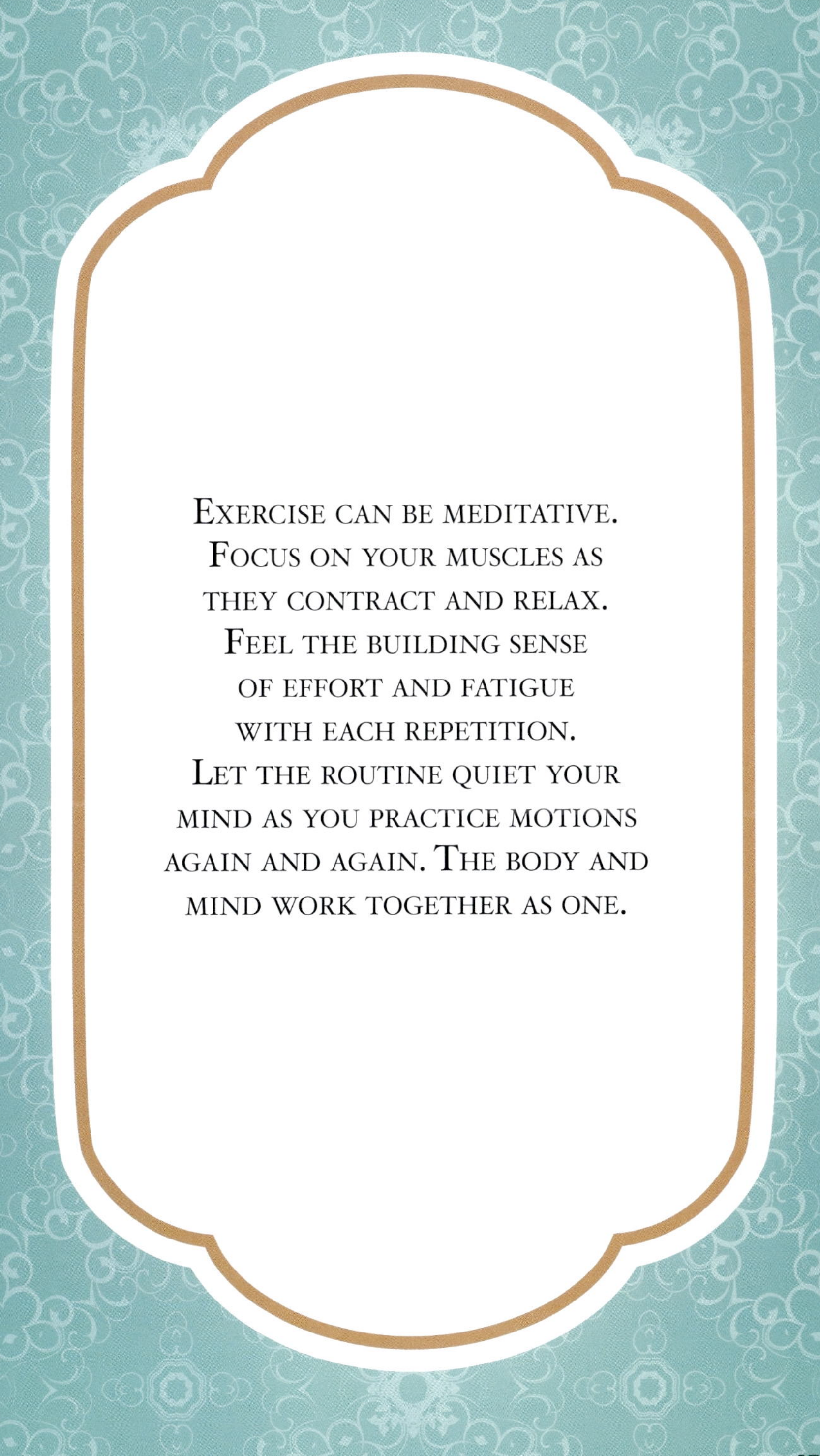

Exercise can be meditative. Focus on your muscles as they contract and relax. Feel the building sense of effort and fatigue with each repetition. Let the routine quiet your mind as you practice motions again and again. The body and mind work together as one.

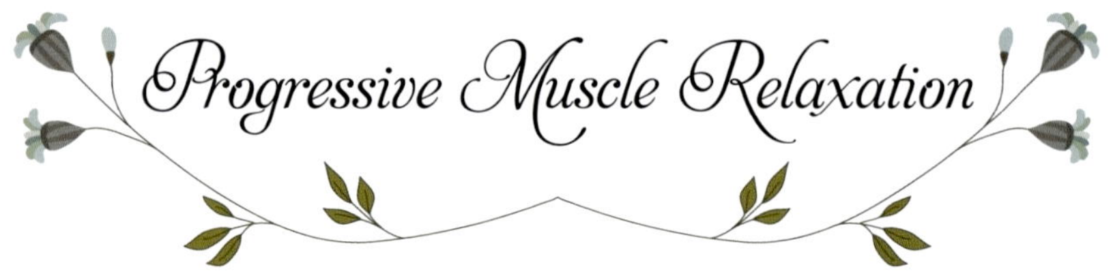

Progressive Muscle Relaxation

Progressive muscle relaxation is a technique many people use to combat stress, anxiety, insomnia, digestive issues, high blood pressure, cancer pain, headaches, and a lot of other issues. Basically, you go through your body one muscle group at a time, tensing and releasing each group. The process helps the muscles relax and, as your body relaxes, your mind follows. Some people begin the process with their hands, moving up to the forehead then down to the feet. Others move from the feet to the head.

Time

A full run-through takes about 10 to 20 minutes. Try this technique without setting a timer, though, and focus more on how your body feels rather than how much time has passed.

Posture

Most people lie down for the duration of this exercise, especially when they're using it to help them fall asleep. You can also sit up on a chair or other support. Just make sure you're comfortable and have a little space to move around.

Remember

Your mind will wander, and that's ok. When it wanders, acknowledge that it has. Then gently bring your attention back to the sound. Tense your muscles hard, but not so hard that you feel pain. You can tense and release a muscle group more than once, until you feel your muscles truly relaxing. You can also go through your entire body, then start over again.

Step 1

As you inhale, tense your hands by making fists. Stay here for 5 to 10 seconds.

Step 2

Exhale slowly, completely releasing the tension.

Step 3

Take about 30 seconds to take stock of any physical changes in your hands and forearms. How do the muscles feel?

Step 4

Inhale, bringing your hands to your shoulders and tensing your biceps. Stay here for 5 to 10 seconds. Then exhale and release the tension. Notice any changes in your upper arms.

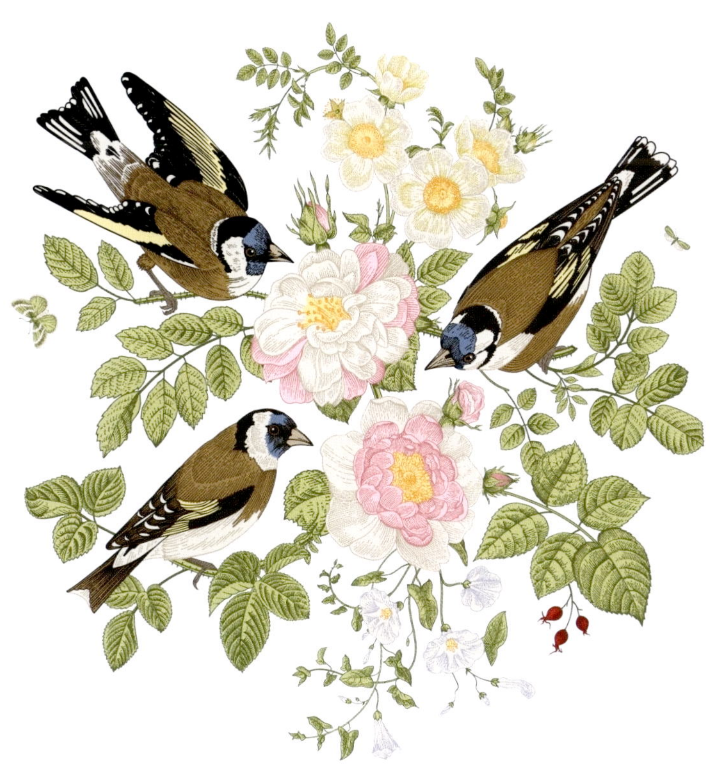

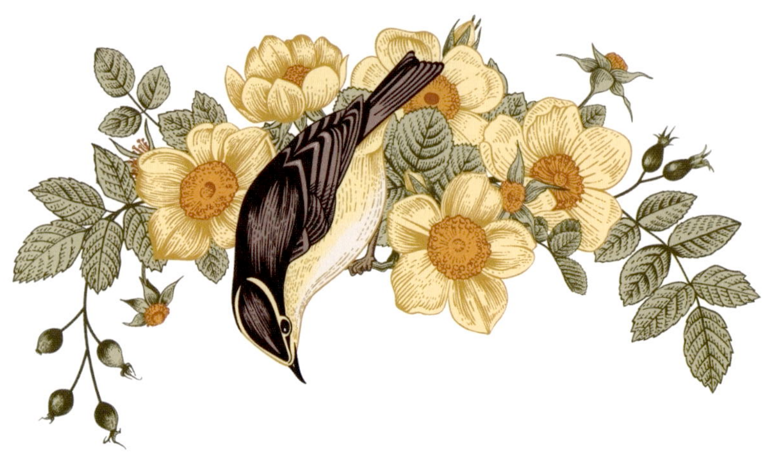

Step 5

Continue down through each muscle group.
Shoulders: Shrug, holding the shoulders up around your ears.
Forehead: Raise your eyebrows as high as you can.
Eyes and cheeks: Squeeze your eyes shut.
Jaw: Smile as widely as possible.
Lips: Tightly purse your lips.
Back of the neck: Press the back of the head into the floor, or place a hand on the back of your head and use your neck muscles to press against the hand.

Step 6

Front of the neck: Place a hand on your forehead and use your neck muscles to press into the hand.
Upper back: Roll your shoulders back to press your shoulder blades together, pushing your chest out.
Chest: Breathe in and hold your breath for a moment.
Stomach: Suck your belly in tightly.
Hips and buttocks: Squeeze your buttock muscles together.
Thighs: Clench your thigh muscles.
Calves: Curl your toes back.
Feet: Point your toes away from you, curling the foot.

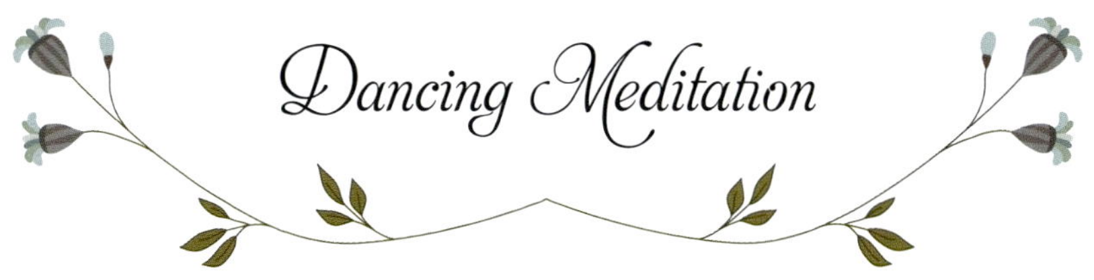

Dancing Meditation

Dancing is as old and as multifaceted as the human species. People dance alone, with a partner, or with a group. There might be strict choreography, a set of steps to be mixed and matched, or something entirely improvised. It can be worship, self-expression, celebration, performance, social interaction, and exercise. It can also be meditation. Any dance requires a certain amount of mental focus. Your primary attention is usually on your body, while additional attention can be given to the music, a partner, or some choreography. When using dance as a method of meditation, all your attention is on your body and the music, just as you would focus everything on the breath or a mantra in other meditations.

Dance meditation is adaptable to a range of abilities and interests. You can dance across the floor on your feet, swing your arms from a seated position, or just bob your head or tap your toe to the music. The important part is to bring your attention to your movement and how it feels. The music can be anything you want it to be, from hymns, to opera, to EDM. Choose a style of music that naturally speaks to you and, preferably, inspires some positive feeling.

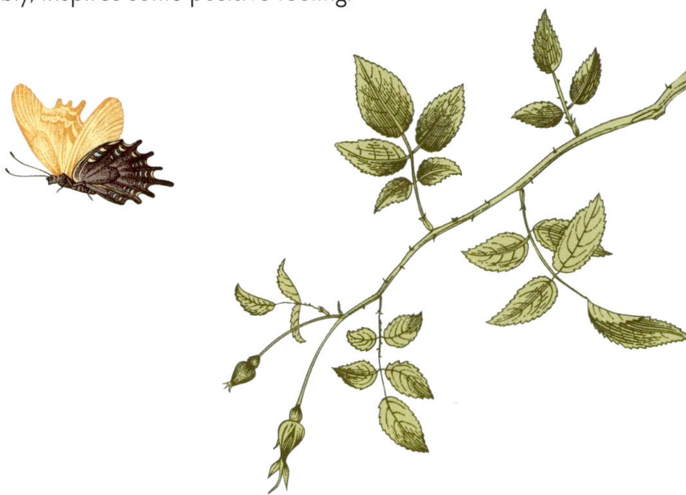

Time

If you're new to dance meditation, try spending 10 to 15 minutes with it at first. That time can be extended to 30 or more minutes as you become more comfortable.

Space

Make sure you have the space needed to move freely. If you'll be on your feet, make sure the floor is clear of obstacles.

Remember

Your mind will wander, and that's ok. When it wanders, acknowledge that it has. Then gently bring your attention back to the music and your movement. Dance freely and without judgement. Dance meditation is not about beauty or skill; it's just about moving.

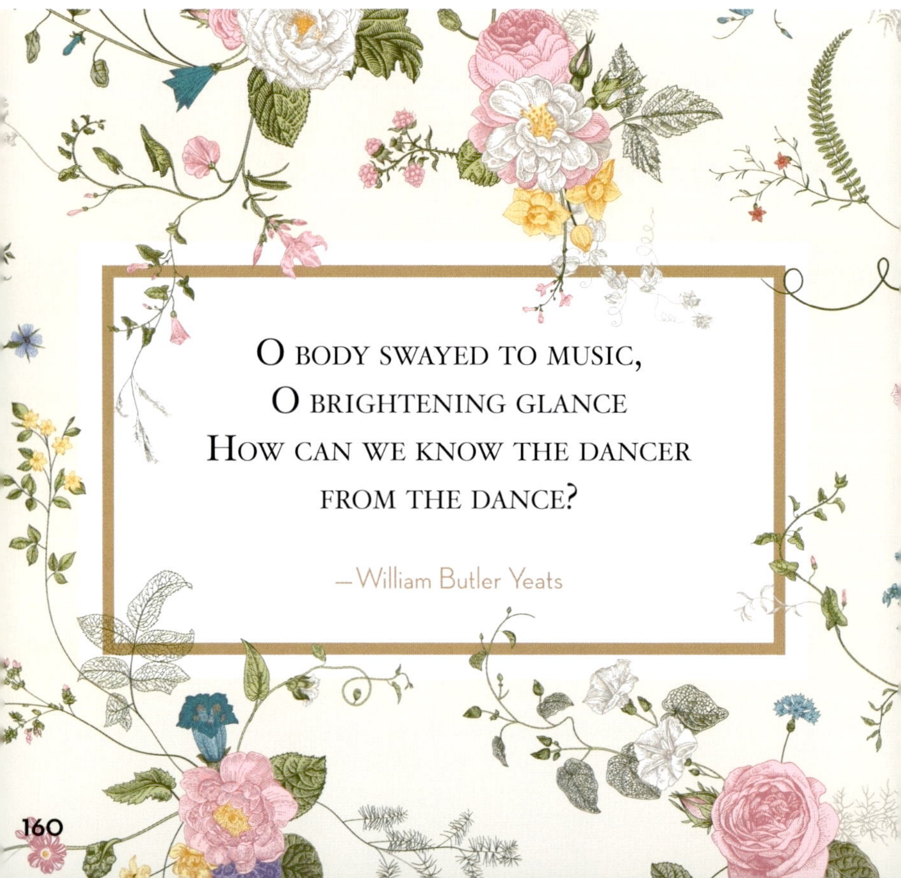

O body swayed to music,
O brightening glance
How can we know the dancer
from the dance?

—William Butler Yeats

STEP 1
Start the music. Take a few deep breaths to ground yourself. Then return to natural breathing.

STEP 2
Bring your focus to the rhythm of the music. Imagine it pulsing within your body. It can help to lightly nod, tap a toe, or tap a finger to the rhythm.

STEP 3
Shift your attention to the melody of the music. Notice each note as it passes by.

STEP 4
Turn that melody into movement. For example, as the melody goes up, you can raise your arms. As it goes down, you can reach toward the floor. (These are just examples; there's no need for you to follow them.) Move your body by instinct, if you can, without too much thought.

STEP 5
Bring your focus to your body as it moves. Note each muscle that drives the movement, and each bone and tendon that supports it.

STEP 6
If there is harmony in the music, turn your focus to that. Notice how the harmony interacts with the melody. Incorporate this added complexity to your movement.

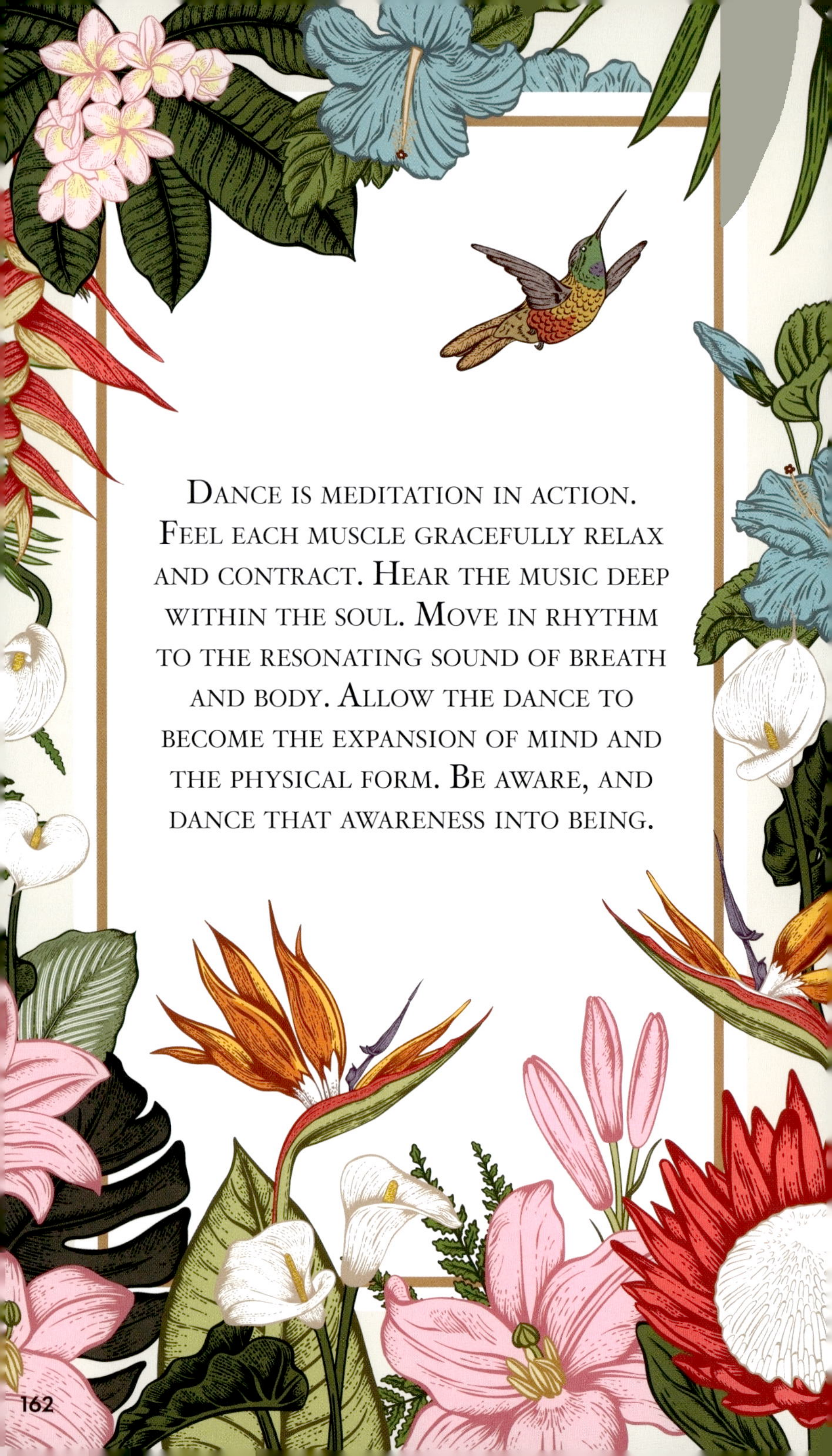

Dance is meditation in action. Feel each muscle gracefully relax and contract. Hear the music deep within the soul. Move in rhythm to the resonating sound of breath and body. Allow the dance to become the expansion of mind and the physical form. Be aware, and dance that awareness into being.

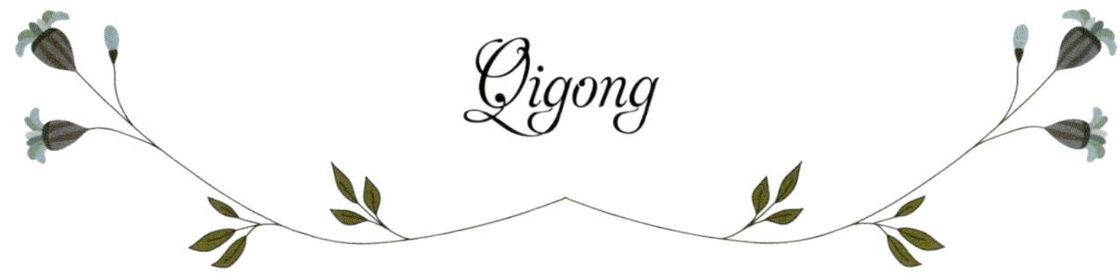

Qigong

Qigong first developed thousands of years ago in China. Its careful combination of movement, breath, and focused intention is designed to open up and control the body's flow of qi, which can be roughly defined as breath or life energy.

Practitioners who've harnessed their qi can use it in healing, in martial arts, or as a spiritual path. Different movements can also affect the body differently: some movements calm, while others invigorate.

Qigong is generally performed by repeating one cyclical movement several times before moving on to the next. As you practice, move gradually, feeling the energy within each moment. Breathe deeply from the belly. Pay attention to how each inhale and exhale fits into the movement. Feel free to adapt the movements as you need to so they suit your body.

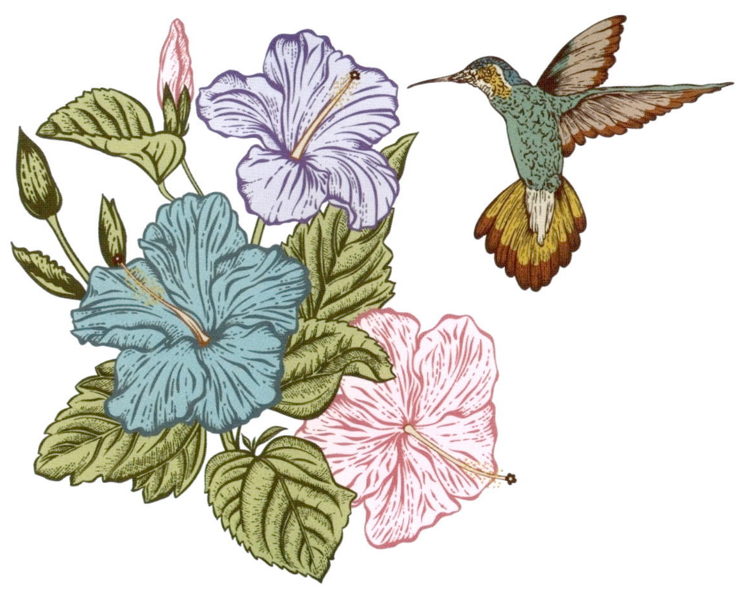

Raising Arms

Step 1

Begin in a relaxed but upright standing posture. Feet are hip-width apart, toes pointing forward. Let your arms hang at your sides, palms facing in. Your gaze should be relaxed and unfocused.

Step 2

As you exhale slowly, bend your knees slightly to sink down a little. Rotate your wrists so your palms face to the back.

Step 3

Inhale slowly, straightening your legs to rise back up. Lift your arms in front of you to about shoulder height. Keep your elbows and wrists slightly bent, your fingers relaxed, and palms facing down.

Step 4

Exhale, lowering your arms to your sides and bending your knees.

Step 5

Repeat the cycle of raising with an inhale and lowering with an exhale.

Step 6

When you're ready to end the movement, return to your standing posture in Step 1.

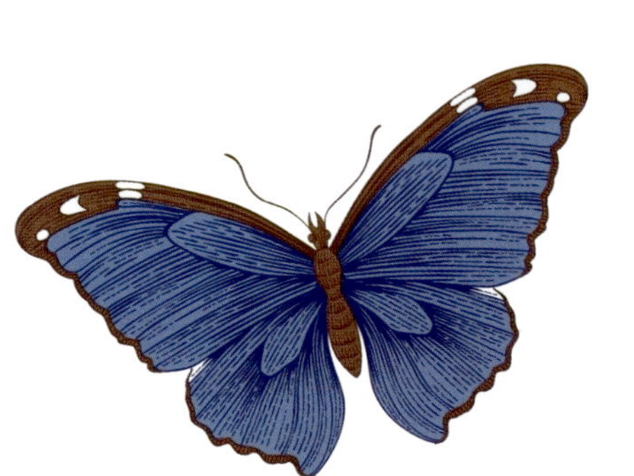

Cloud Hands

Step 1

Begin in a relaxed but upright standing posture. Feet are hip-width apart, toes pointing forward. Let your arms hang at your sides, palms facing in. Your gaze should be relaxed and unfocused.

Step 2

Shift your weight to your right leg. Bend the right knee a little as you do so.

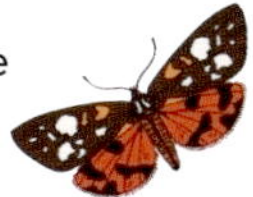

Step 3

Extend the left leg out to the side. Gently set the left foot down a few inches from its starting position.

Step 4

Shift your weight to the center, between your feet, and straighten your legs.

Step 5

Lift your left arm, elbow bent, so the elbow points left and your forearm reaches in front of you. Your palm is in front of the center of your chest, facing down.

Step 6

Lift your right arm to waist height, rounded but not fully bent at the elbow. Reach it out in front of you, palm facing left.

Step 7

Inhale and transfer your weight to the left leg, bending your left knee a little as you do so. Allow your arms to flow to the left as you move, left arm straightening and right elbow bending.

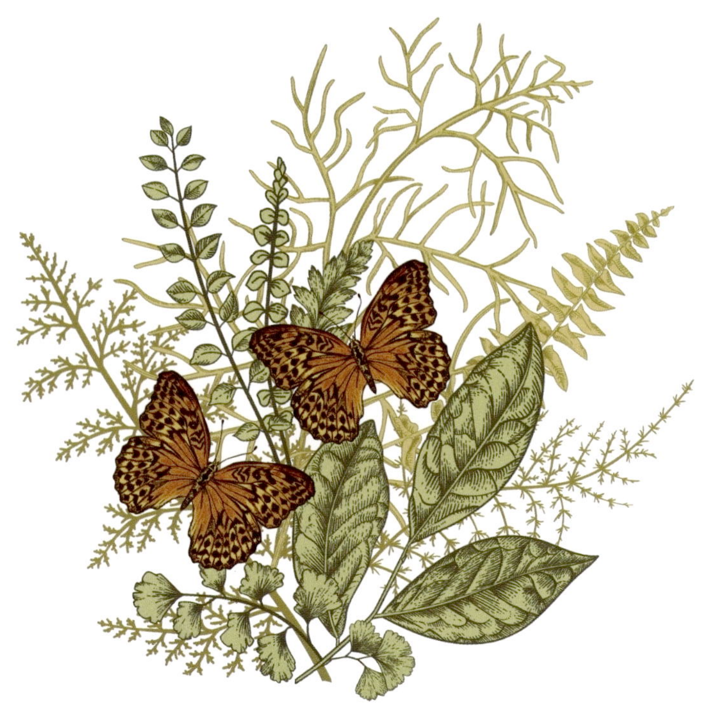

Step 8
Shift your arms so the left is straightened at waist height, while the right is bent at chest height.

Step 9
Exhale as you shift your weight to the center, then inhale and continue to the right.

Step 10
Switch your arms again (right straight at waist, left bent at chest). Exhale as you shift your weight to the center, then inhale as you continue to the left.

Step 11
Continue swaying from left to right, moving your arms in graceful circles. When you're done, return to your standing posture.

Tai Chi

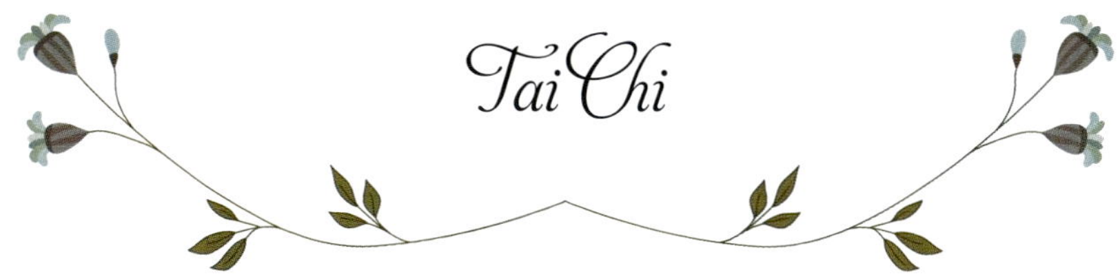

Tai Chi, sometimes called Taijiquan or Tai Chi Chuan, is closely related to Qigong. The major differences between the two lay in their complexity, approaches to movement, and application. Tai Chi practice consists of sequences of movements, rather than Qigong's usual repetition of single movements, and this means Tai Chi can take a lot longer to learn.

Technique is also more rigid in Tai Chi. As for application, Tai Chi is considered a martial art. Qigong is usually more of a wellness-focused practice. That said, Qigong movements and philosophies are often used in Tai Chi, and many people today use Tai Chi purely as a method of meditation or exercise, rather than a martial art.

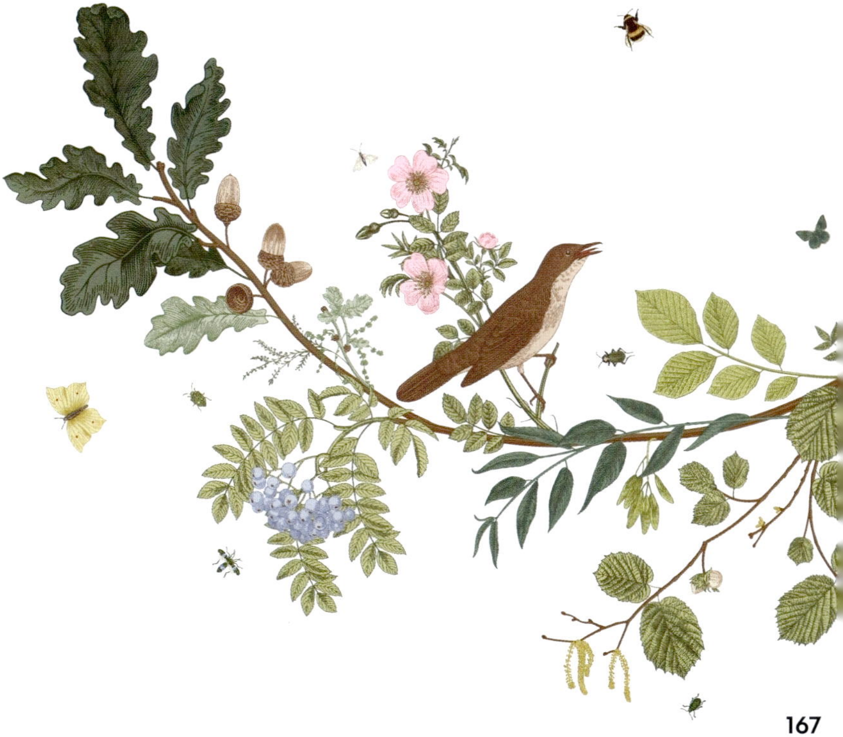

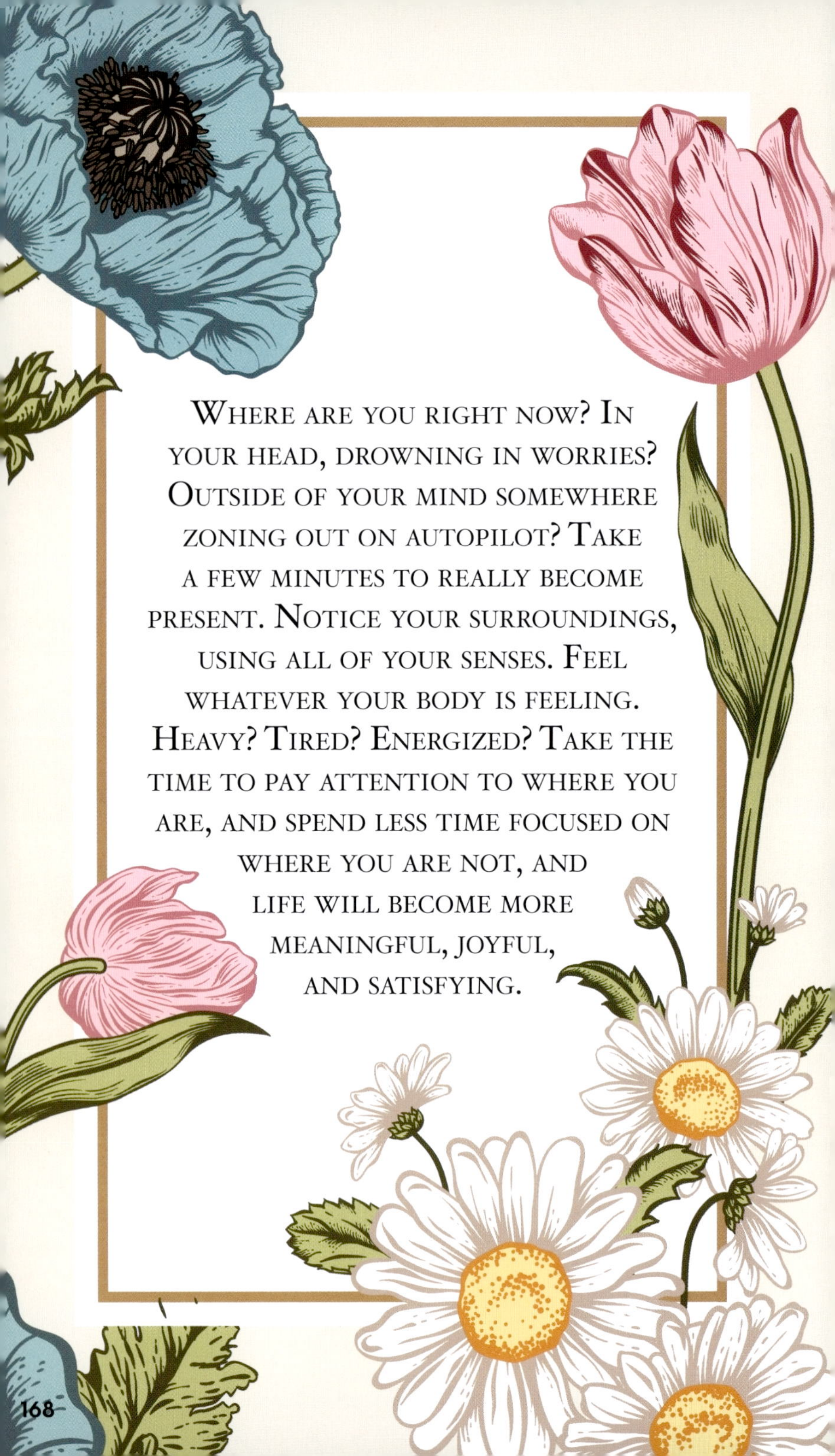

Where are you right now? In your head, drowning in worries? Outside of your mind somewhere zoning out on autopilot? Take a few minutes to really become present. Notice your surroundings, using all of your senses. Feel whatever your body is feeling. Heavy? Tired? Energized? Take the time to pay attention to where you are, and spend less time focused on where you are not, and life will become more meaningful, joyful, and satisfying.

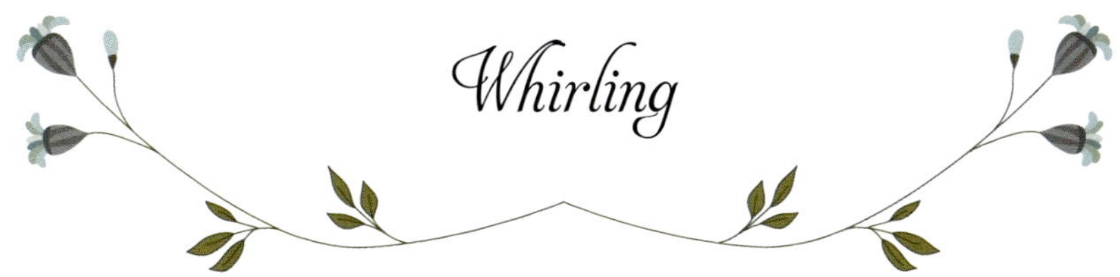

Whirling

Sema, often called whirling in English, is a meditative dance practiced in the Mevlevi order of Sufism. The meditation practice is centered on the act of spinning, as music plays in the background. Formal practitioners receive a huge amount of training—perhaps 1,000 days—before becoming fully involved in the Sema ceremony as dervishes. When practicing Sema, trained dervishes can spin continuously for as long as an hour, without ever feeling dizzy.

As they practice, dervishes strive toward ecstasy and a direct connection to God, as well as ridding themselves of their individual egos. Their clothing reflects this last point: the tall, conical hat represents the ego's tombstone, and the long white robe is the ego's death shroud.

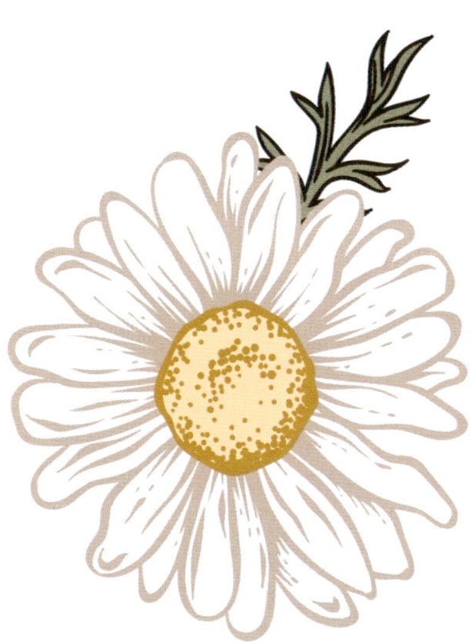

Step 1

Cross your arms in front of you, right over left, so each hand rests on the opposite shoulder. Bow to the space where you'll be whirling, and to the divine.

Step 2

Begin to whirl slowly, counterclockwise, pivoting on your right foot. Your gaze should be relaxed and unfocused.

Step 3

Start to unfurl your arms from their crossed positions, raising them gradually until they arch up.

Step 4

Speed up gradually.

Step 5

When you're ready to end the practice, slow your spin gradually. Stand a moment, then kneel and touch your forehead to the floor.

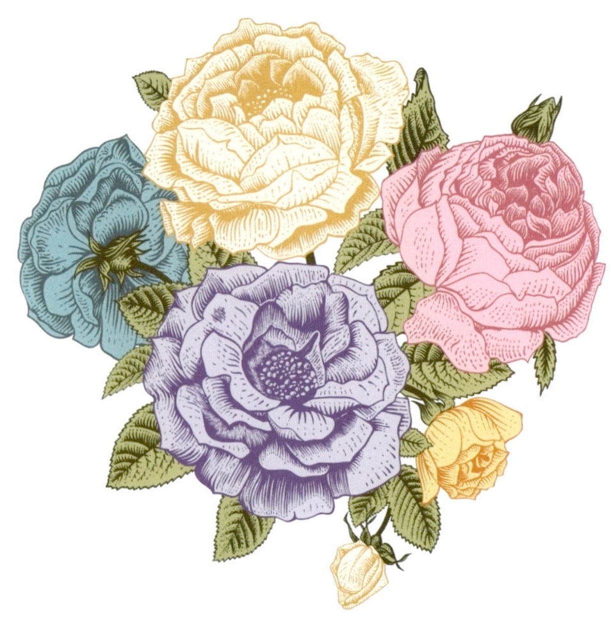

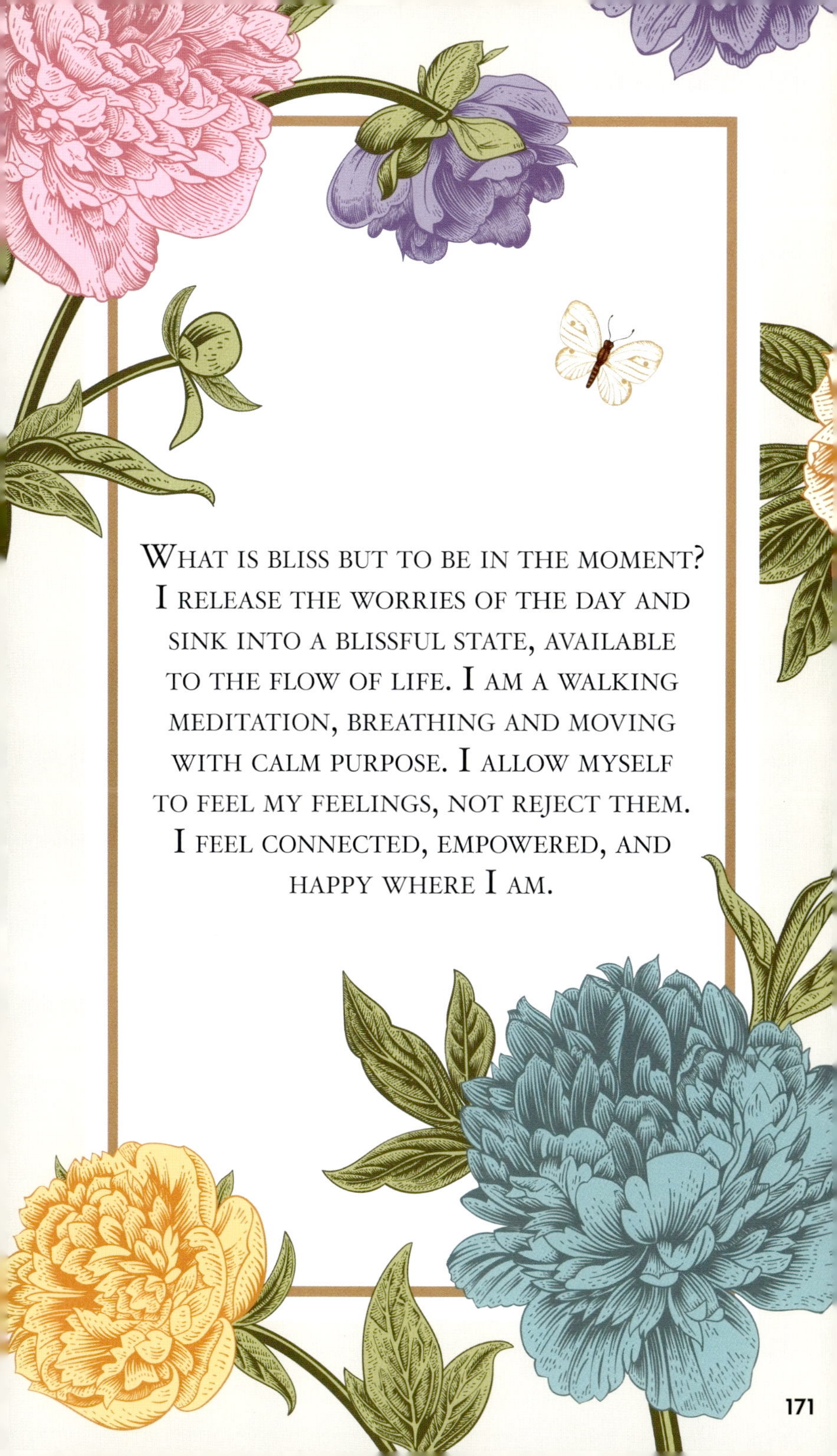

What is bliss but to be in the moment? I release the worries of the day and sink into a blissful state, available to the flow of life. I am a walking meditation, breathing and moving with calm purpose. I allow myself to feel my feelings, not reject them. I feel connected, empowered, and happy where I am.

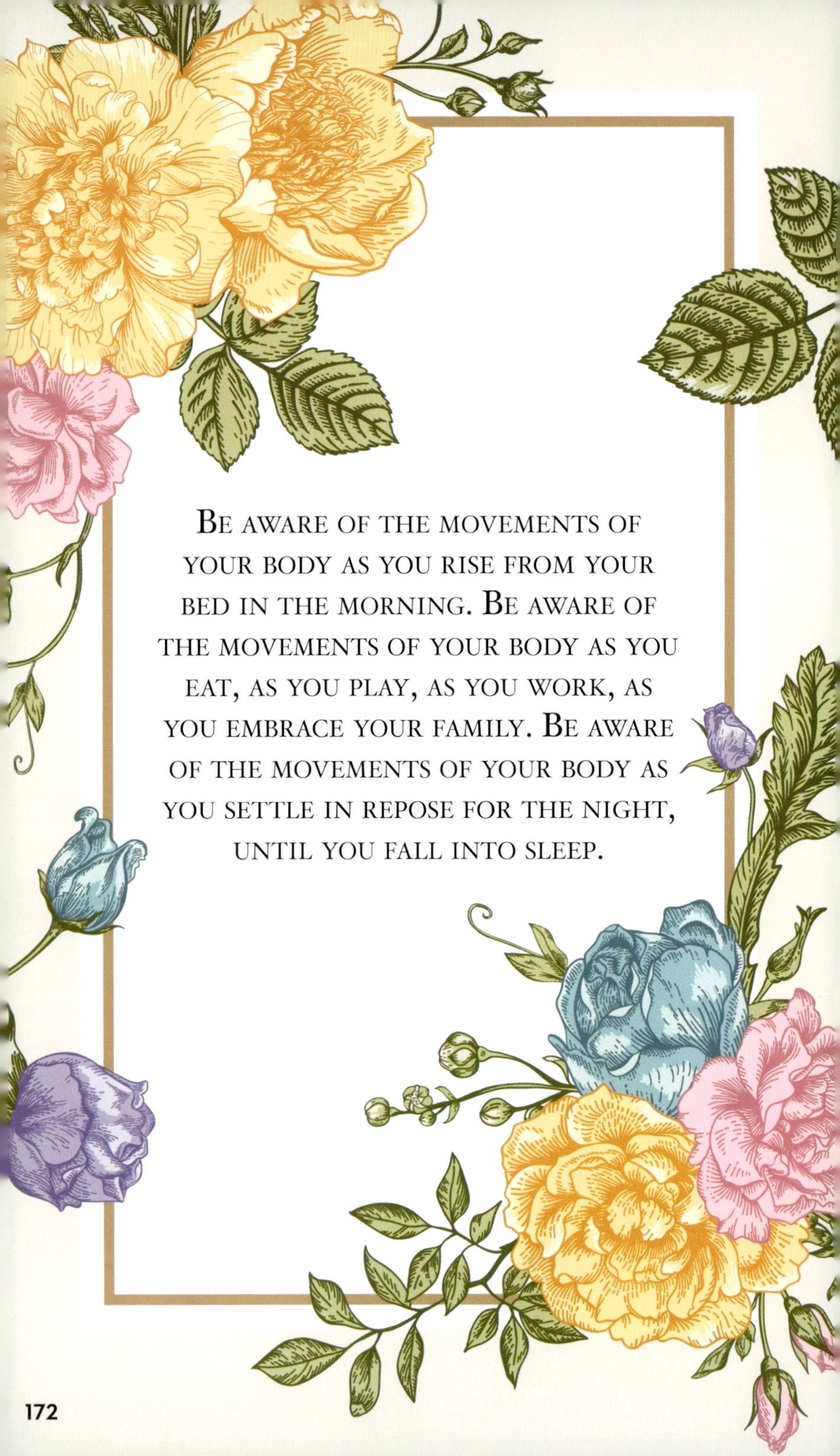

Be aware of the movements of your body as you rise from your bed in the morning. Be aware of the movements of your body as you eat, as you play, as you work, as you embrace your family. Be aware of the movements of your body as you settle in repose for the night, until you fall into sleep.

In this busy life, blocks of time to yourself can be difficult to come by. Learn to snatch tidbits—a solitary cup of coffee, a lunchtime walk, an extra-long shower.

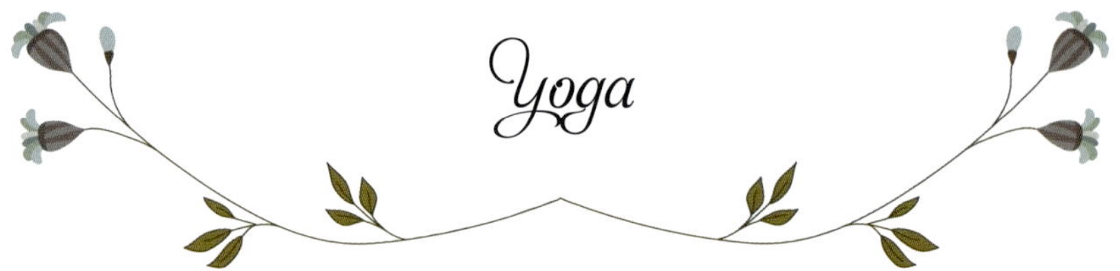

Yoga

What we often think of as yoga today is an adaptation of a Hindu practice first written about millennia ago. Classical yoga is defined by disciplined physical, mental, and spiritual exercises. These are practiced to help the practitioner achieve oneness with the divine or supreme knowledge.

Today, yoga encompasses a range of paths to follow, each of which focuses on different techniques. There are yogas that use sounds or images. Some paths make more use of breath control, while others prioritize mental concentration. There are also the practices that focus most on physical exercises.

People also come to yoga with a variety of goals. Nowadays, not all yogis are working toward union with the divine. Some people come for relaxation, others for improvements to their strength, flexibility, or mental discipline. If you explore yoga, ask yourself what your intentions are with the practice. Some paths will serve those intentions better than others. Of course, you can also switch from one practice to another, or combine them for the best fit.

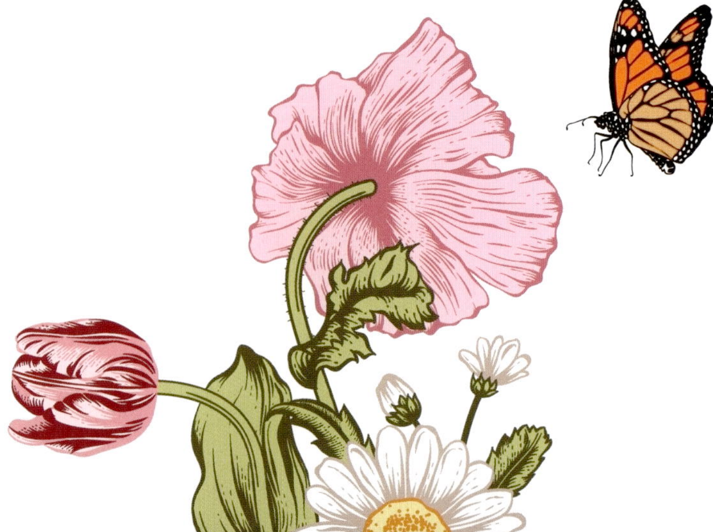

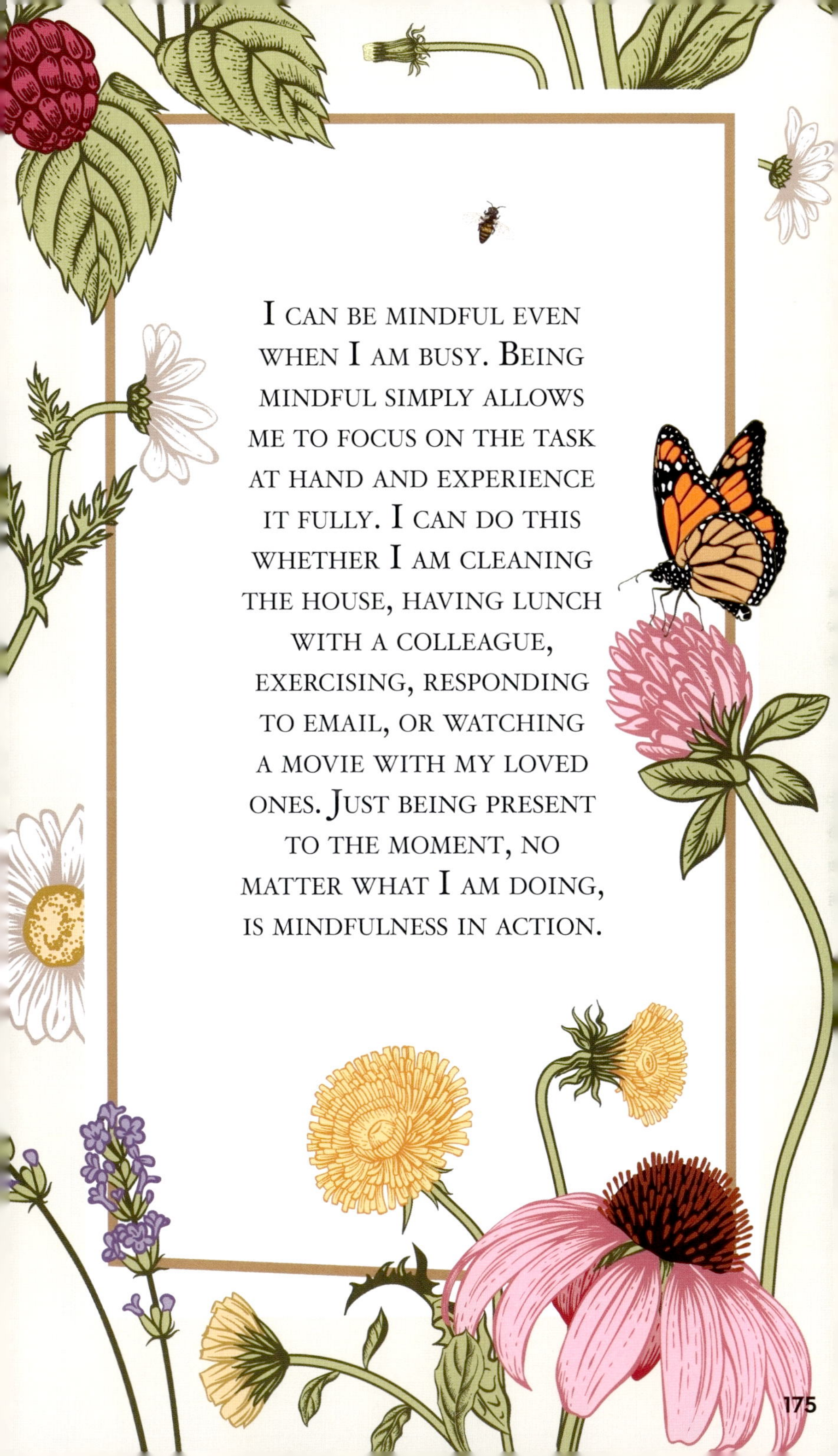

I can be mindful even when I am busy. Being mindful simply allows me to focus on the task at hand and experience it fully. I can do this whether I am cleaning the house, having lunch with a colleague, exercising, responding to email, or watching a movie with my loved ones. Just being present to the moment, no matter what I am doing, is mindfulness in action.

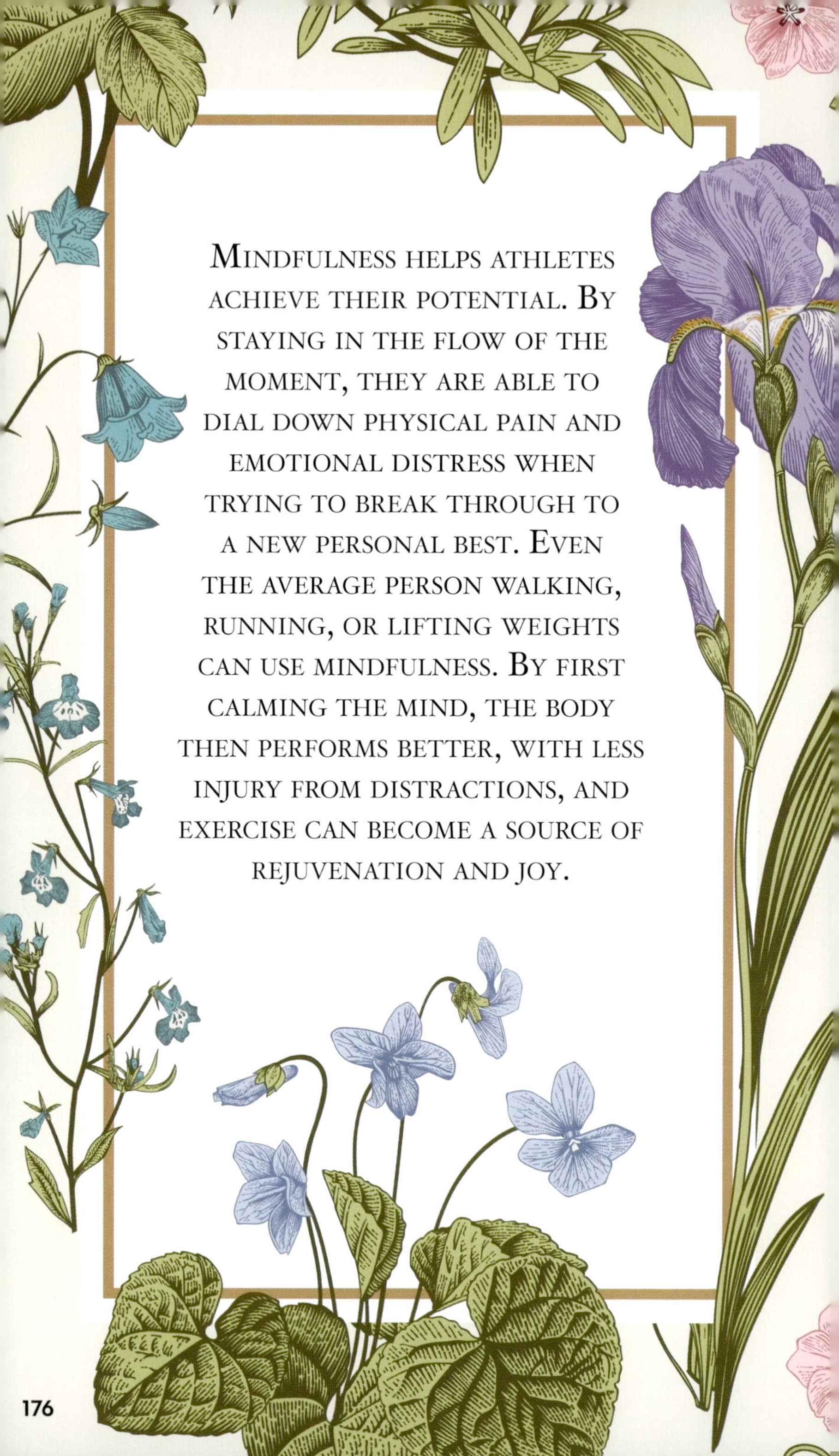

MINDFULNESS HELPS ATHLETES ACHIEVE THEIR POTENTIAL. BY STAYING IN THE FLOW OF THE MOMENT, THEY ARE ABLE TO DIAL DOWN PHYSICAL PAIN AND EMOTIONAL DISTRESS WHEN TRYING TO BREAK THROUGH TO A NEW PERSONAL BEST. EVEN THE AVERAGE PERSON WALKING, RUNNING, OR LIFTING WEIGHTS CAN USE MINDFULNESS. BY FIRST CALMING THE MIND, THE BODY THEN PERFORMS BETTER, WITH LESS INJURY FROM DISTRACTIONS, AND EXERCISE CAN BECOME A SOURCE OF REJUVENATION AND JOY.

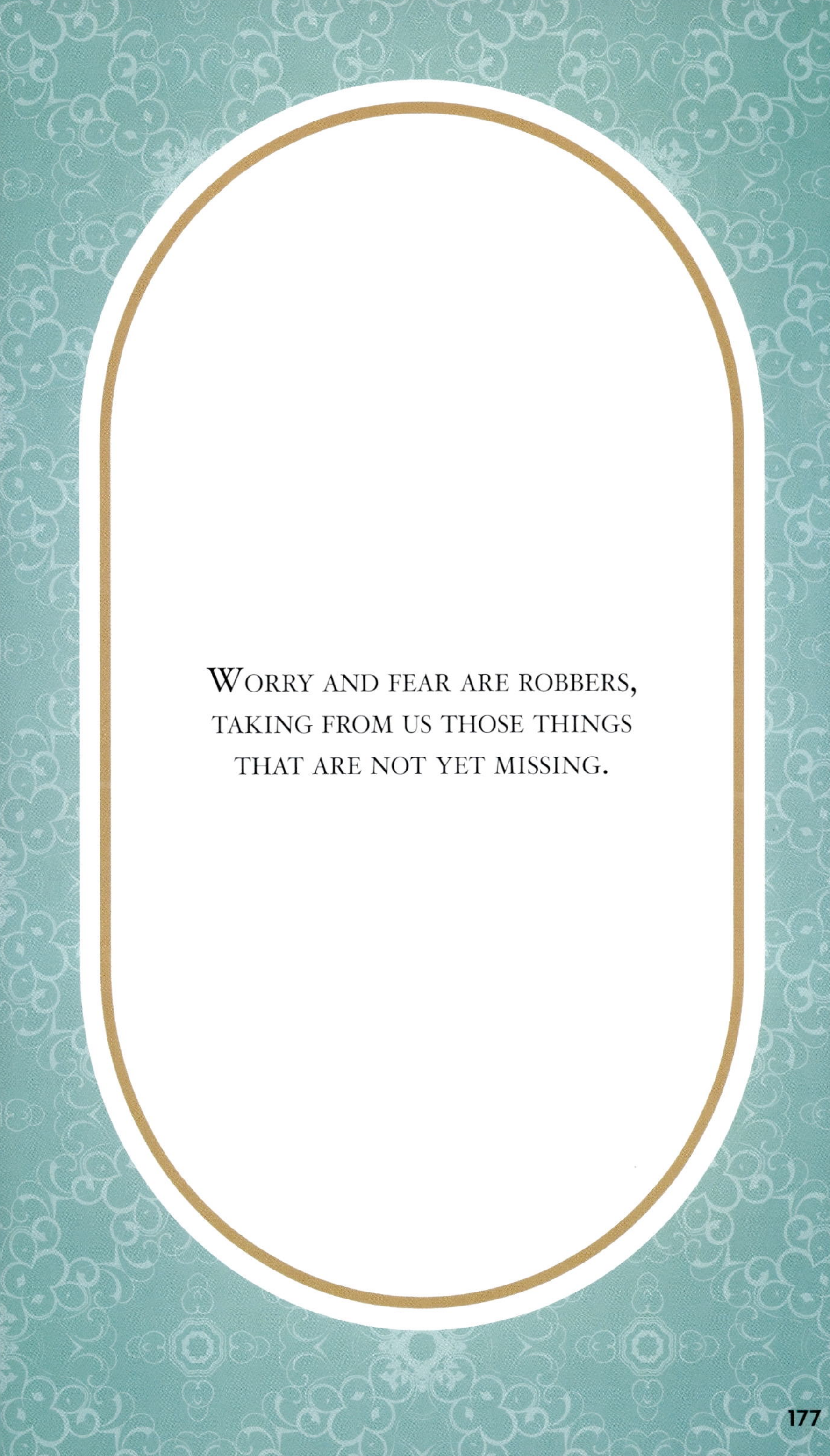

WORRY AND FEAR ARE ROBBERS,
TAKING FROM US THOSE THINGS
THAT ARE NOT YET MISSING.

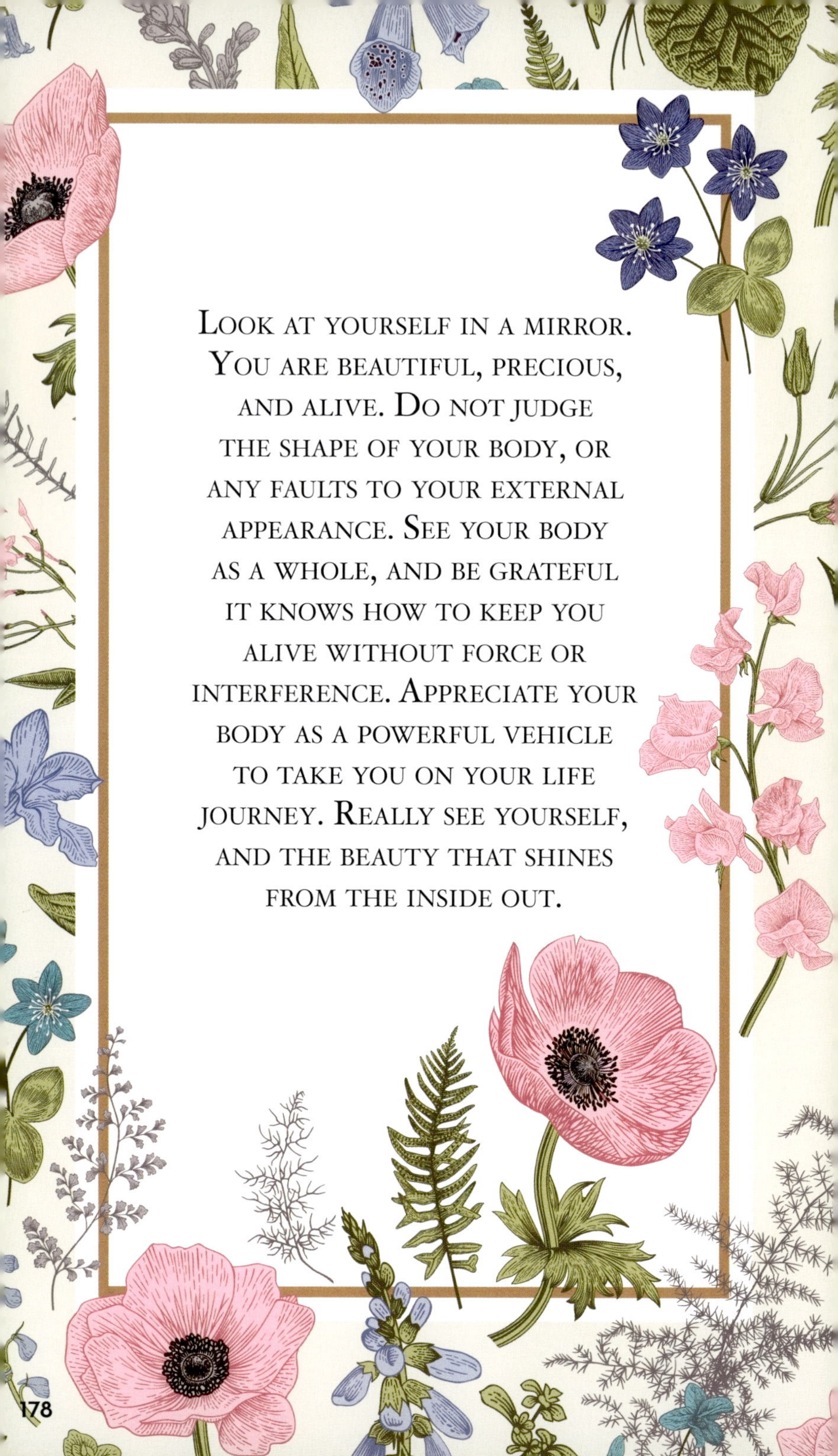

Look at yourself in a mirror. You are beautiful, precious, and alive. Do not judge the shape of your body, or any faults to your external appearance. See your body as a whole, and be grateful it knows how to keep you alive without force or interference. Appreciate your body as a powerful vehicle to take you on your life journey. Really see yourself, and the beauty that shines from the inside out.

The Calming Effects of Nature

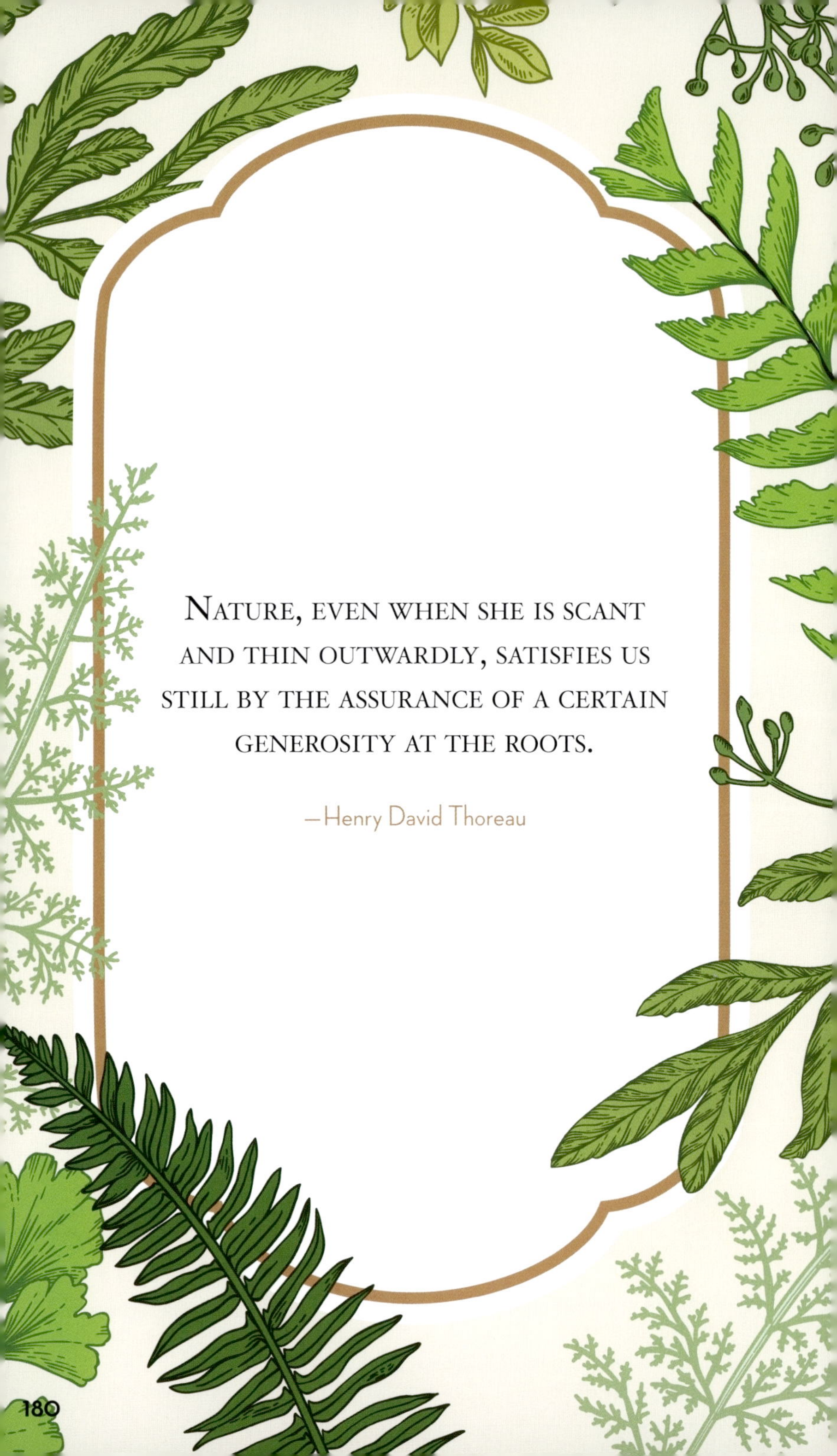

Nature, even when she is scant and thin outwardly, satisfies us still by the assurance of a certain generosity at the roots.

—Henry David Thoreau

Nature

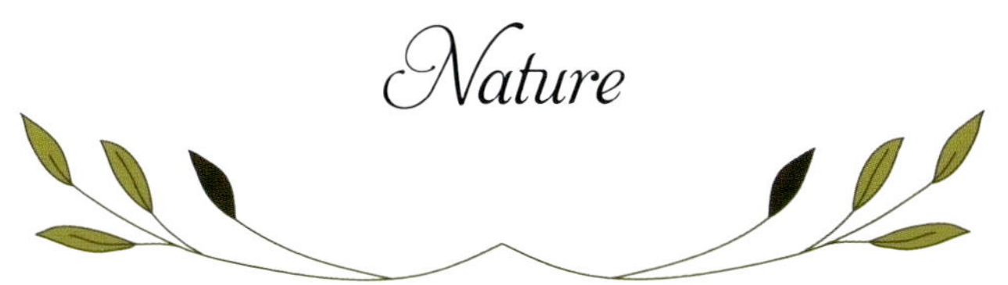

My mind is in a quiet place deep in nature, warmed by an inner sun. A gentle breeze moves across my body. Eyes closed, I allow myself to be in this magical place, with no expectations or goals. I become both the warm sun and the gentle breeze. I am at one with my surroundings. I am at peace.

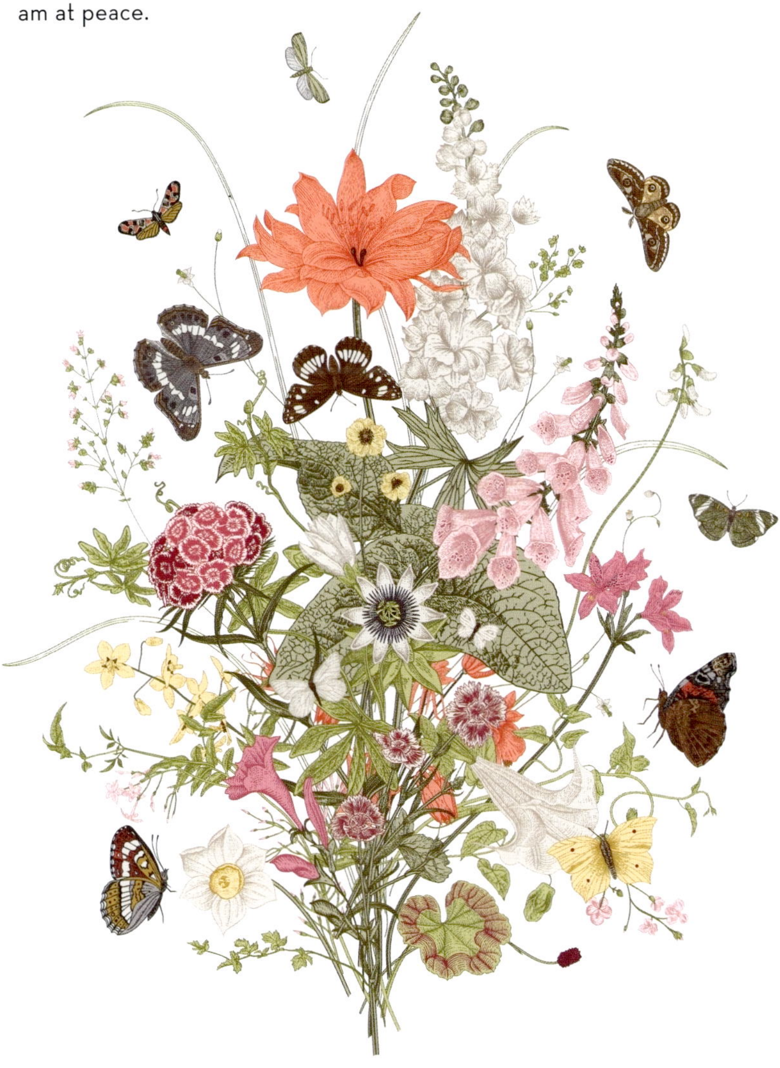

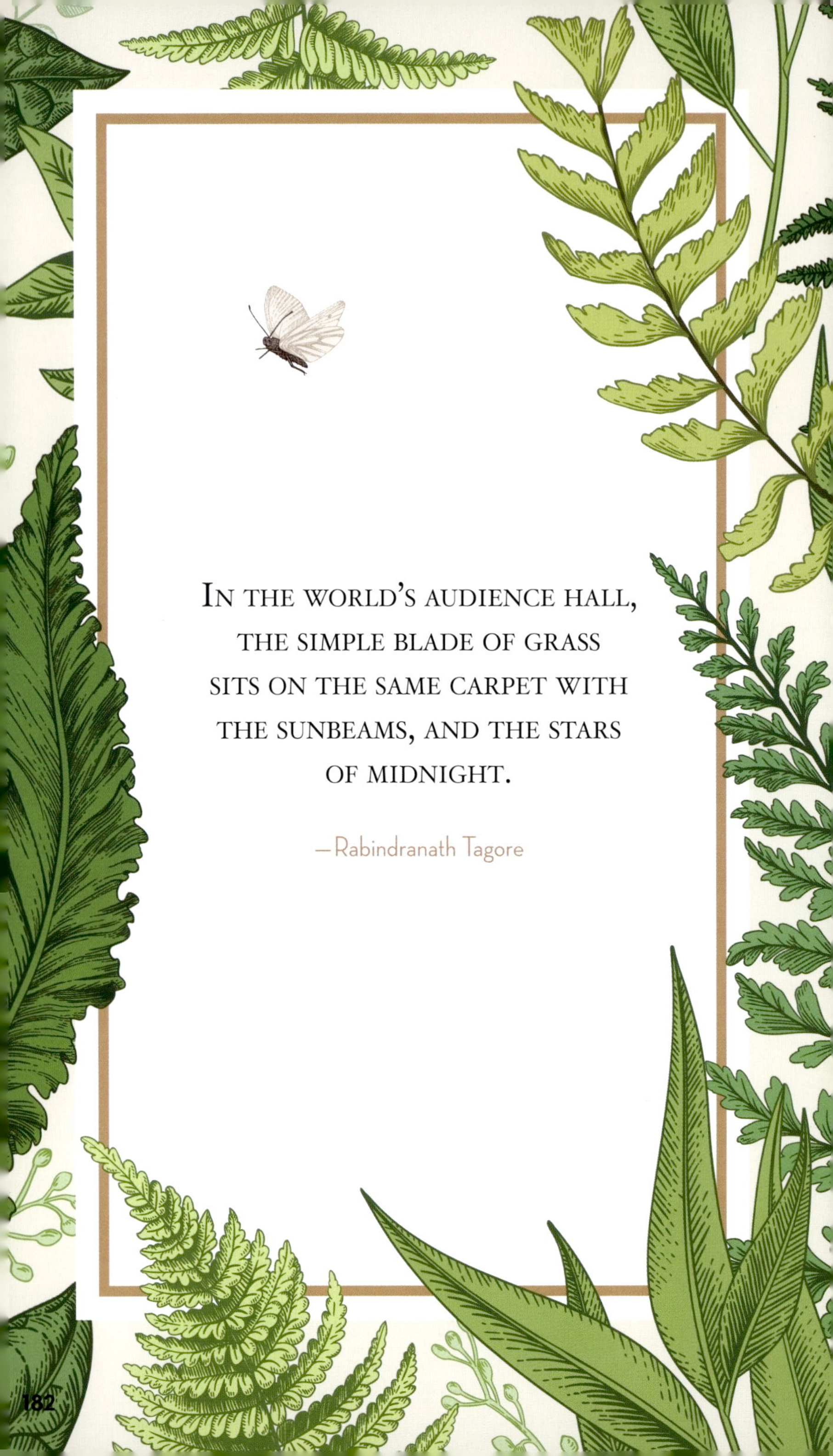

In the world's audience hall,
the simple blade of grass
sits on the same carpet with
the sunbeams, and the stars
of midnight.

—Rabindranath Tagore

The gentle breeze softly
caressing my face

The softness of a sweater draped
around my shoulders

Sounds of nature filling the
empty spaces in my mind

Nourishing breath moving in
and out of my lungs

Sweet calm washing away the
chaos of the day

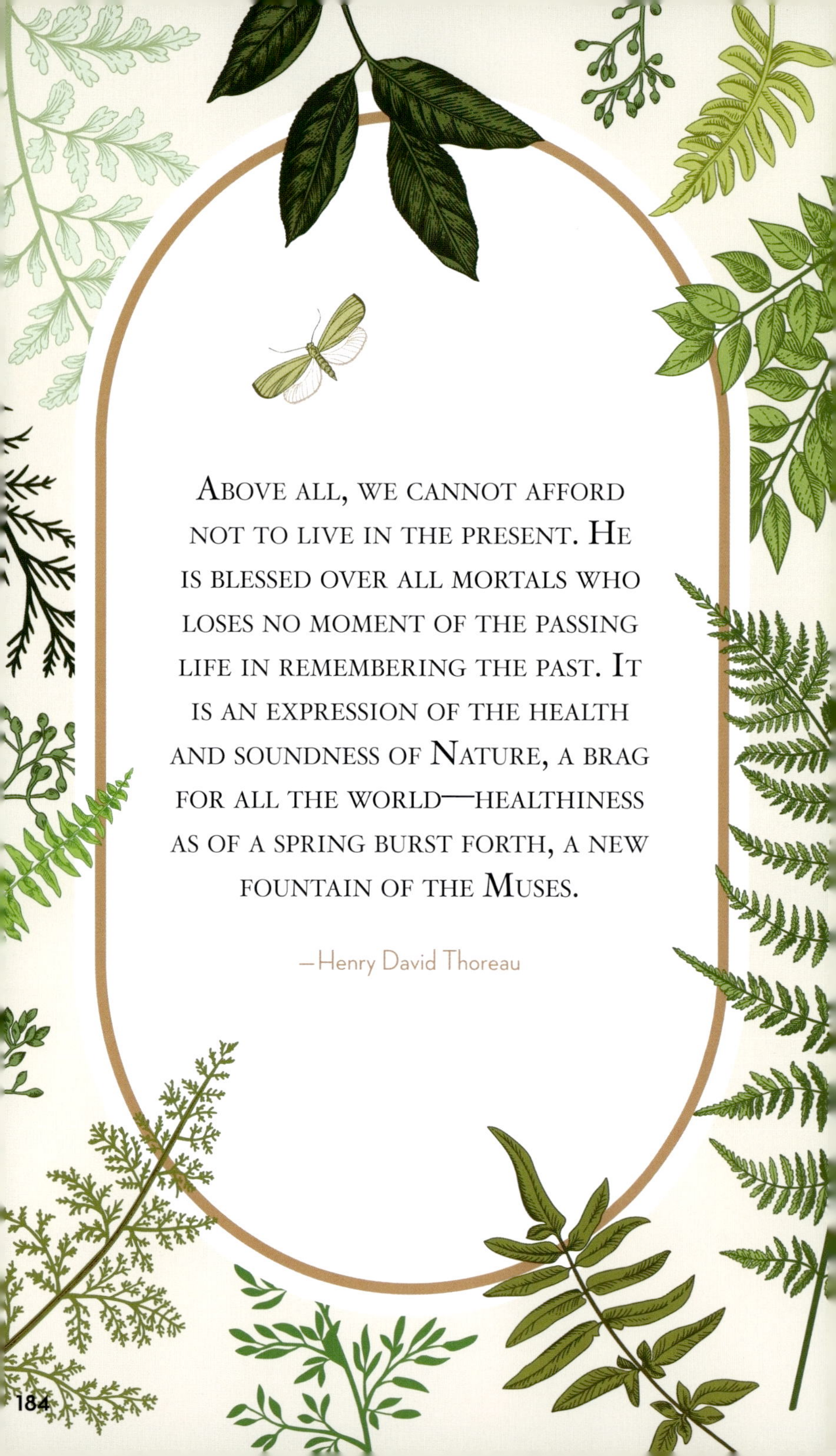

Above all, we cannot afford not to live in the present. He is blessed over all mortals who loses no moment of the passing life in remembering the past. It is an expression of the health and soundness of Nature, a brag for all the world—healthiness as of a spring burst forth, a new fountain of the Muses.

—Henry David Thoreau

A bird in flight is a meditation in beauty and freedom: lifting, diving, floating on air. A bird sometimes flies to find food or shelter, but sometimes just for the sheer joy of it. With wings spread to catch cloud and sun and sky, a bird has no limits, no hindrances—just a moment upon the wind, soaring.

The mind is a bird in flight.

Visualization

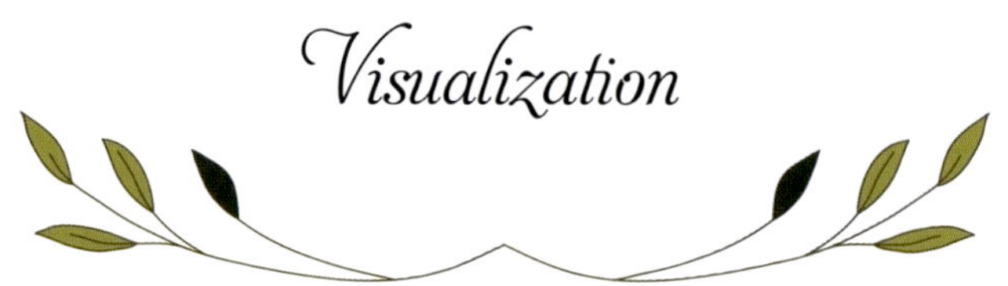

Visualize a lovely bench at the edge of a field of wildflowers. Sit down, in your mind, and look at the colors spread across the field like a painter's palette. Feel the sun and the breeze and relax, basking in the warmth and beauty of nature. Listen to birds in the trees bordering the field. Stay here awhile, among the flowers, among the birds.

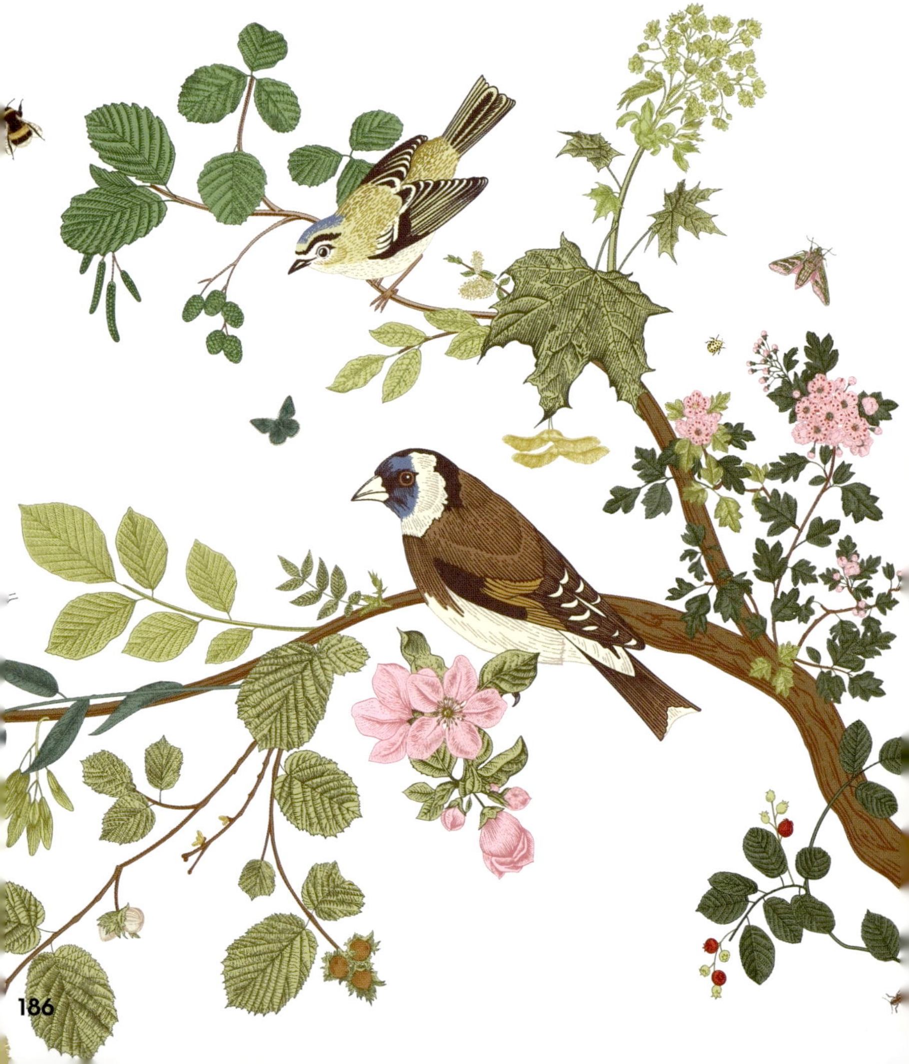

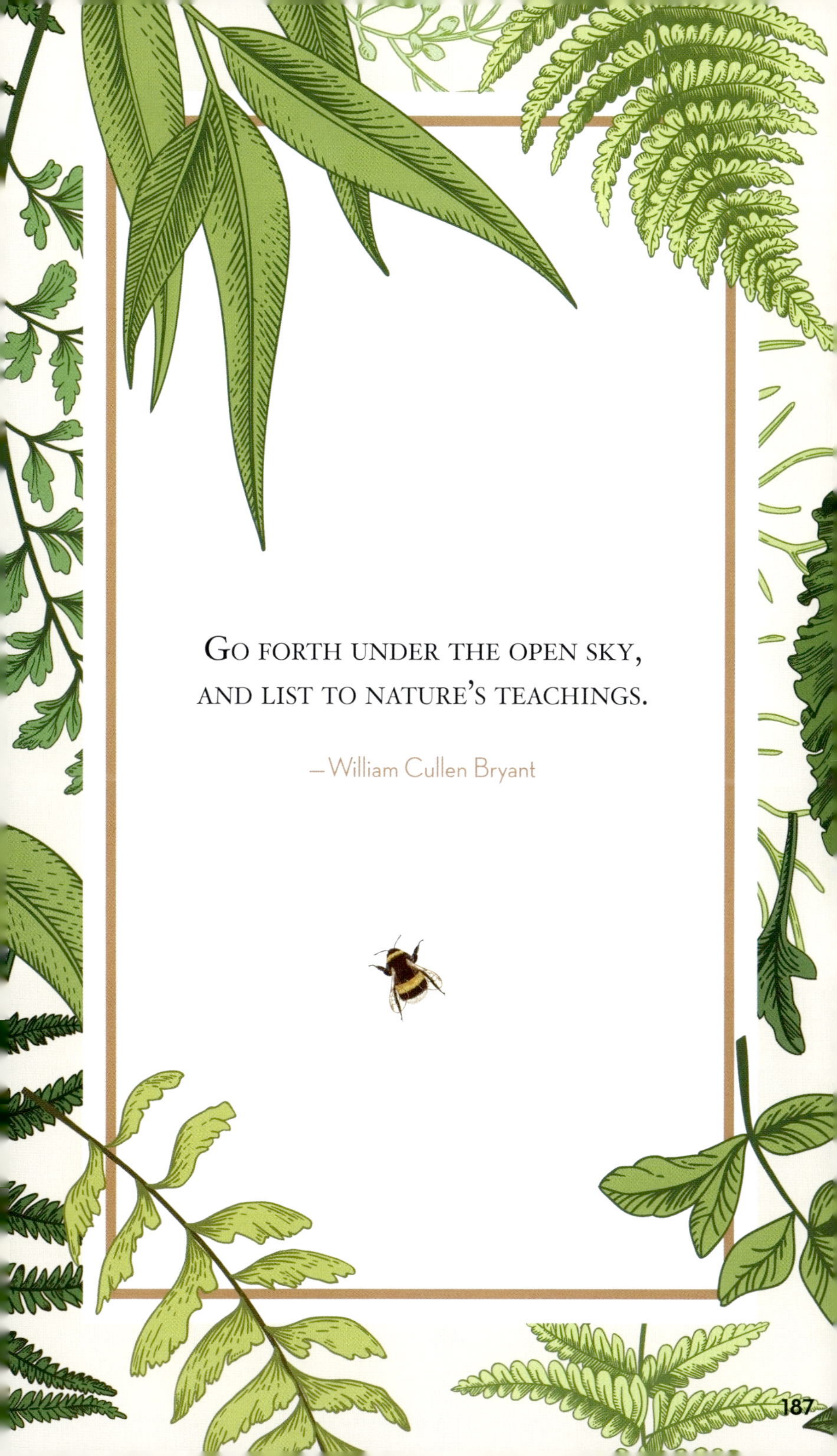

Go forth under the open sky,
and list to nature's teachings.

—William Cullen Bryant

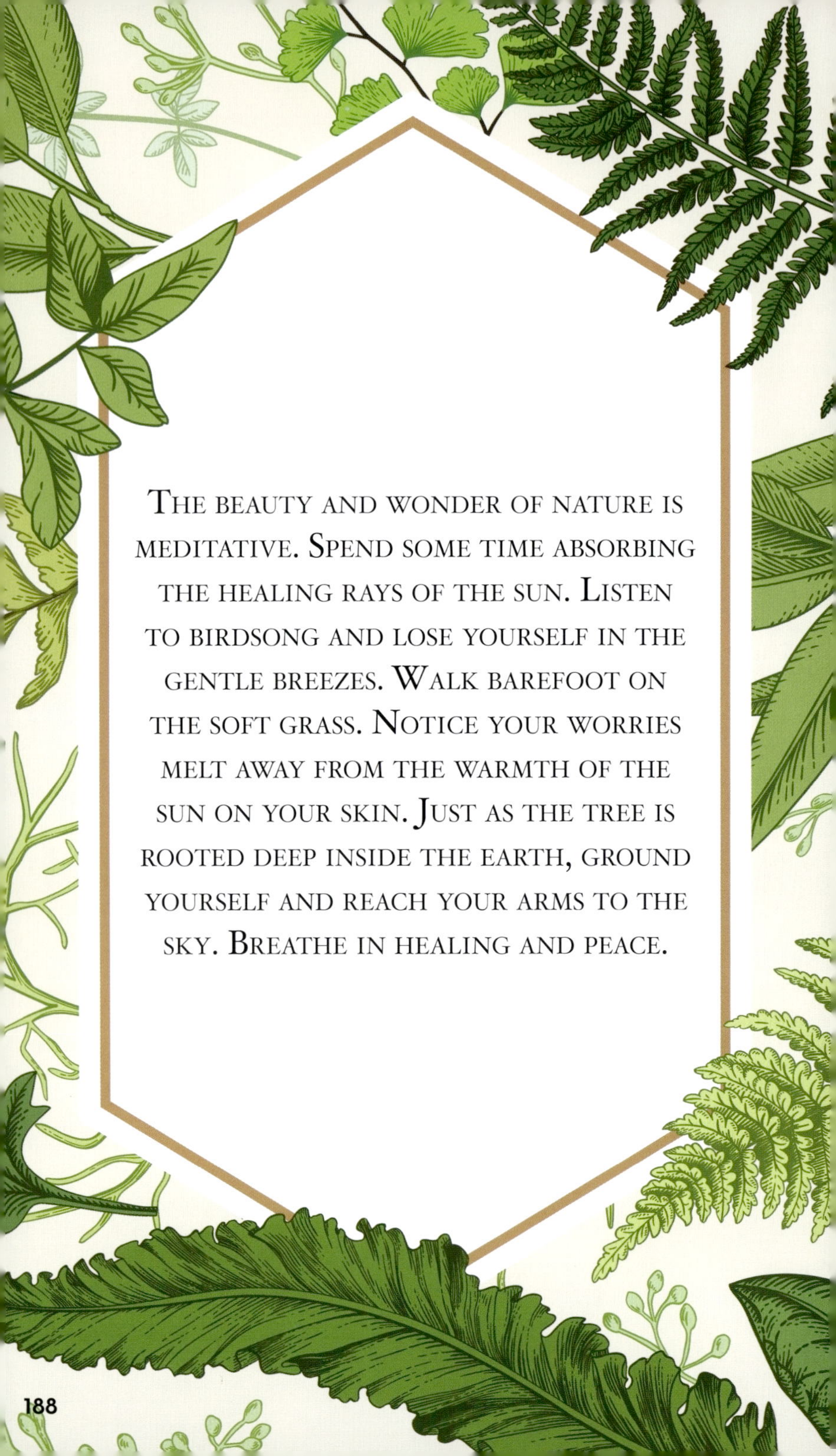

The beauty and wonder of nature is meditative. Spend some time absorbing the healing rays of the sun. Listen to birdsong and lose yourself in the gentle breezes. Walk barefoot on the soft grass. Notice your worries melt away from the warmth of the sun on your skin. Just as the tree is rooted deep inside the earth, ground yourself and reach your arms to the sky. Breathe in healing and peace.

A Bird's Flight

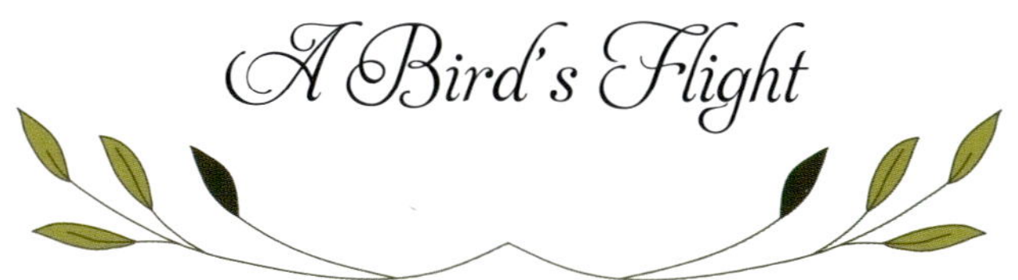

Watching a bird soar in the blue sky, I feel my body begin to relax. My mind clears, thinking only of the flight of the bird. I imagine the wind lifting my body and the view of the earth below me. I sense the motion of soaring, diving, and climbing. My breathing slows, deep and steady, as I observe, detached from the rest of the world around me. I am one with the bird.

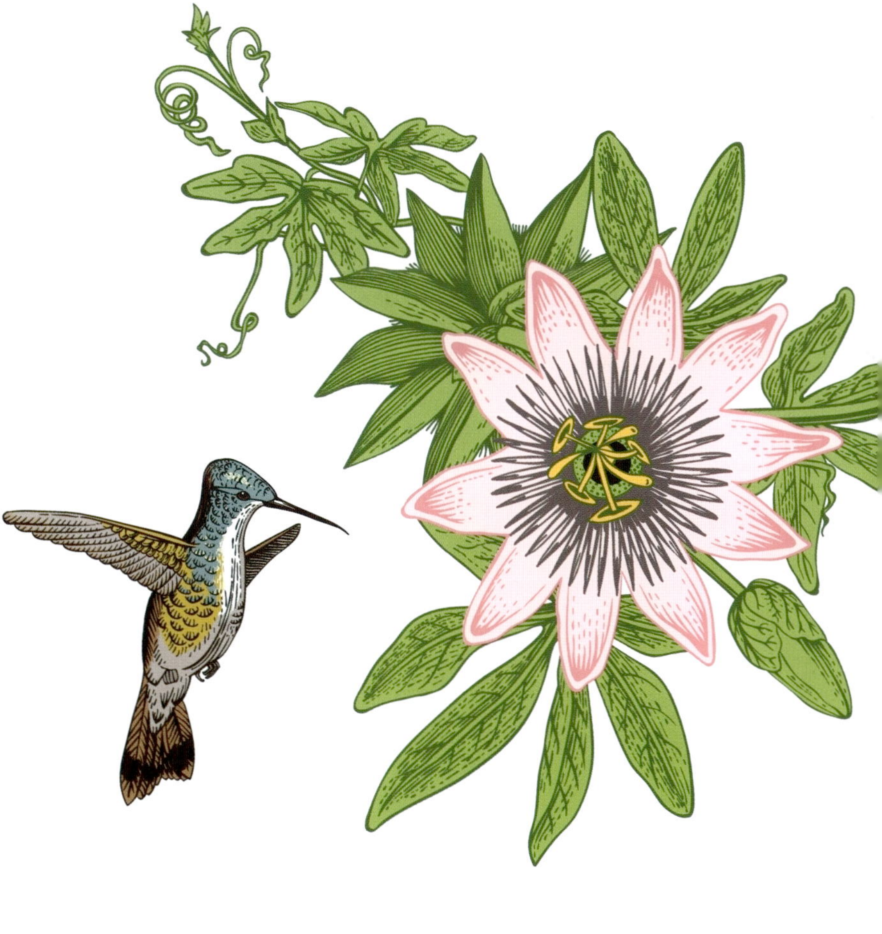

Notice a flower in bloom as you go about your day, or picture one in your mind. Look closely at the intricacy of the petals. Imagine scents that soothe the mind and delight the soul. Remember peaceful walks in parks and gardens. We are nourished by the sun's warm rays. We raise our faces toward the sky.

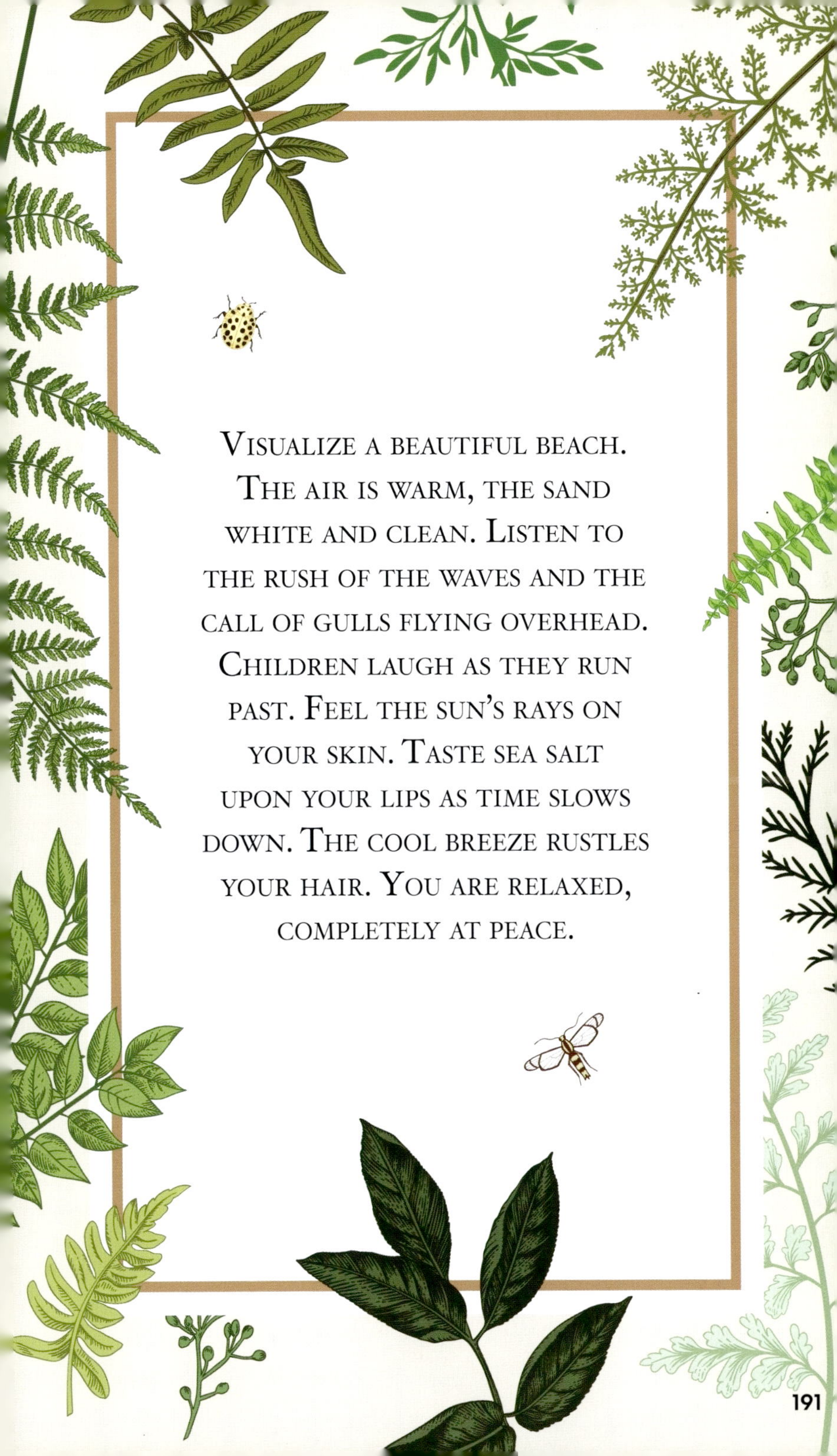

Visualize a beautiful beach. The air is warm, the sand white and clean. Listen to the rush of the waves and the call of gulls flying overhead. Children laugh as they run past. Feel the sun's rays on your skin. Taste sea salt upon your lips as time slows down. The cool breeze rustles your hair. You are relaxed, completely at peace.

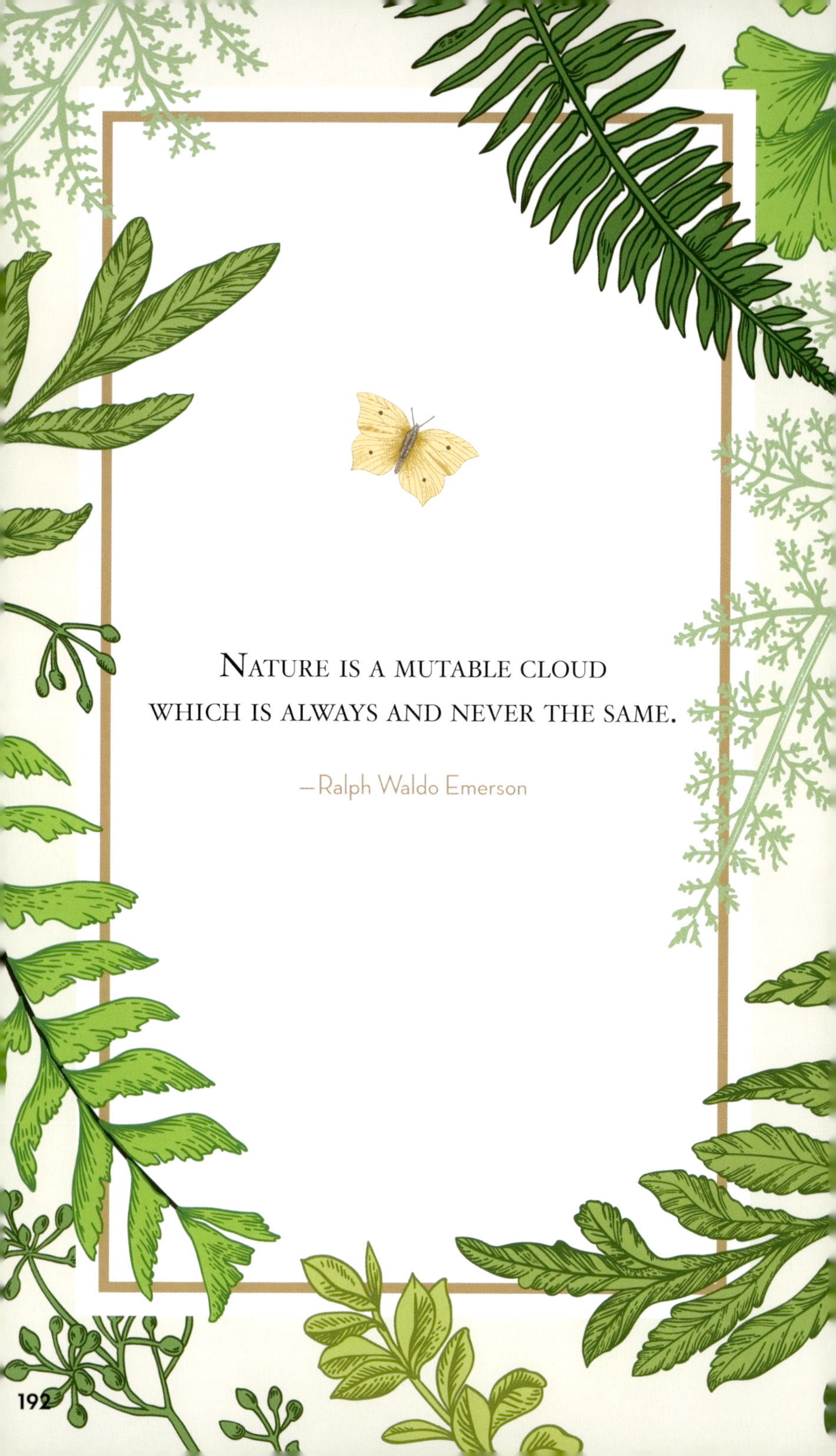

Nature is a mutable cloud
which is always and never the same.

—Ralph Waldo Emerson

Human beings are the only creatures that strive to be something they are not. Perhaps we should take a lesson from the birds of the sky, who never ache to be anything other than creatures able to fly on a lifting breeze. Or learn from the fish of the sea, who don't doubt their own ability to glide through blue waters dappled with sunlight. Or spend some time watching wild horses thunder over the open plains, and we would see that not once do they stop to wish they were anything more than glorious, beautiful, and free.

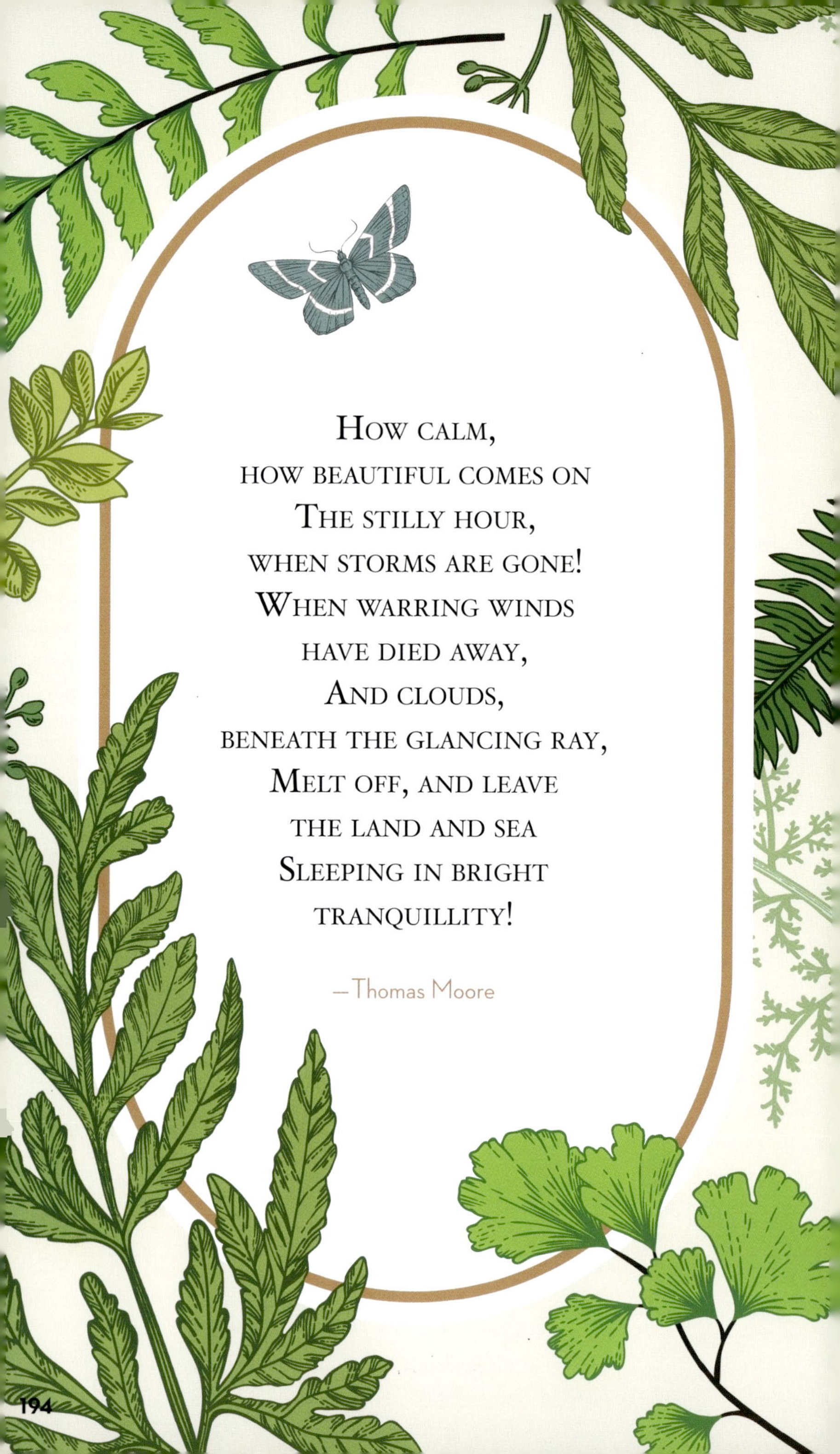

How calm,
how beautiful comes on
The stilly hour,
when storms are gone!
When warring winds
have died away,
And clouds,
beneath the glancing ray,
Melt off, and leave
the land and sea
Sleeping in bright
tranquillity!

—Thomas Moore

THE EARTH IS ASLEEP. THE BUDS OF SPRING LIE IN WAIT. THE WONDER OF THE WORLD SEEMS IN A HOLDING PATTERN, WAITING FOR THE GO-AHEAD TO GROW. LET WINTER TEACH YOU THE VALUE OF STILLNESS, OF SILENCE, AND OF MEDITATION. NATURE'S QUIET TIME OF REGENERATION MAY SPARK THE SAME IN YOU.

Rainy Day Meditation

Be mindful of a rainy day and let your stress slip away. Listen to the falling rain and lose yourself in the patter on the window. Breathe deeply the smell of nourished soil. Let your worry wash away with the rain, leaving your mind cleansed. Sit with the sights, sounds, and smells of rainfall and allow them to renew and refresh your spirit.

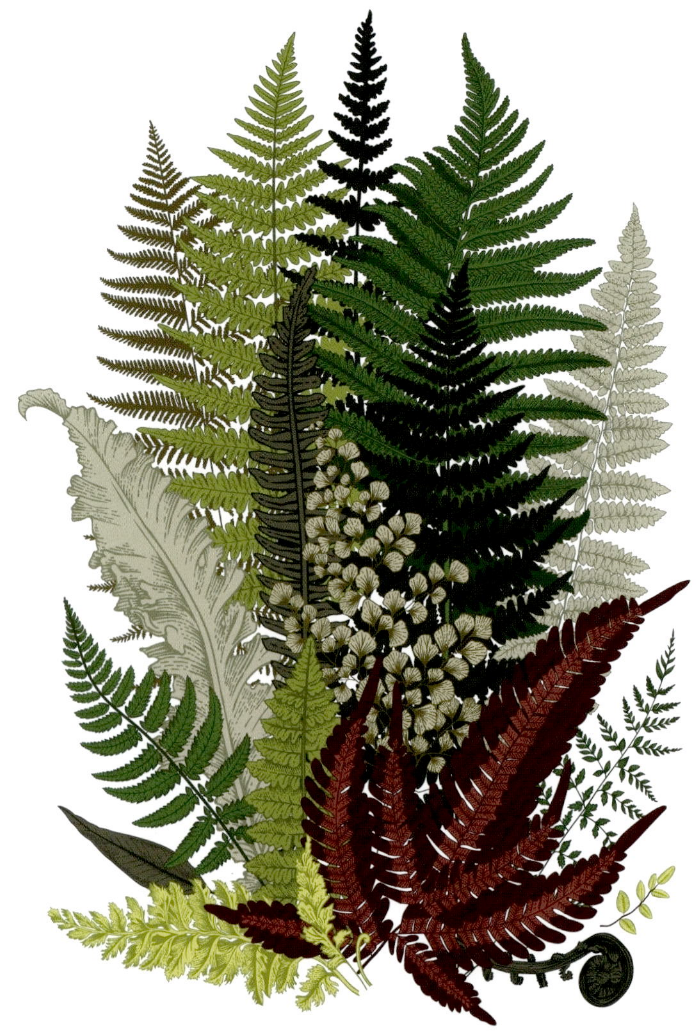

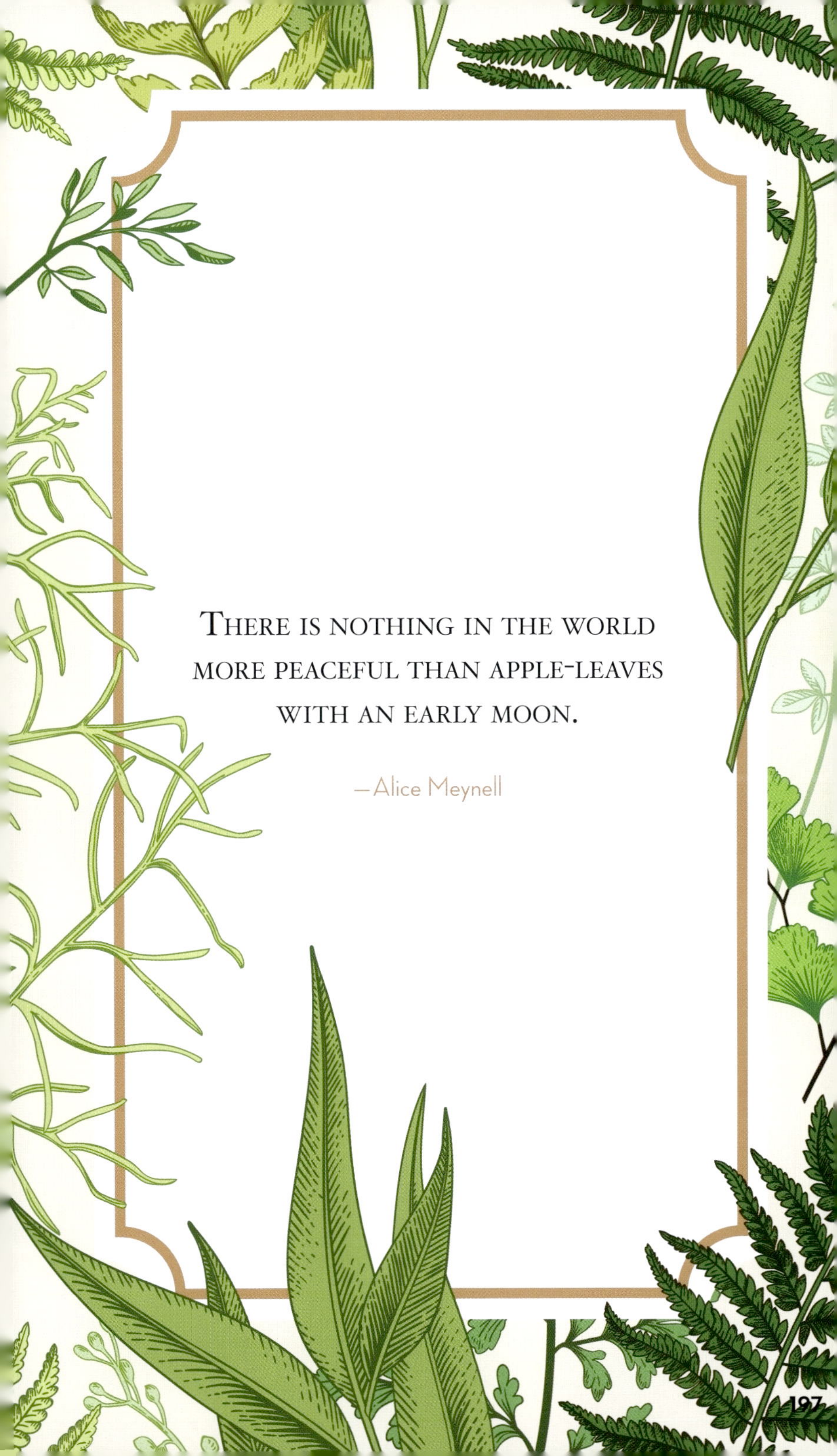

There is nothing in the world more peaceful than apple-leaves with an early moon.

—Alice Meynell

In the solitude of a natural setting, the heart discovers serenity, the soul knows abiding peace, and the spirit finds renewal. Surround yourself with the serenity of nature, and you will feel more at peace with yourself and your world.

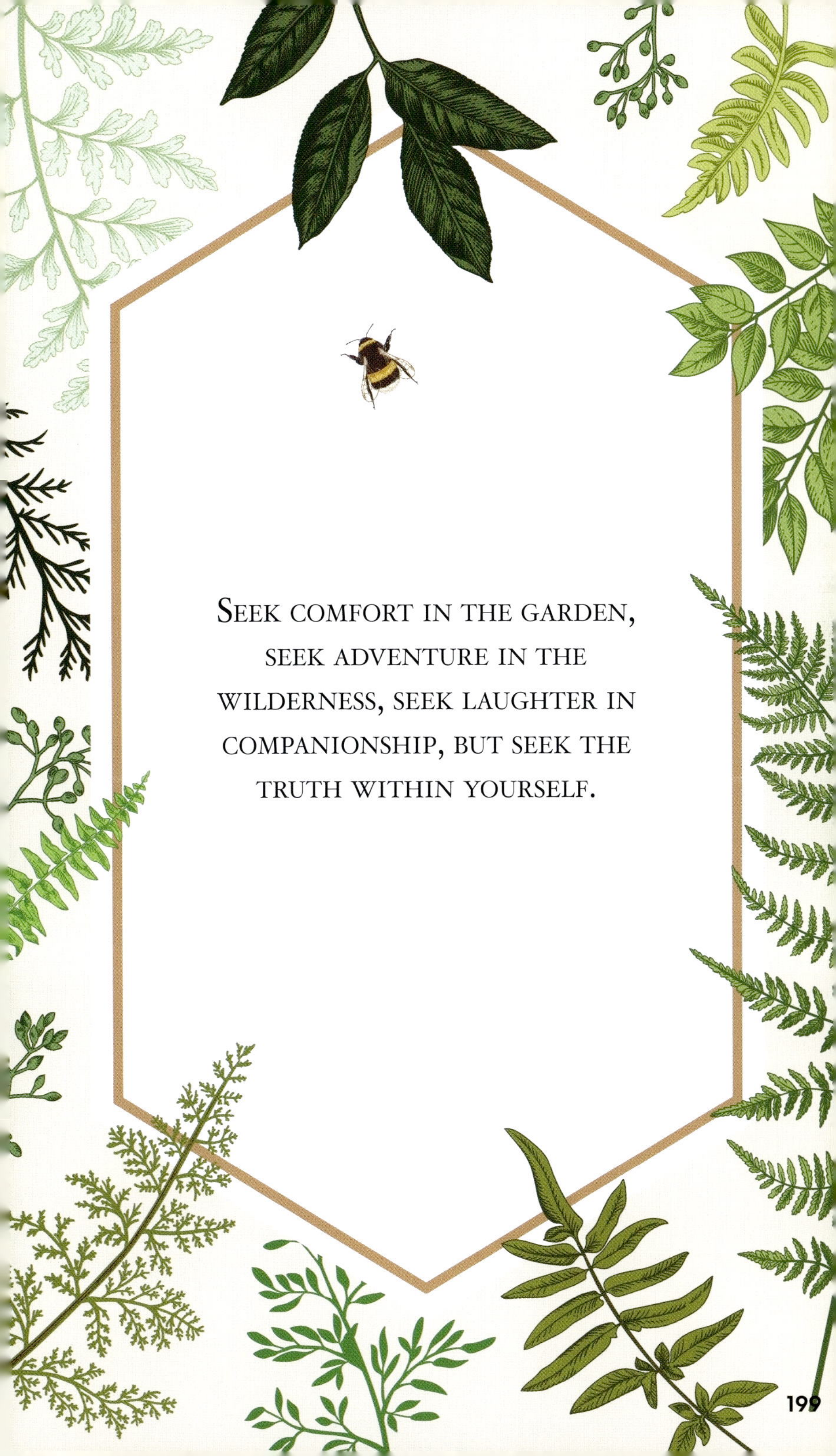

Seek comfort in the garden, seek adventure in the wilderness, seek laughter in companionship, but seek the truth within yourself.

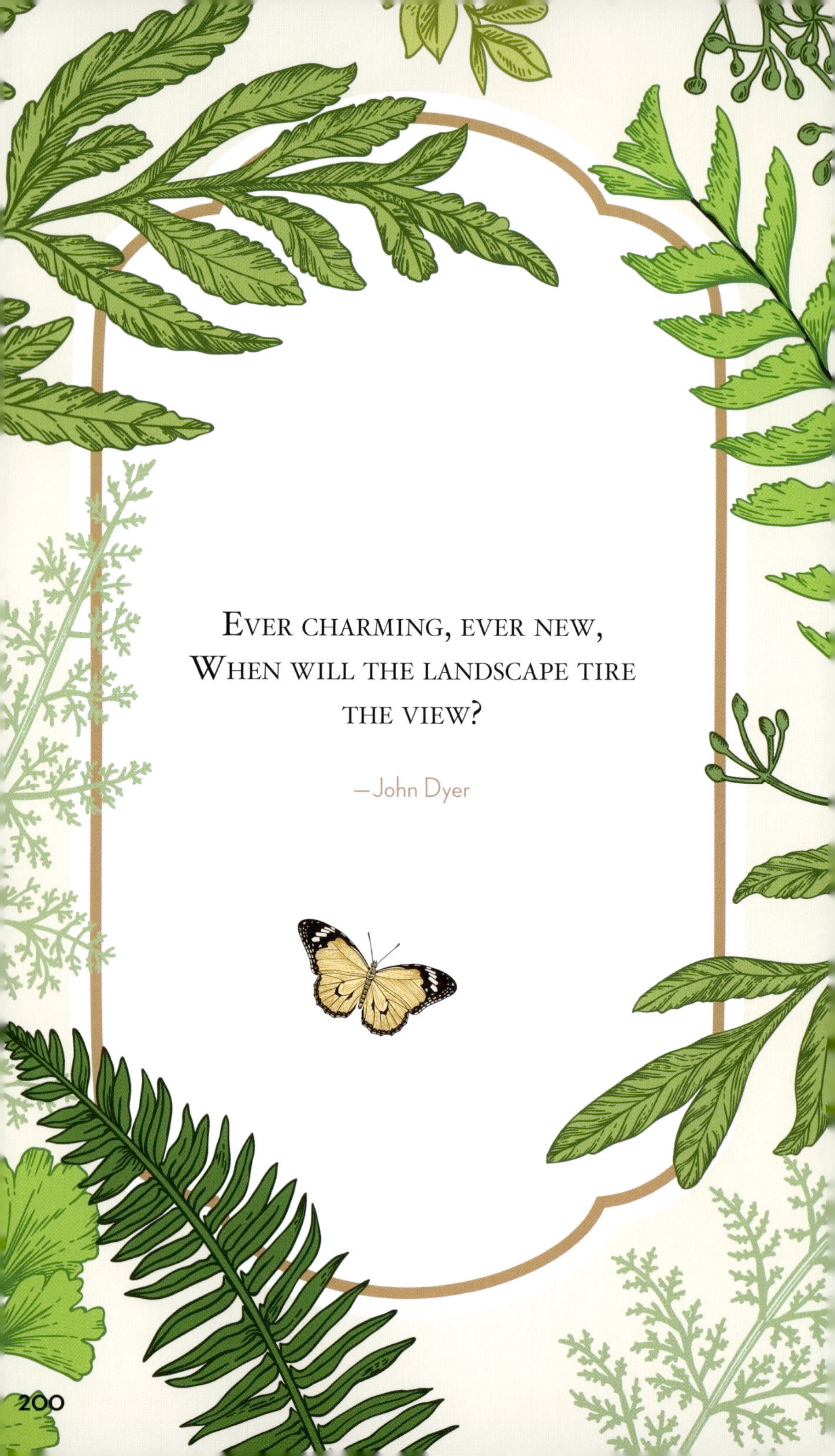

EVER CHARMING, EVER NEW,
WHEN WILL THE LANDSCAPE TIRE
THE VIEW?

—John Dyer

A Water Lily

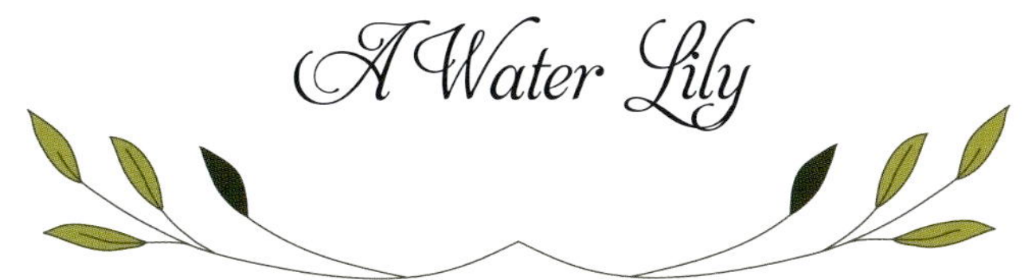

We can take a lesson from the precious water lily. For no matter what outside force or pressure is put upon the lily, it always rises back to the water's surface again to feel the nurturing sunlight upon its leaves and petals. We must be like the lily, steadfast and true in the face of every difficulty, that we too may rise above our problems and feel the light on our faces again.

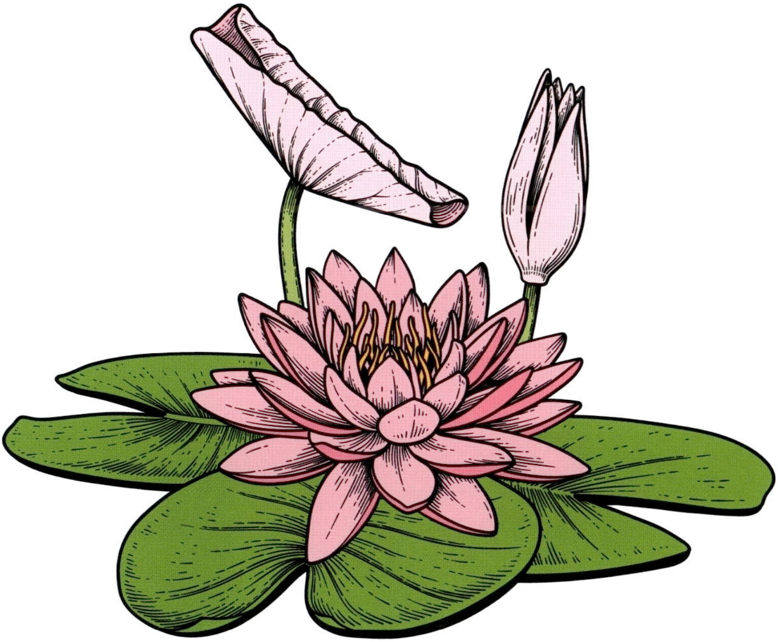

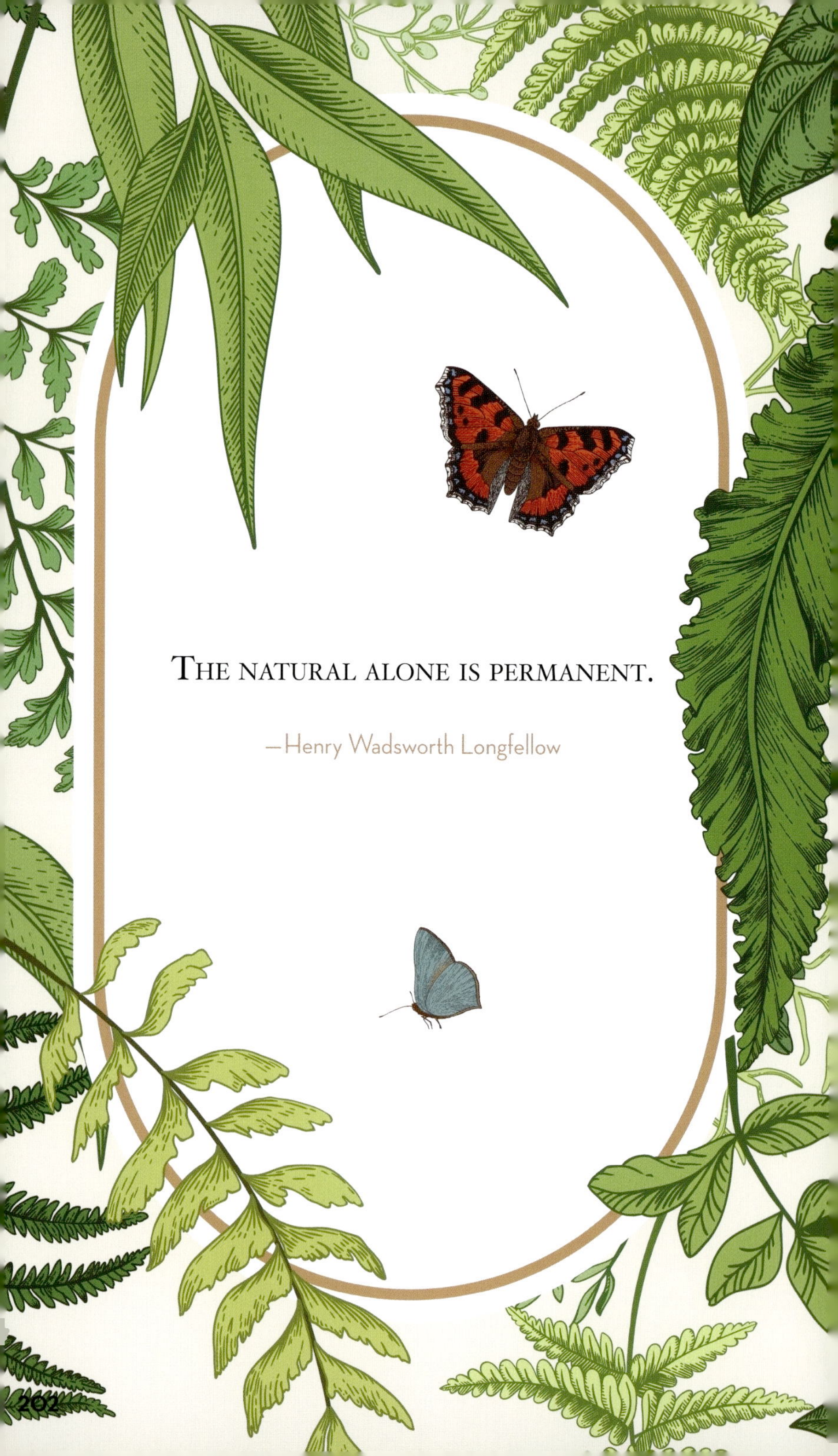

THE NATURAL ALONE IS PERMANENT.

—Henry Wadsworth Longfellow

And joy is everywhere; it is in the earth's green covering of grass; in the blue serenity of the sky; in the reckless exuberance of spring; in the severe abstinence of grey winter; in the living flesh that animates our bodily frame; in the perfect poise of the human figure, noble and upright; in living; in the exercise of all our powers; in the acquisition of knowledge; in fighting evils; in dying for gains we never can share. Joy is there everywhere; it is superfluous, unnecessary; nay, it very often contradicts the most peremptory behests of necessity. It exists to show that the bonds of law can only be explained by love; they are like body and soul. Joy is the realisation of the truth of oneness, the oneness of our soul with the world and of the world-soul with the supreme lover.

—Rabindranath Tagore

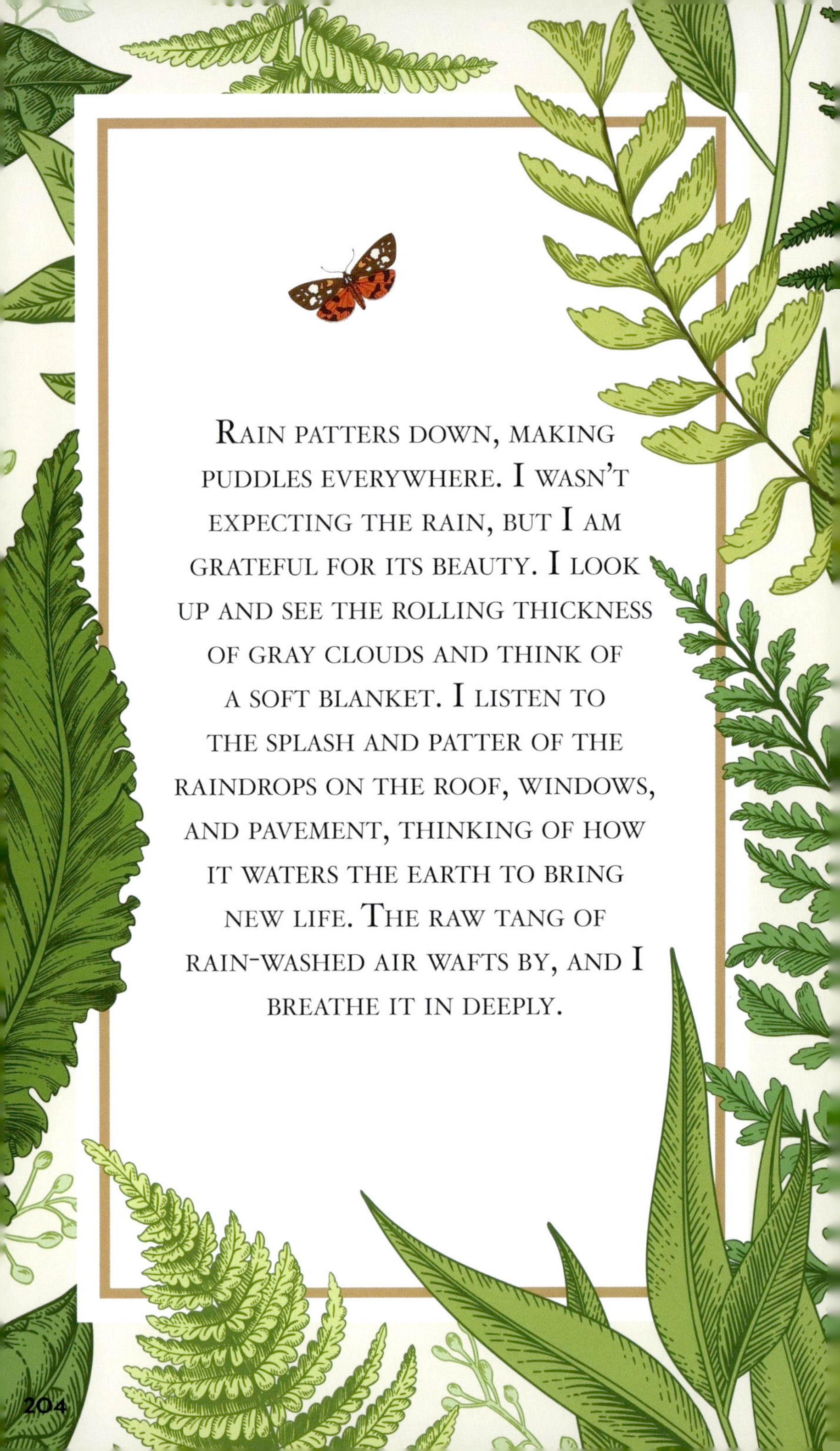

Rain patters down, making puddles everywhere. I wasn't expecting the rain, but I am grateful for its beauty. I look up and see the rolling thickness of gray clouds and think of a soft blanket. I listen to the splash and patter of the raindrops on the roof, windows, and pavement, thinking of how it waters the earth to bring new life. The raw tang of rain-washed air wafts by, and I breathe it in deeply.

Today I am thinking of something simple yet wonderful: wind. The sound of it, its promise of change, the feeling of excitement it creates—wind is indeed a mysterious thing. When a storm marches in from the west, I like watching how invisible wind arrives first, making itself visible in the movement of trees and scuttle of leaves. The wind tells me that anything is possible!

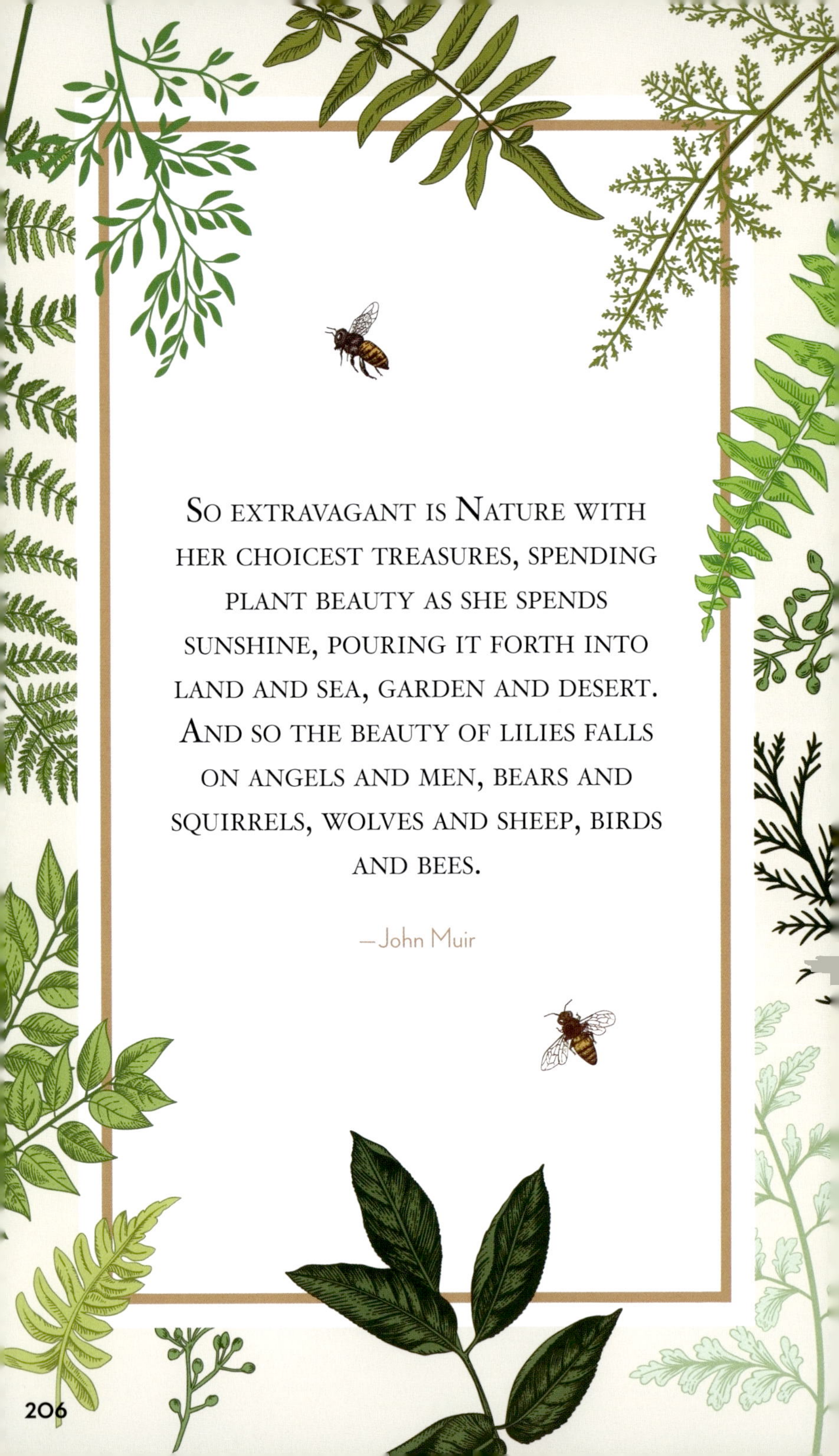

So extravagant is Nature with her choicest treasures, spending plant beauty as she spends sunshine, pouring it forth into land and sea, garden and desert. And so the beauty of lilies falls on angels and men, bears and squirrels, wolves and sheep, birds and bees.

—John Muir

I feel the warmth of the sun on my face and the breeze against my skin. I hear the sound of birds in the trees calling to each other. In nature, I come back to the fullness of life in the moment. All my worries drift away as I lift my eyes to the blue sky. I am calm and centered amidst the sights and sounds around me, becoming one with them, and with the world.

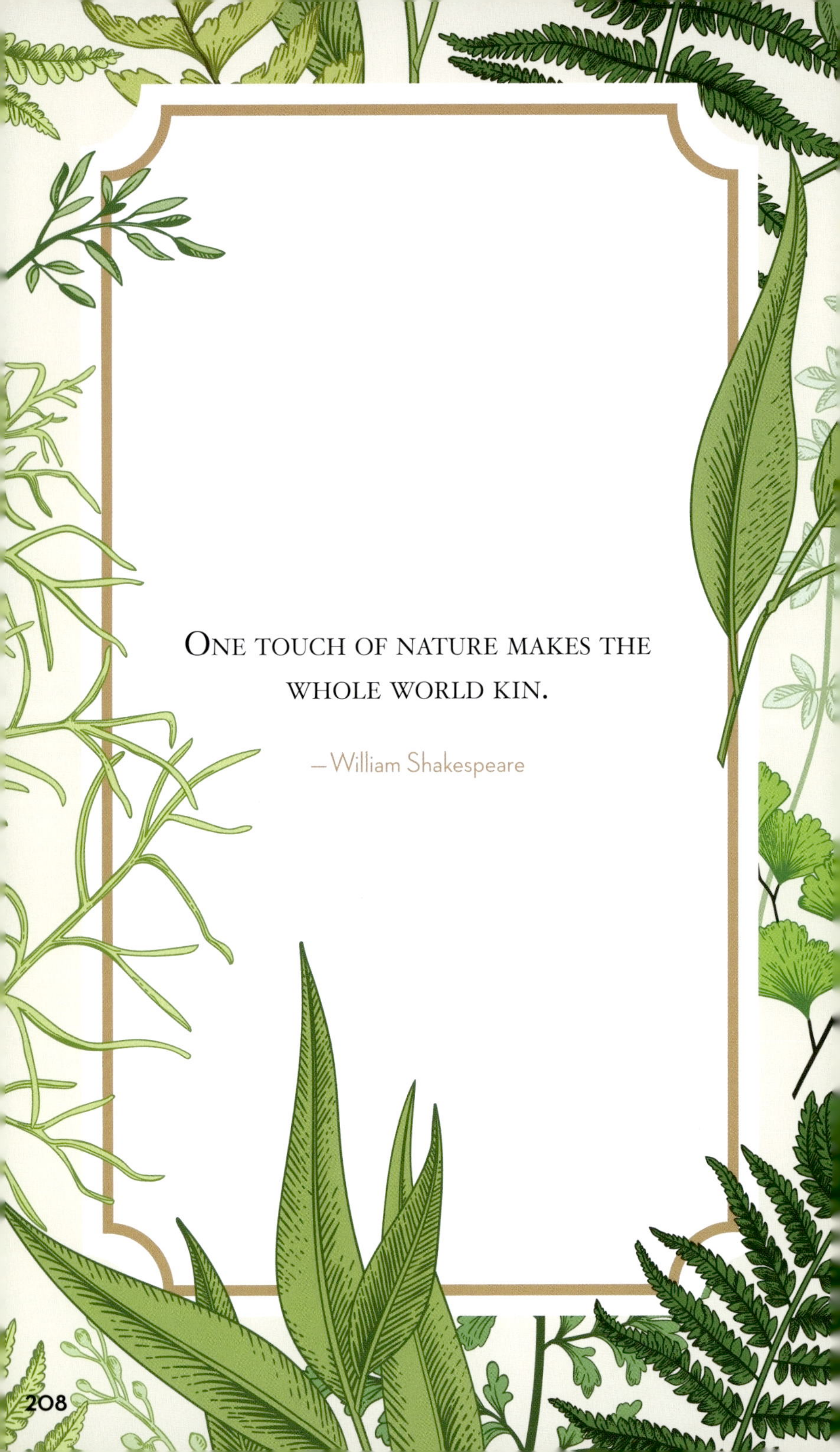

One touch of nature makes the whole world kin.

—William Shakespeare

The key to finding the good in life is paying attention to the beautiful details. Nature provides us with the perfect opportunity to see perfection in action. Look at a flower, and how delicate it is. Watch a hawk glide in an azure blue sky, majestic and free. Run your hand through the coolness of a flowing creek. Smell a rosebush deeply. It's the simple things that ground us to the gifts of the present.

Not all being alone is loneliness.
Not all solitude is a problem to solve.
With others far away, bask in the blessings of quietness.

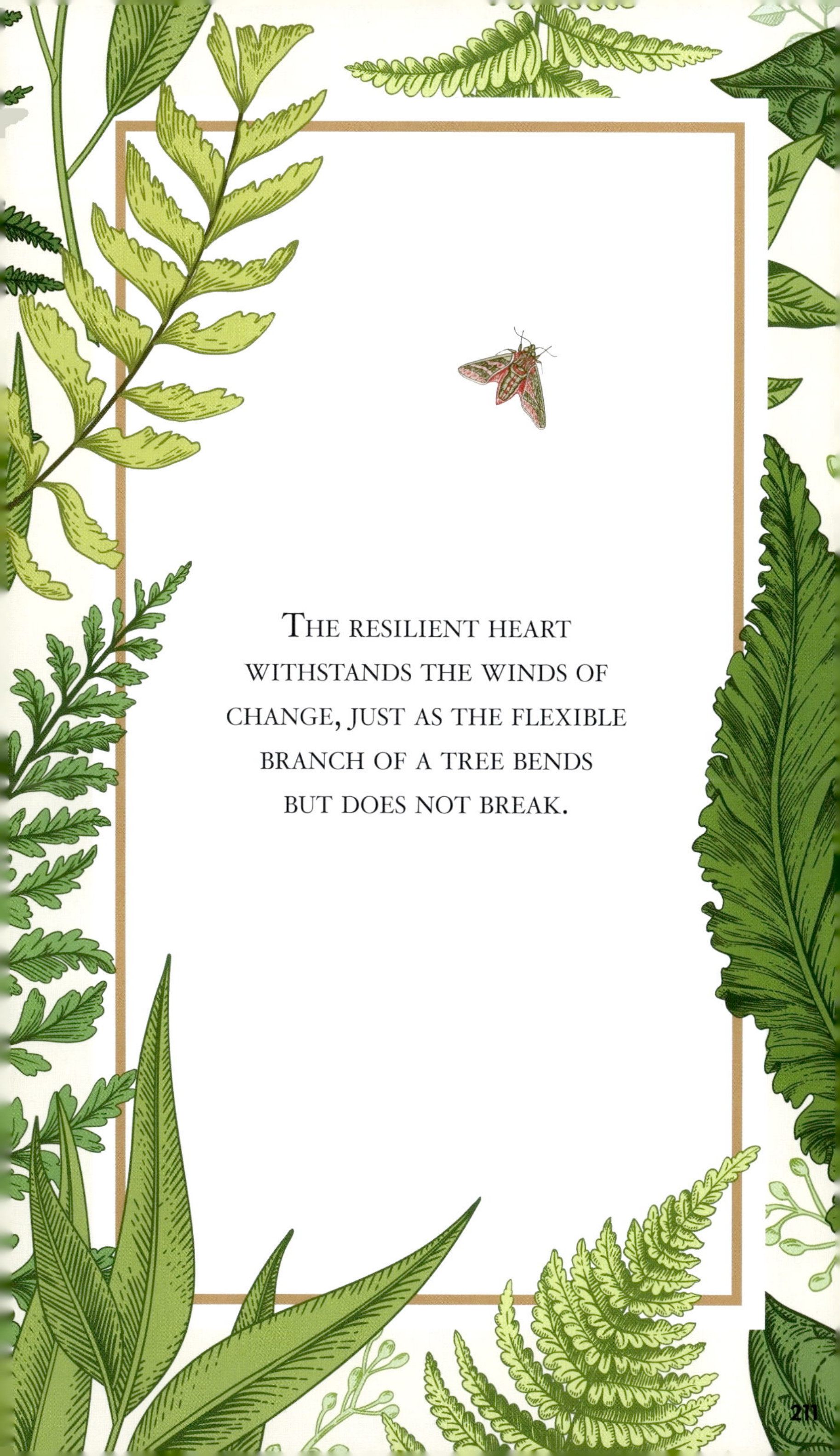

THE RESILIENT HEART WITHSTANDS THE WINDS OF CHANGE, JUST AS THE FLEXIBLE BRANCH OF A TREE BENDS BUT DOES NOT BREAK.

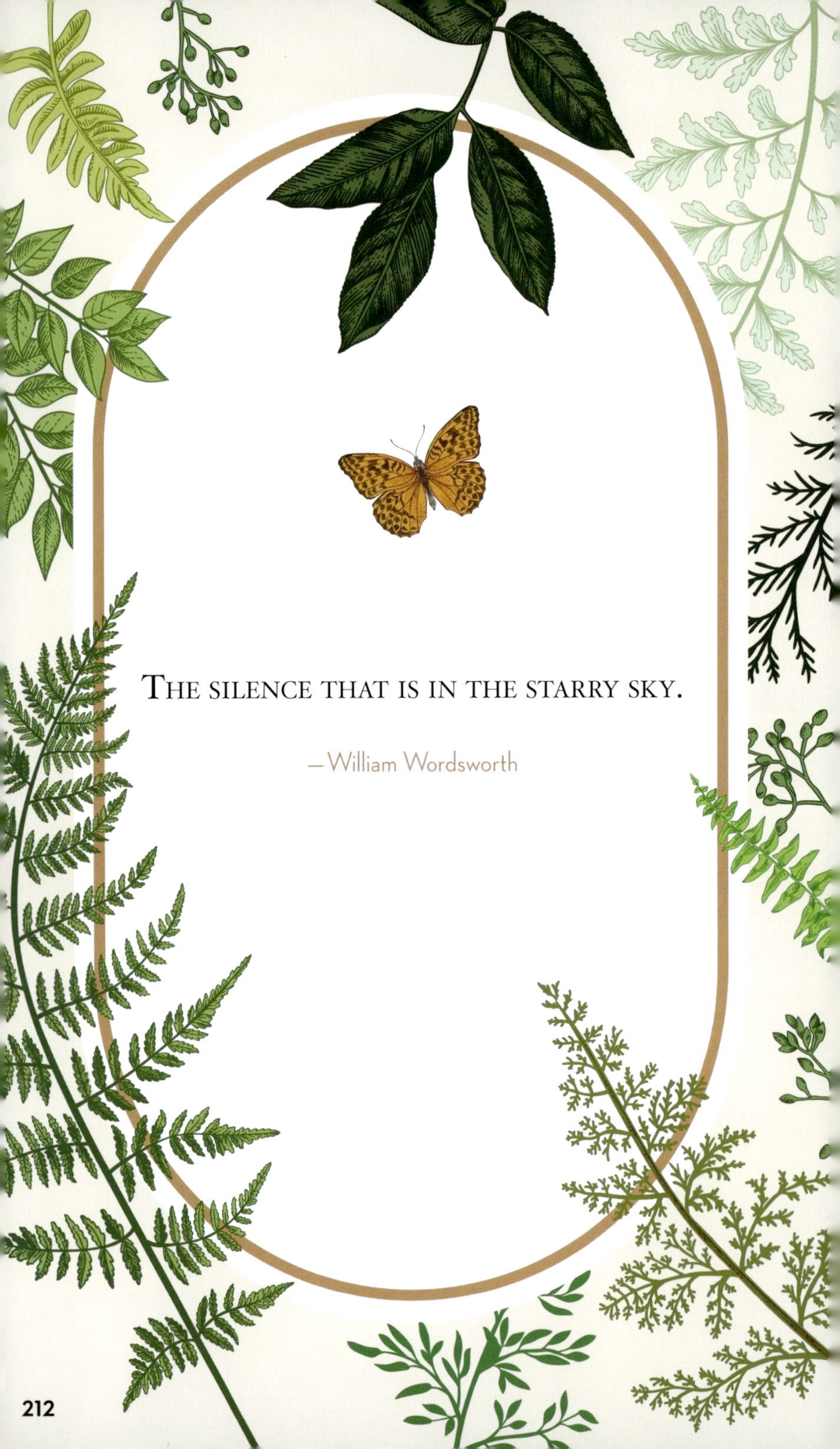

THE SILENCE THAT IS IN THE STARRY SKY.

—William Wordsworth

Seeing What's There

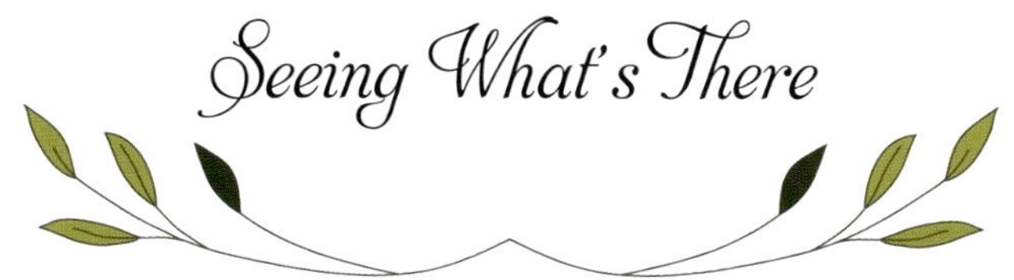

Do you look at an object, but not really see it? So much of life's blessings and miracles are evident when we stop long enough to truly see what is in front of us. The delicate beauty of a rose is only visible to those who take the time to fully pay attention to the color and shape of the petals, the sharpness of the thorns, the deep green of the leaves. Mindfulness lets us experience the fullness of life.

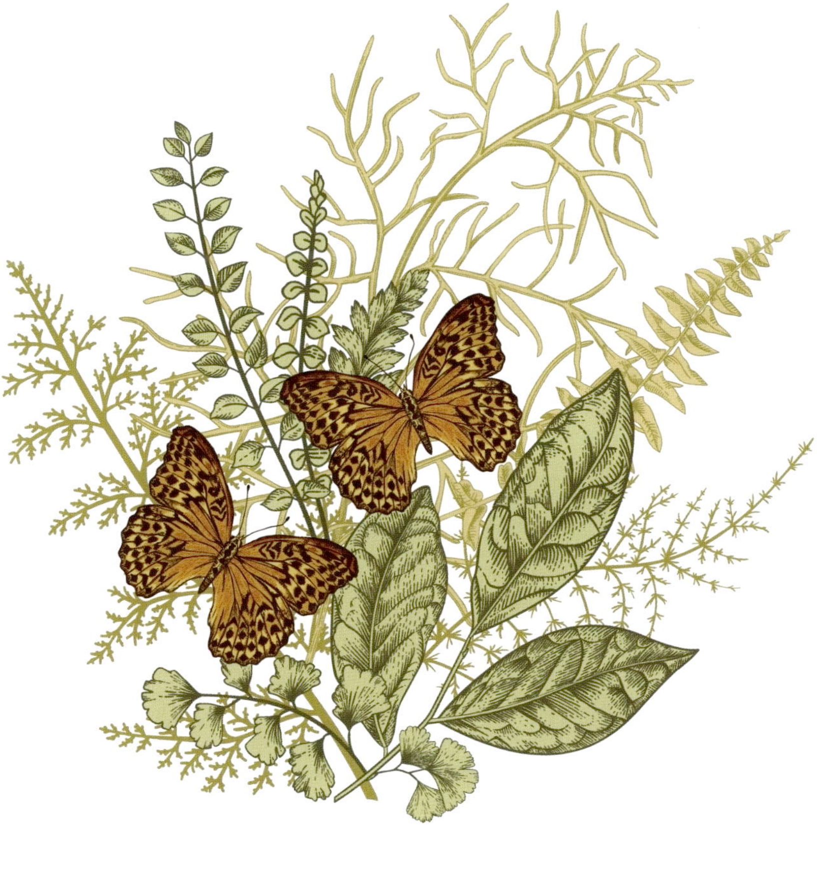

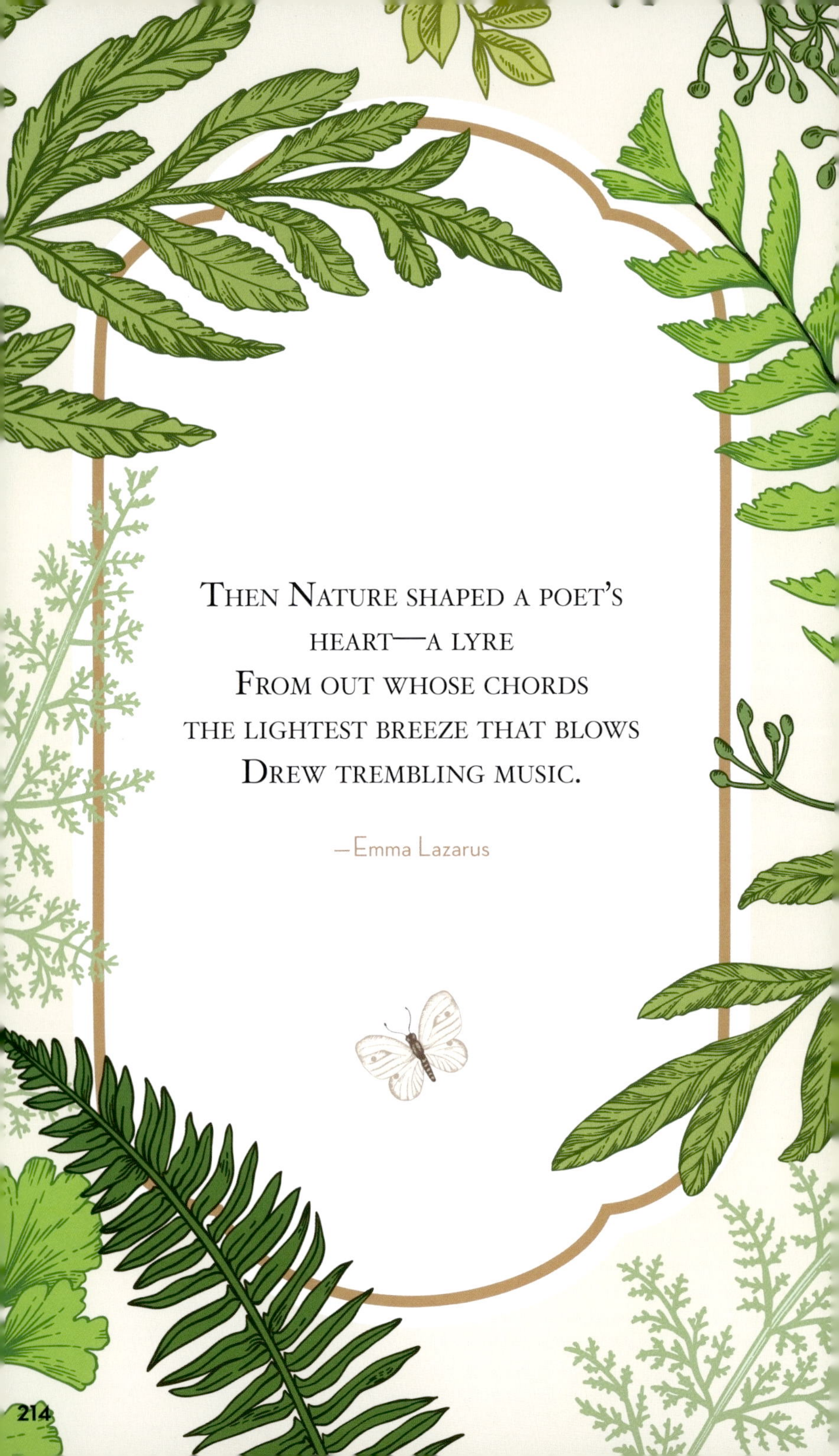

Then Nature shaped a poet's heart—a lyre
From out whose chords
the lightest breeze that blows
Drew trembling music.

—Emma Lazarus

Sitting quietly, let the noises of the outside world fade into the background. Notice your breath. Listen to the air that is life-giving and nourishing. Breathe in through your nose and hold, then release. Be so present to the moment that you become one with your breath. Become aware of the external noises around you now, but do not let them drown out the sound of your breath as you go about your day awakened.

A flower is a delight to the senses. One simple object can fill us with joy and make us smile. The problem is, we miss out on the miracles of the world around us, because we are focused on achievement, doing, having, and rushing here and there. Stop. Look at the sky, a tree, and a bird flying. Don't just watch it; really see it with the fullness of presence. This is how we notice the many miracles that make up our lives.

The Joys of Nature

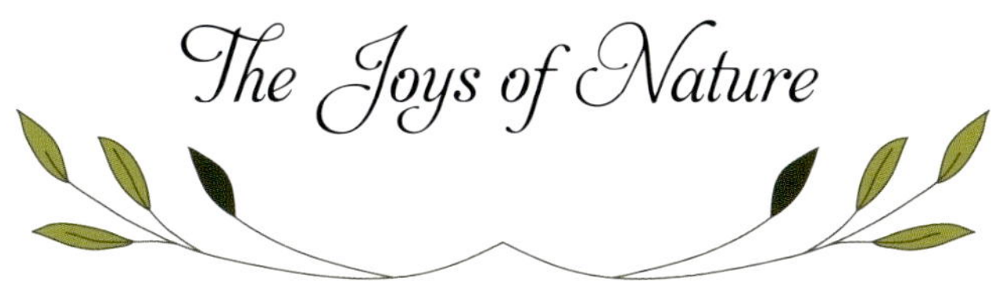

Getting out into nature is a wonderful way to stay mindful and connect our spirits to the power of the present. The call of wild birds, the sight of a beautiful mountain vista, or the trickle of a gently running stream serve to dissipate worries and anxieties and bring us back into the current of life. In nature, we find ourselves and lose the labels and perceptions we have taken on from others. Nature returns us to our source.

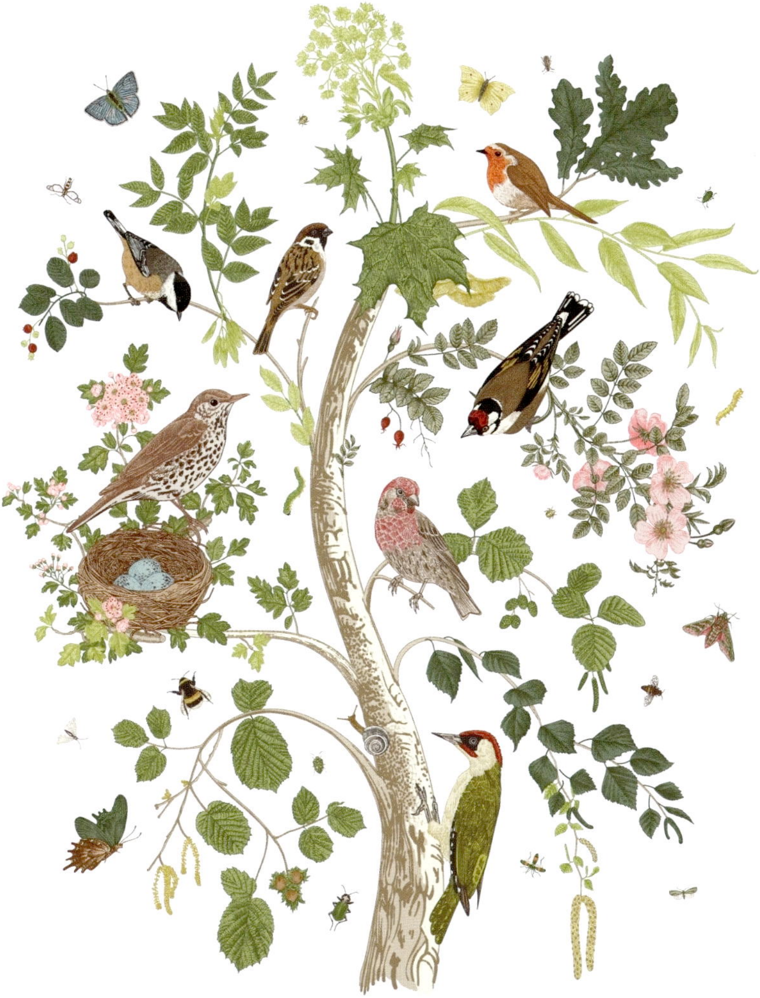

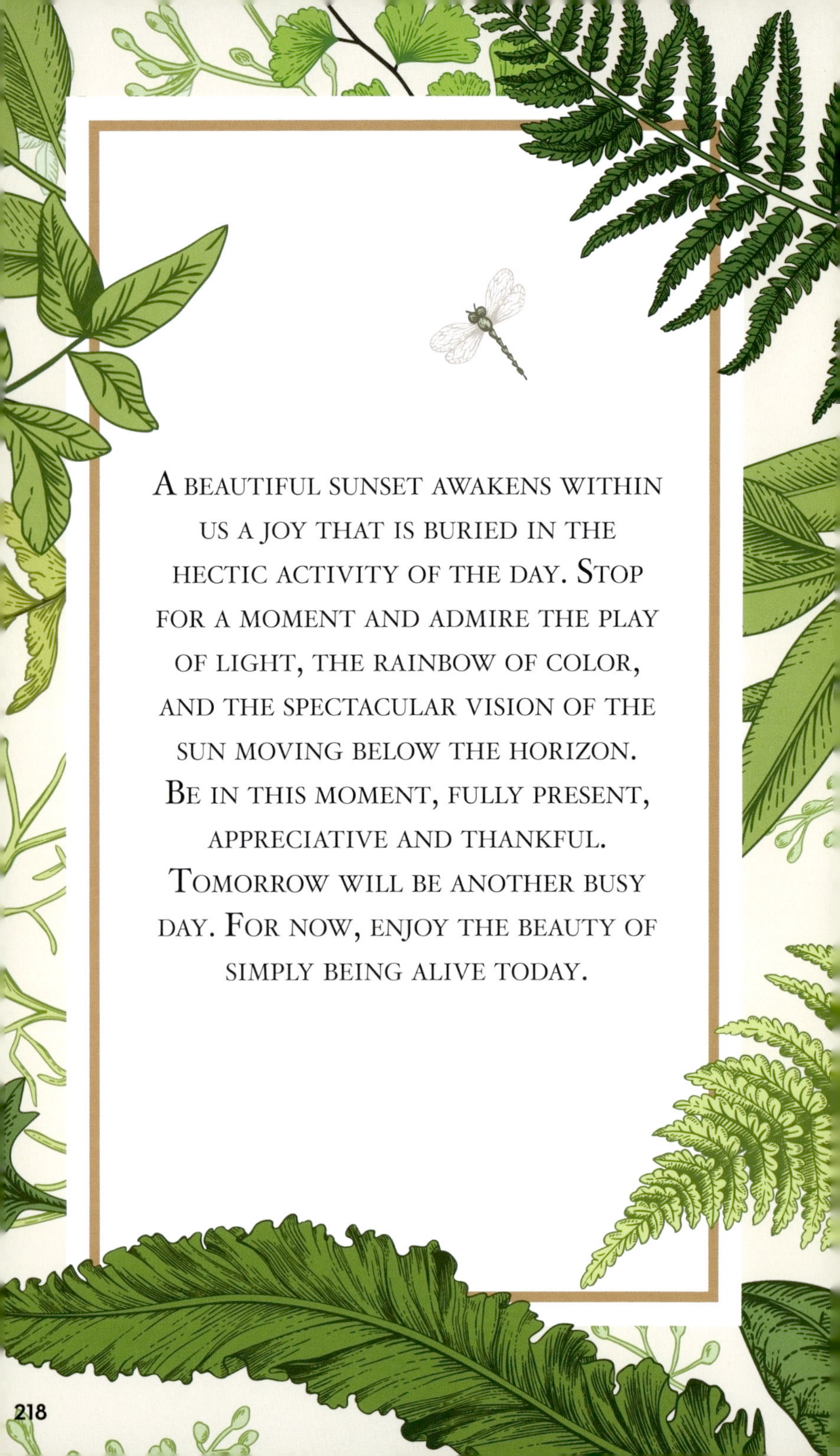

A beautiful sunset awakens within us a joy that is buried in the hectic activity of the day. Stop for a moment and admire the play of light, the rainbow of color, and the spectacular vision of the sun moving below the horizon. Be in this moment, fully present, appreciative and thankful. Tomorrow will be another busy day. For now, enjoy the beauty of simply being alive today.

THE LAUGHTER OF A CHILD IS SOOTHING FOR THE SPIRIT. IT REMINDS US HOW, AS CHILDREN, WE LIVED FOR THE MOMENT AND LET OUR PARENTS WORRY ABOUT EVERYTHING FOR US. WE HAD FUN, OFTEN WITH NOTHING BUT OUR OWN COMPANY, WATCHING BIRDS FLY OR LOOKING FOR CLOUD SHAPES. WE DIDN'T NEED TECHNOLOGY OR OTHER DIVERSIONS TO EXPERIENCE AWE AND WONDER. NATURE WAS OUR PLAYGROUND AND WE SPENT EACH MOMENT IN CAREFREE ABANDON, FULLY ENGAGED WITH LIFE.

Enjoy each lake and mountain, every small stone along the way. Enjoy the view around you, the breeze on your face, and even the insects flitting around you. Each element of nature has its place.

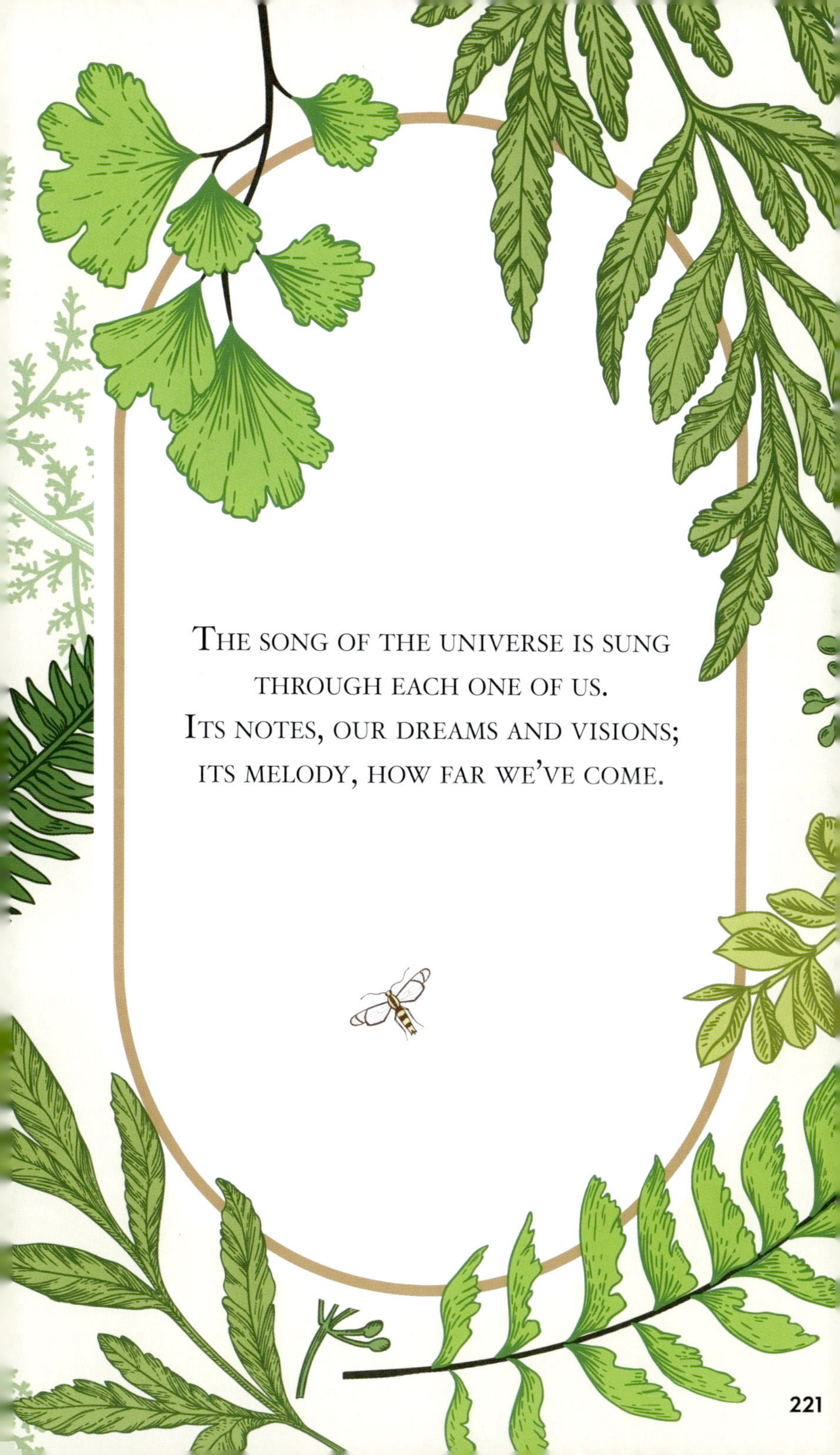

The song of the universe is sung
through each one of us.
Its notes, our dreams and visions;
its melody, how far we've come.

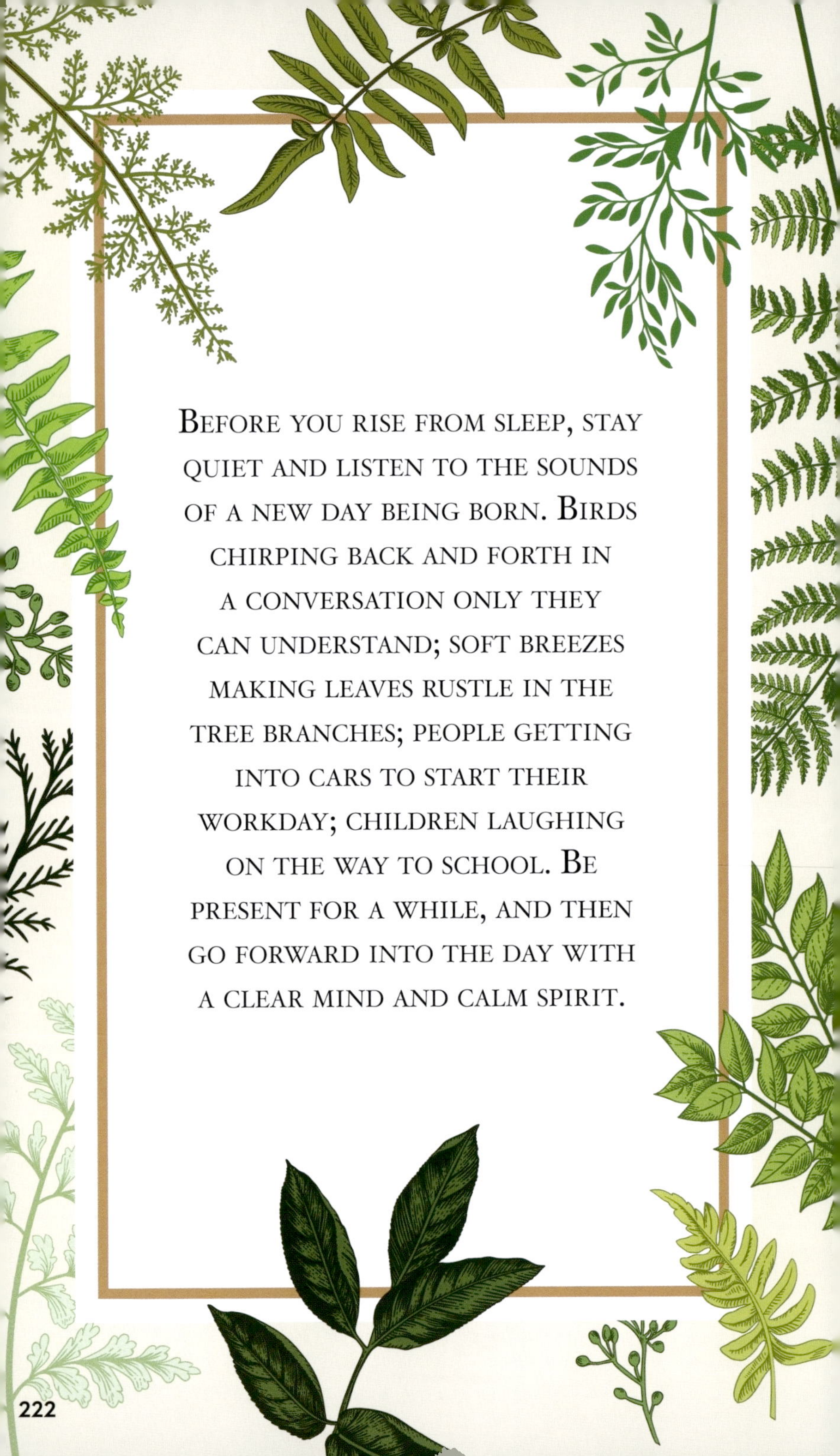

Before you rise from sleep, stay quiet and listen to the sounds of a new day being born. Birds chirping back and forth in a conversation only they can understand; soft breezes making leaves rustle in the tree branches; people getting into cars to start their workday; children laughing on the way to school. Be present for a while, and then go forward into the day with a clear mind and calm spirit.

Today

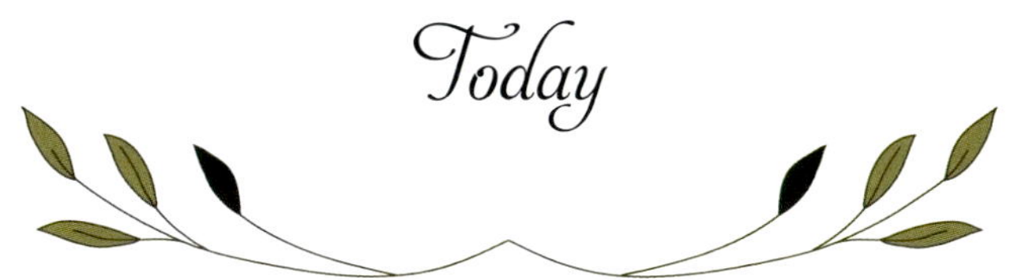

Today I pledge to walk mindfully. I will appreciate the mystery of my body and the way I can move. I will take in the weather around me and really focus on the touch of the wind and the brightness of the sky. I will feel the earth beneath my feet. I will feel gratitude for the simple act of walking.

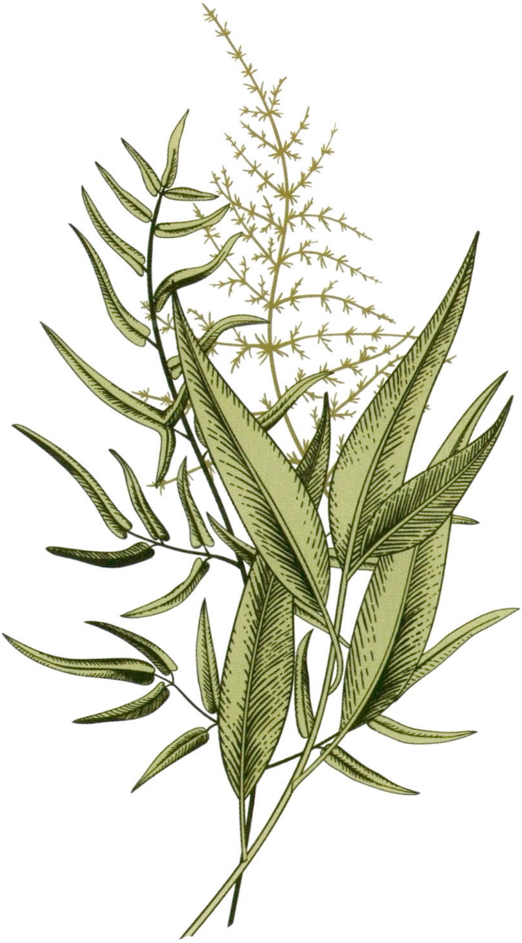

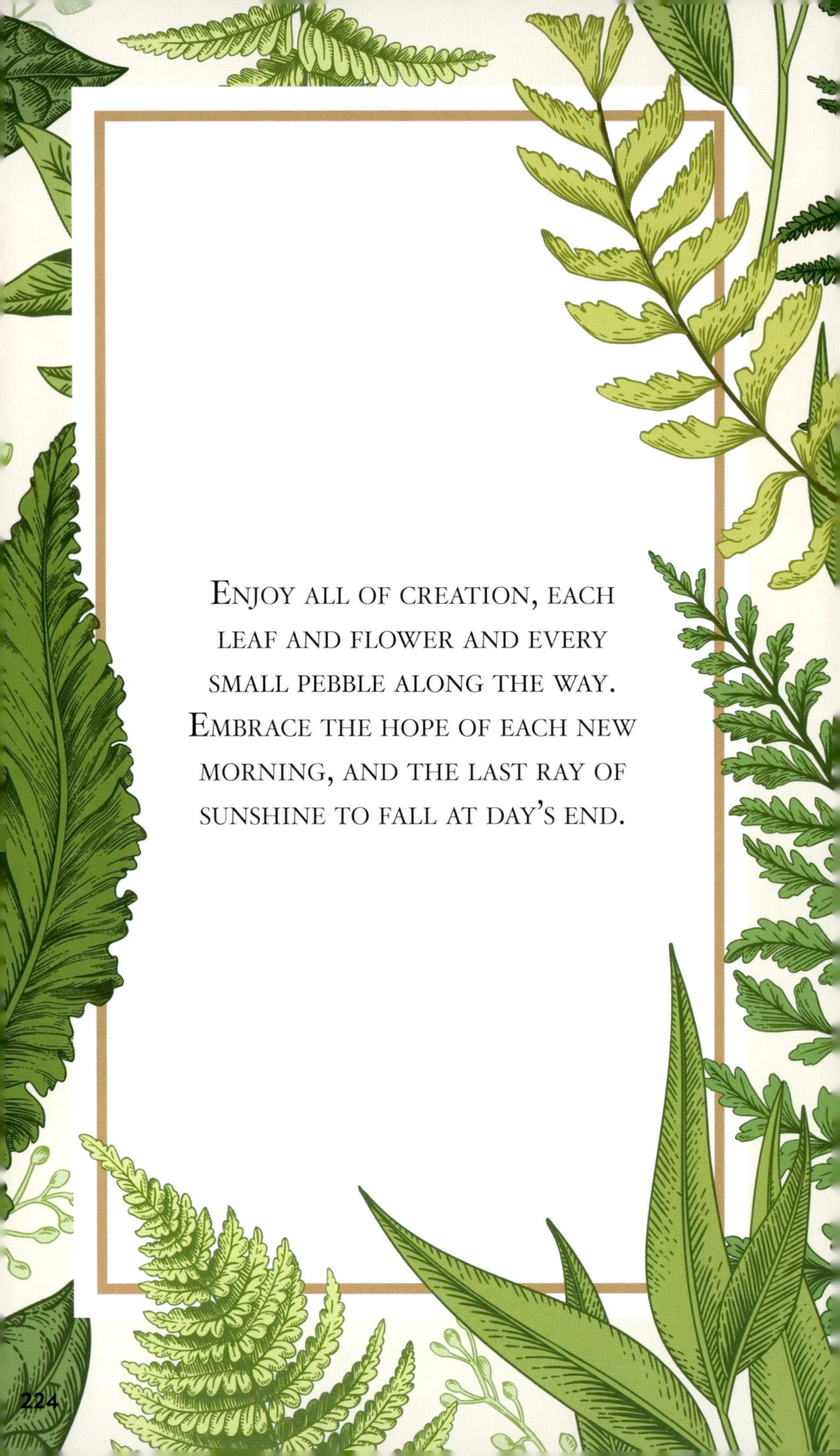

Enjoy all of creation, each leaf and flower and every small pebble along the way. Embrace the hope of each new morning, and the last ray of sunshine to fall at day's end.

Enhancing Calm through the Senses

The Power of the Senses

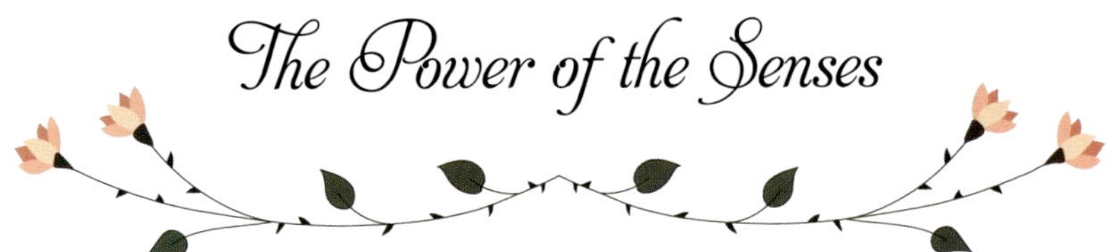

Sounds, sights, and smells can bring us back to special places and times in our lives.

- The nightsong of crickets outside the window
- The distant whistle of a passing train
- The alluring scent of night-blooming jasmine
- The taste of salt on the lips from the ocean waves
- The steady beat of summer rain

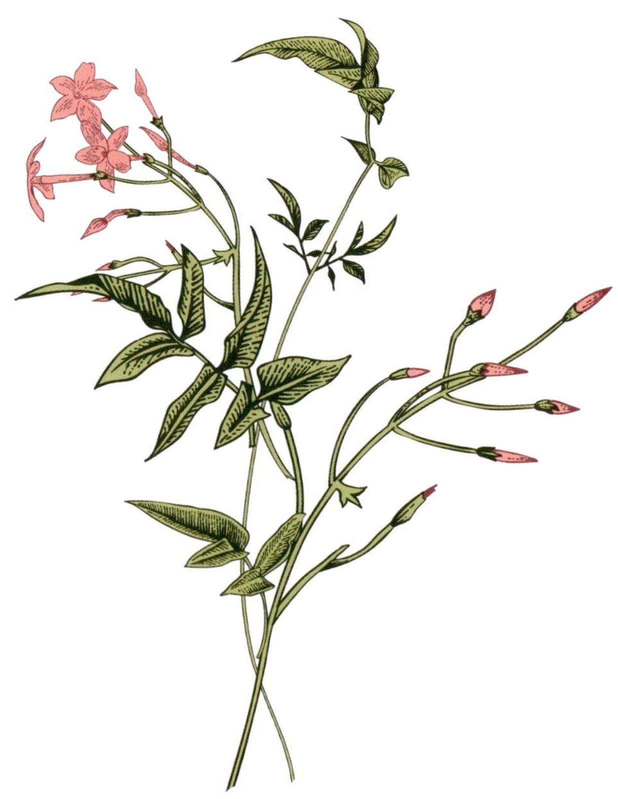

Sense meditation involves the use of one or more senses to still the mind and create focus. For example, imagine stroking the soft fur of a cat or calm dog—in fact, do so if possible. Feel the softness between your fingertips. Let touch guide you, focusing only on the sensation of the nerve endings in your fingers. Forget all other senses for now. Only touch.

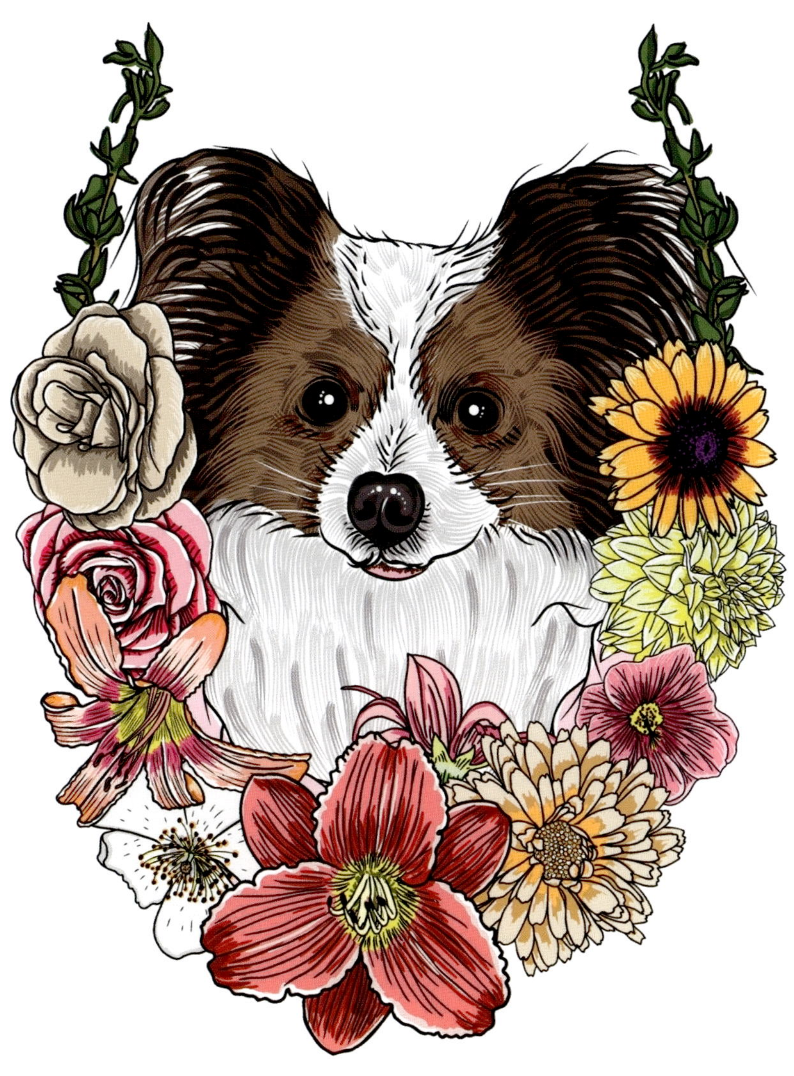

Sounds in Meditation

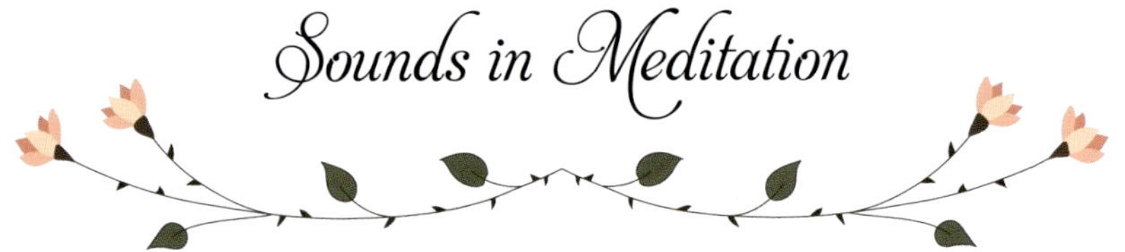

One way to personalize your meditation space is with sound. Experiment to find what best suits your practice; some sounds might be calming or entrancing, while others are just distracting.

Ambient Music

This music is designed to be in the background. You might associate this kind of instrumental music with elevators, but it can also be useful in meditation. It can affect the way you feel without making many demands on your attention.

Chanting

Chanting is a feature in many religions around the world. Listening to chants can help quieten your mind and help you focus.

Instrumental Tones

Gongs, bells, chimes, and didgeridoo sounds can calm your mind, or give you something to focus on.

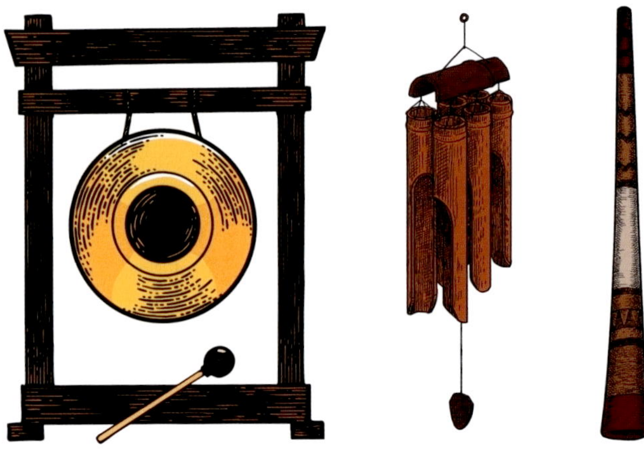

Singing Bowls

A singing bowl is a type of bell that has long been used in Buddhist meditation. You play it by rubbing a mallet around the bowl's outside rim. This produces a clear, constant tone. You can either listen to recordings of singing bowls or play one yourself.

Nature Sounds

There are countless types of nature sounds that can fill your space. Recordings of rain, thunder, or beach waves can be easy to find. There are also a range of animal sounds, from birdsong, to whale song, and various things in between.

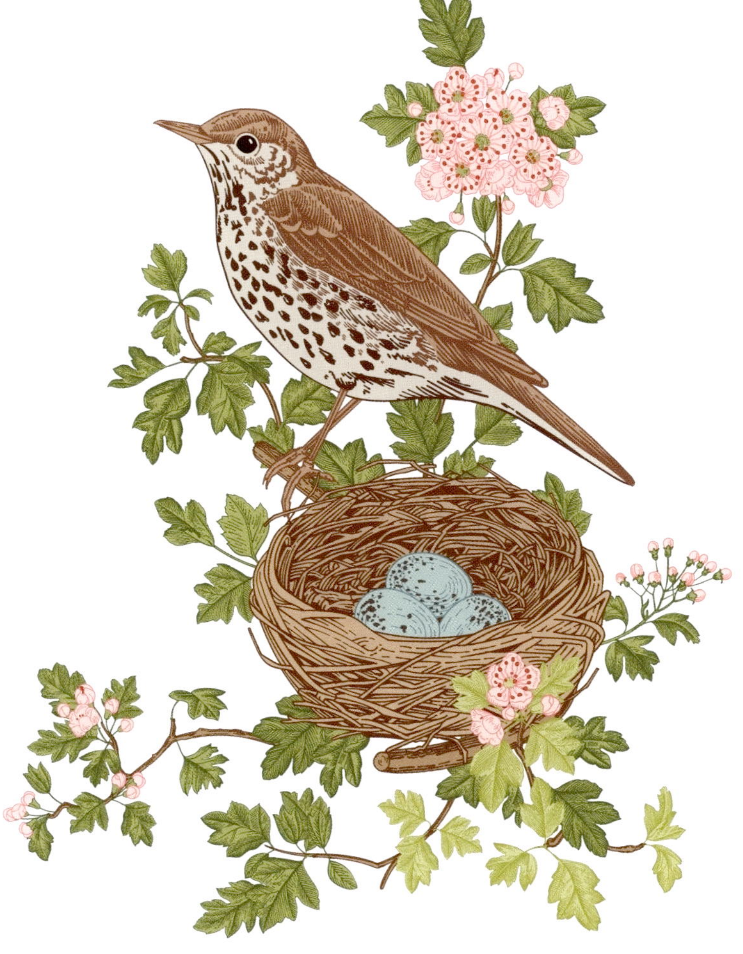

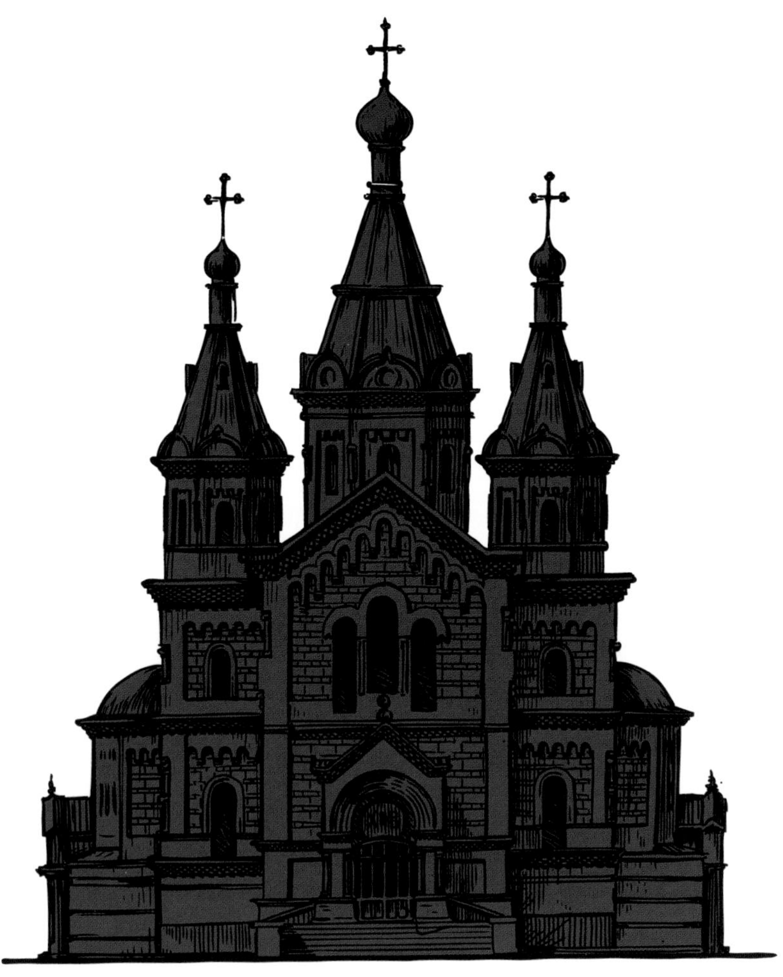

The sound of bells and chimes can be comforting. We live a block away from a church, and at 6 o'clock each night the church bells play a song. The selection is different every night, and I have come to look forward to each reverberant hymn. It is a comforting touchstone in the day. What do bells mean to you?

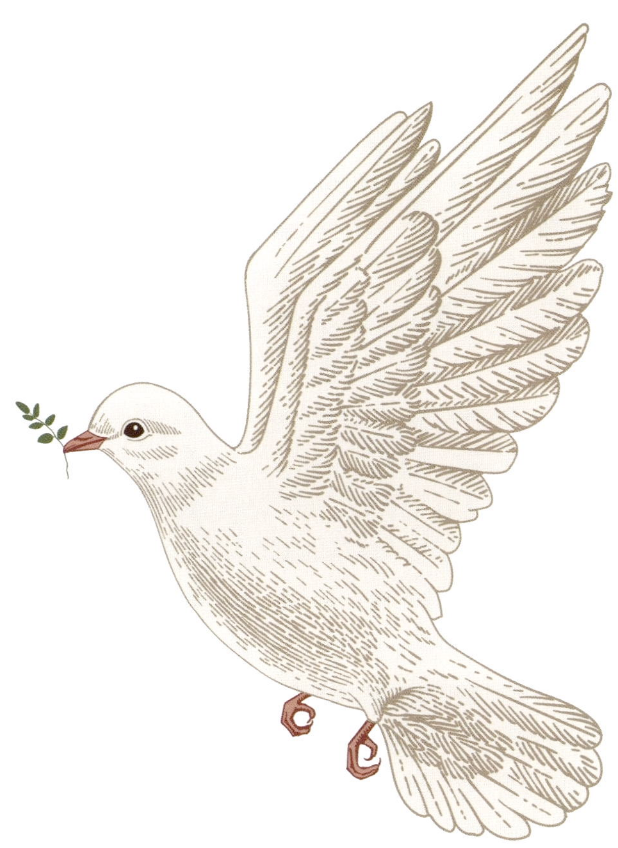

Music is a harmonious meditation that engages our minds and bodies together. Hearing a favorite song energizes us to let go and move our bodies. A beautiful concerto, a fun pop tune, or a loud and boisterous rock song all have the power to make us feel things more deeply. Music is mindful meditation for the soul that loves to dance with life.

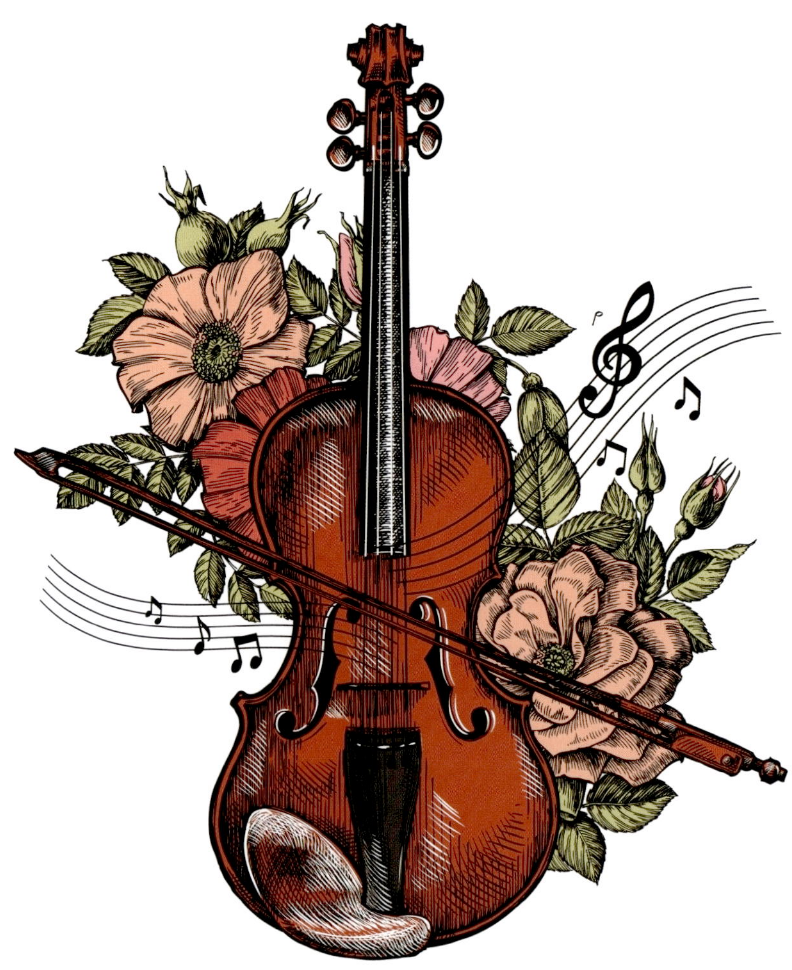

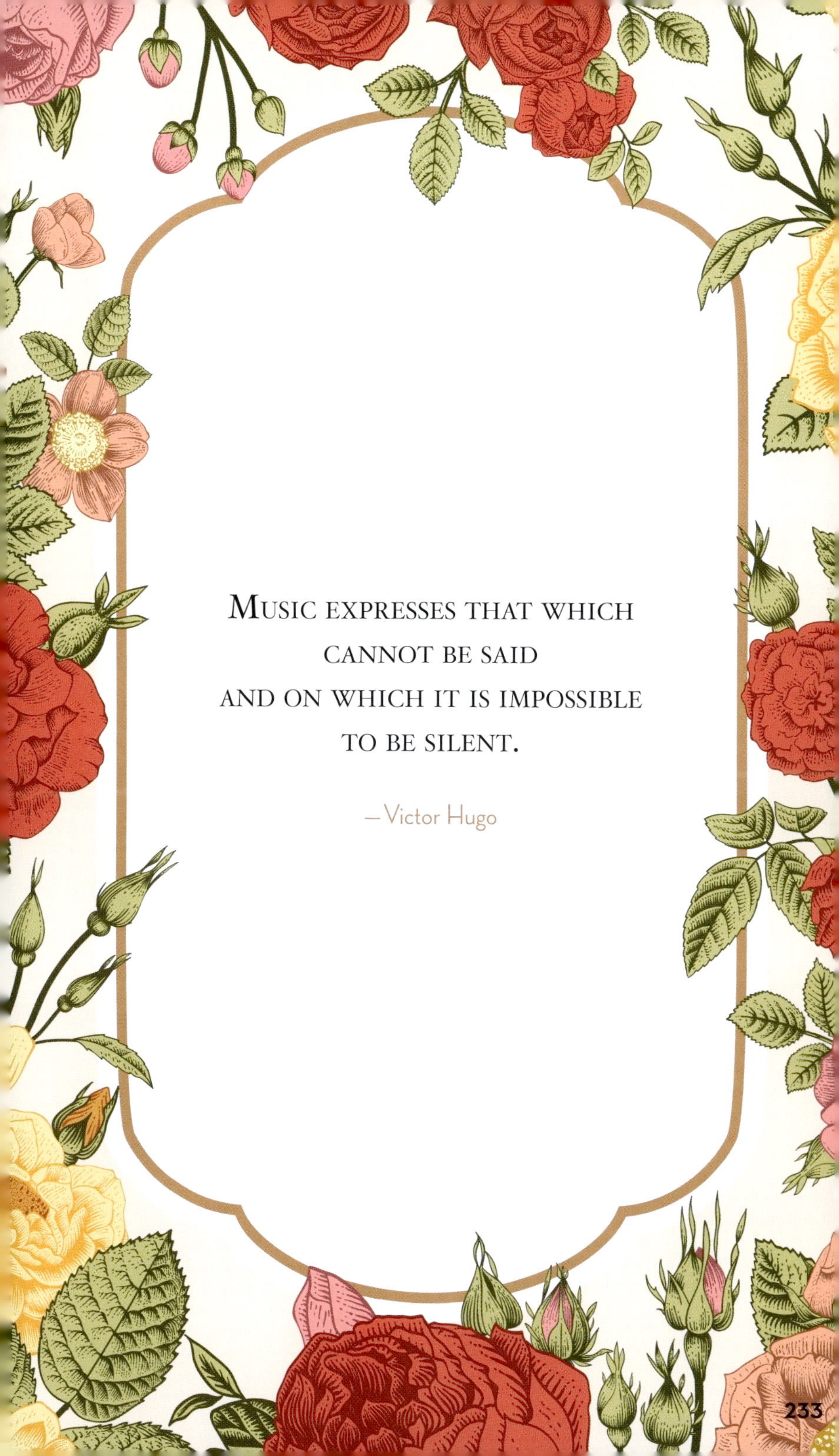

Music expresses that which
cannot be said
and on which it is impossible
to be silent.

—Victor Hugo

Binaural Beats

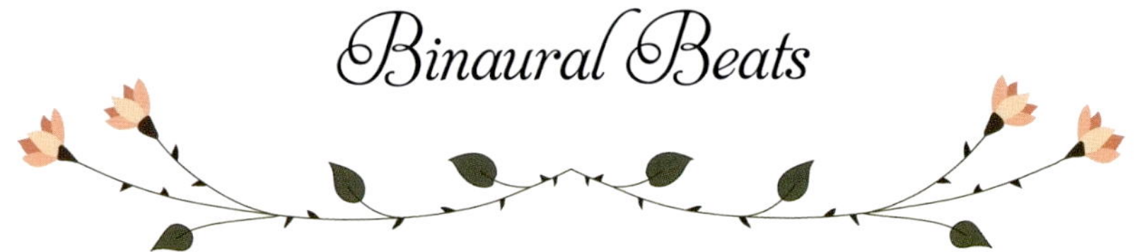

When a tone entering one ear is a certain frequency, and a tone entering your other ear is a slightly different frequency, you start to hear a third tone that isn't really there. That phantom sound, or binaural beat, is pitched at the frequency between the two tones playing in your ears. For example, if one ear hears a tone at 300 Hertz and the other hears one at 305, the binaural beat's frequency is 5 Hertz. It's a phenomenon that researchers are still trying to understand, though there are many theories about what exactly it does to the brain.

There's some evidence that binaural beats affect the way your brain functions, whether by promoting deep sleep, a meditative focus, or a more accurate memory. Different frequencies are also believed to affect the brain differently. It's generally agreed that the longer you spend listening to binaural beats, the more effective they are.

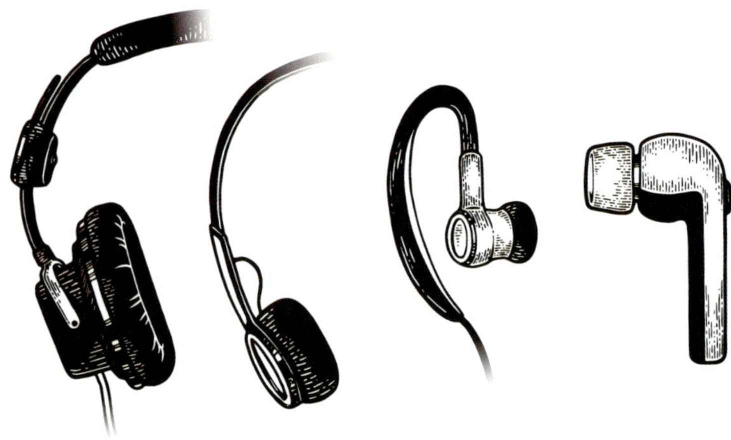

Types	Frequency in Hertz	Effects
Delta	0.5–4	Helps a person enter or stay in deep, dreamless sleep
Theta	4–7	Promotes REM sleep, creative thinking, and meditation
Alpha	7–12	Helps relaxation and lessens anxiety
Beta	12–30	Improves focus, problem-solving, and memory (higher frequencies in this range can increase anxiety)
Gamma	30–50	Helps a person stay alert while awake

Posture

If meditating, assume a posture that suits the form of meditation. Otherwise, you can sit or lie comfortably, or listen as you perform other tasks, such as reading or housework.

Remember

You need headphones to listen to binaural beats. This is the only way to have different tones play in different ears. Don't listen at too loud a volume so you don't end up with damaged hearing. Avoid listening to binaural beats while trying to drive or operate heavy machinery.

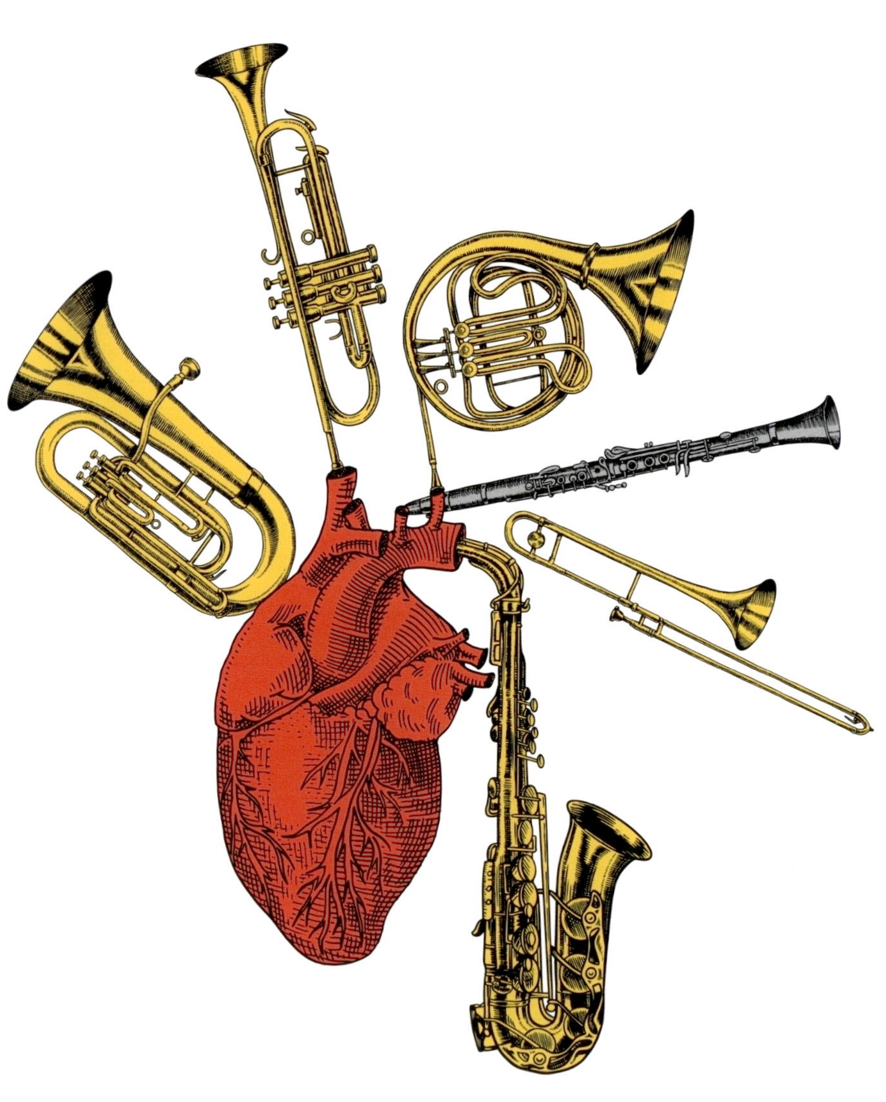

Music is the language of the soul. Let the melody of a favorite song lift your spirit as you allow your body to sink into relaxation. Become the notes. Feel the deep bass, the fairy wings of delicate staccatos. Become one with the music and feel your form melt away. Allow the notes to resonate through every part of your being. Let your spirit dance.

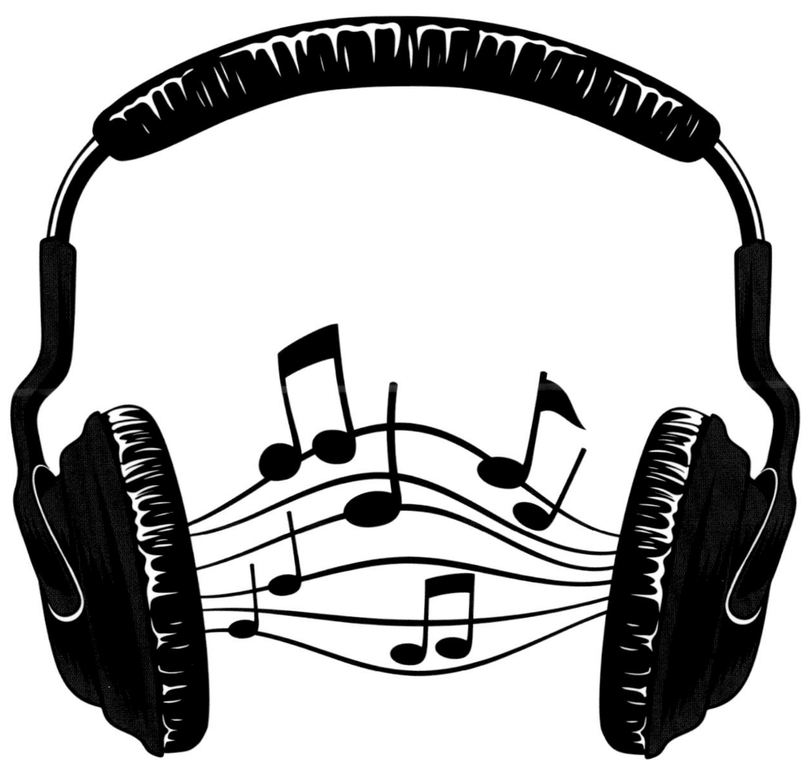

Sound Bath

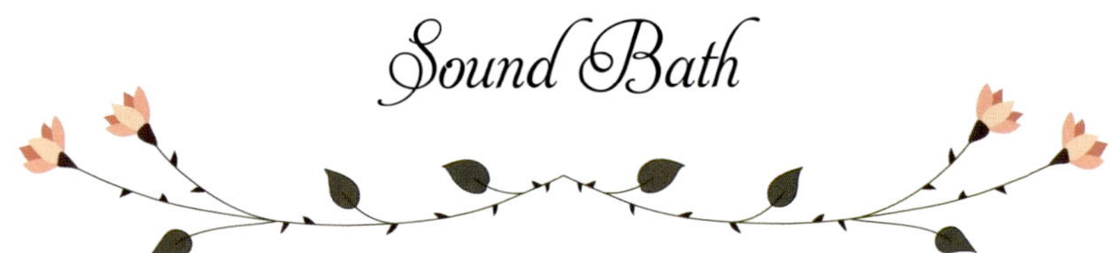

It's well known that music can help us relax. Sound baths strip the idea of calming music down to a non-melodic collection of tones, beats, or other sounds. These sounds often come from singing bowls, gongs, a shruti box (similar to a harmonium), and human vocals. They are called baths because participants often feel surrounded and submerged in the vibrations of the sounds.

Part of a sound bath's effectiveness comes from the basic, calming aspect of the sounds, which give busy minds something to do other than ruminate or plan. Many believe the physical vibrations of the sound waves, moving from the instruments, through the air, and into the body, also help bring relaxation and even healing.

You can listen to sound bath recordings, but the experience pales in comparison to a live event. Group sessions can be found at specialized businesses built around sound baths, as well as some yoga studios and spas. Some people make their own sound baths by playing a singing bowl or other instrument themselves.

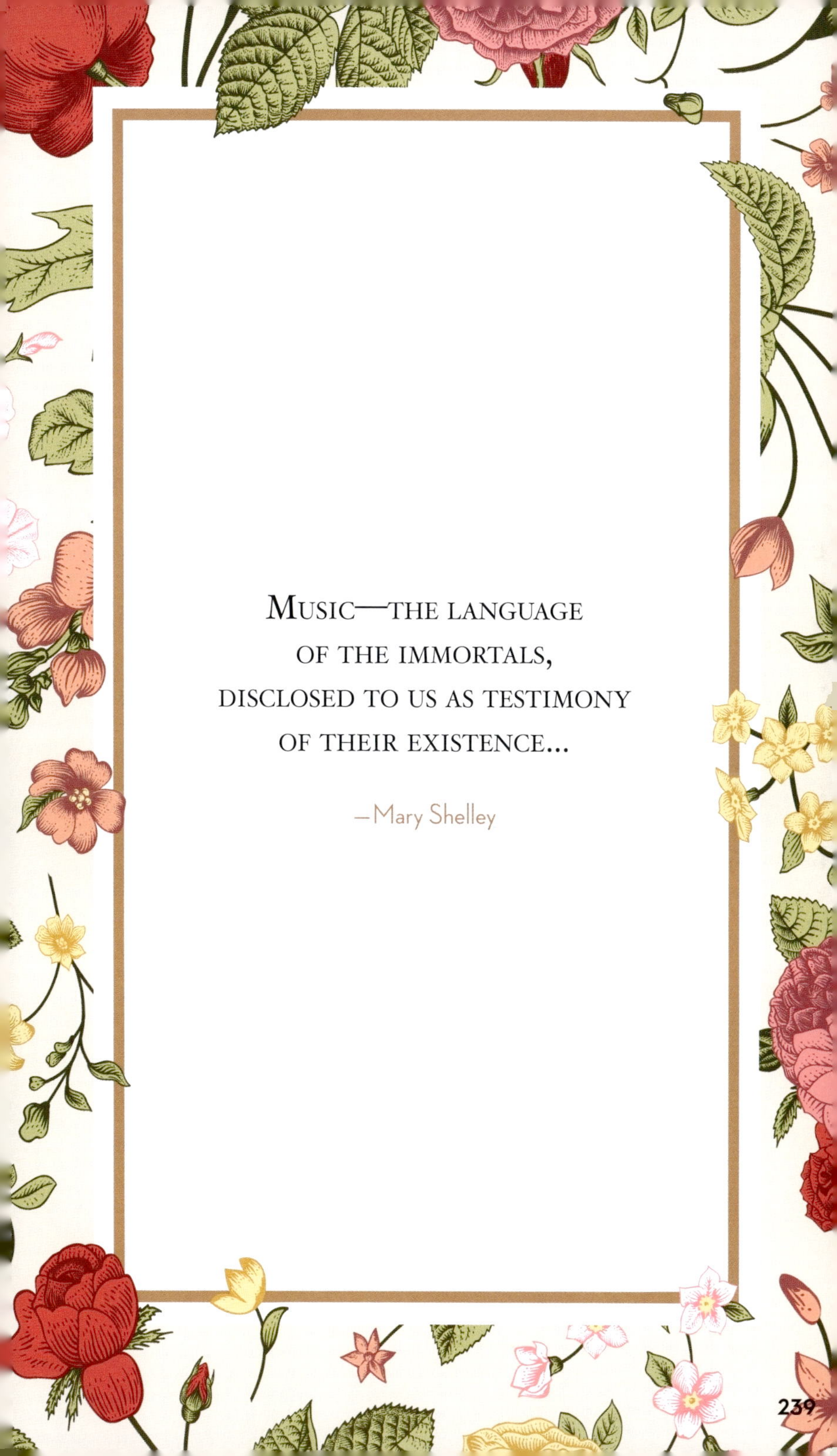

Music—the language of the immortals, disclosed to us as testimony of their existence...

—Mary Shelley

Music is a wonderful way to help free the mind from worries. Meditate on a concerto or other piece of classical music, and let the left brain take a back seat as the right brain opens to creativity and inspiration. Music meditation is about lifting the spirit, not about the song itself, so choose what moves you without fear of judgment. Consciousness shifts and the mind is expanded and awakened.

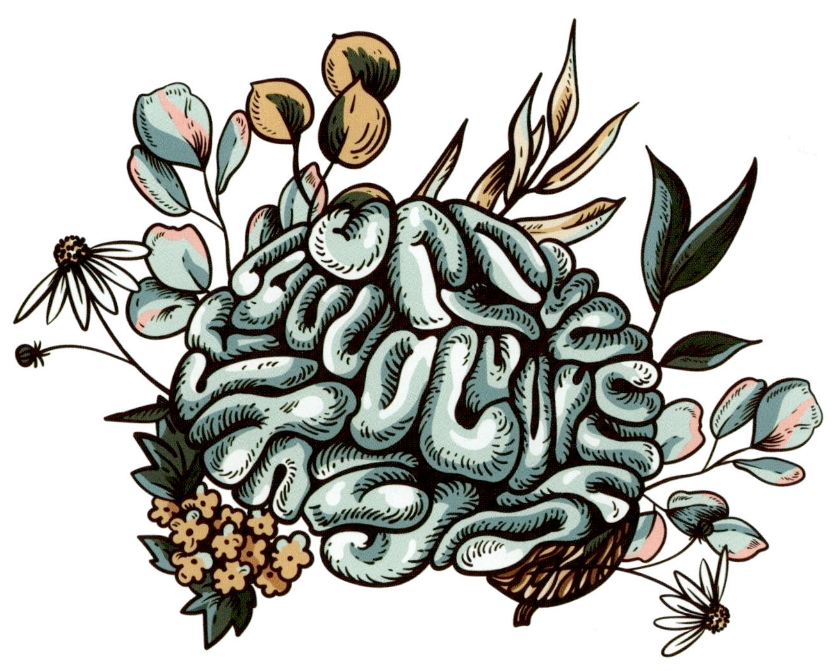

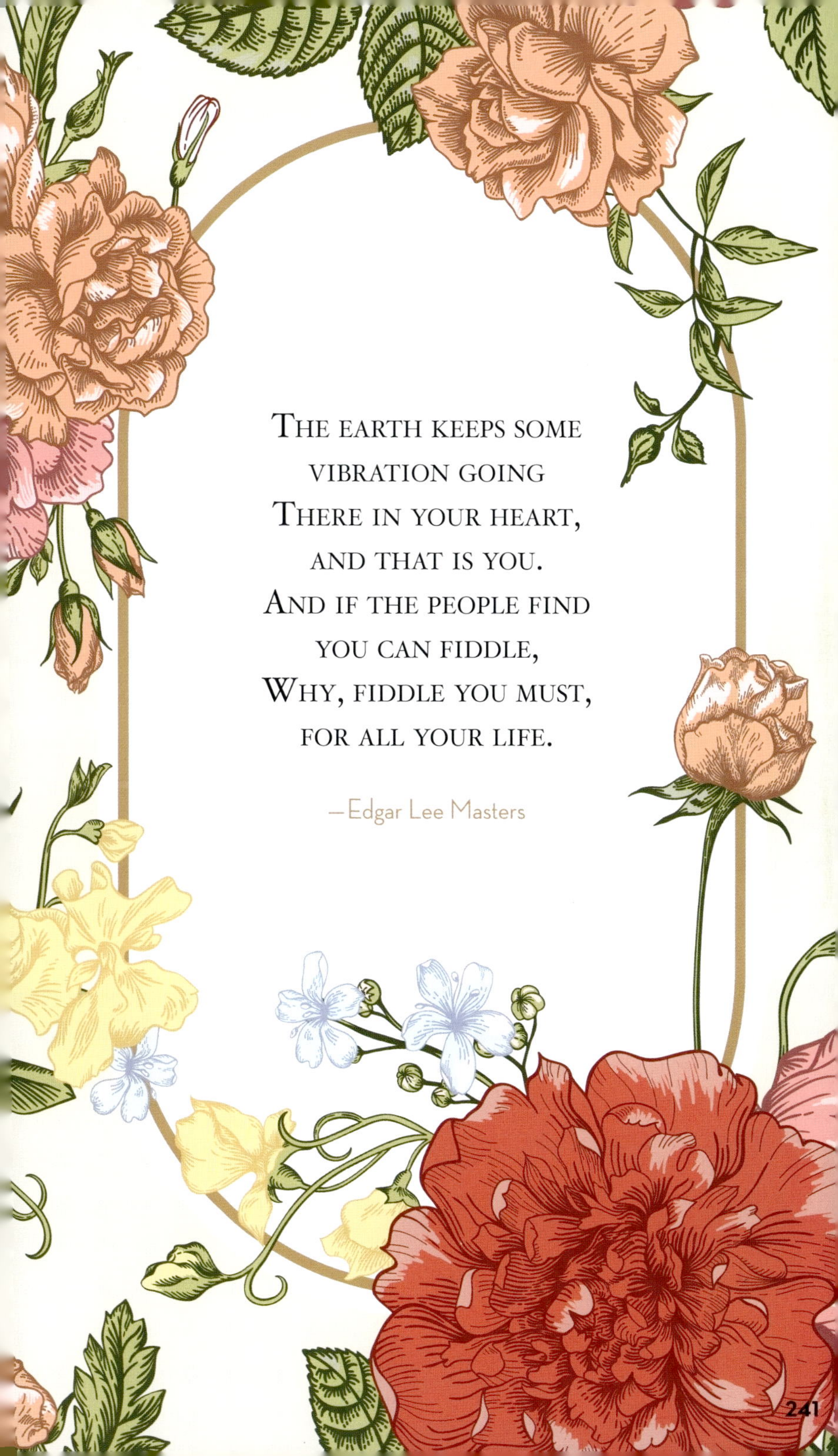

The earth keeps some
vibration going
There in your heart,
and that is you.
And if the people find
you can fiddle,
Why, fiddle you must,
for all your life.

—Edgar Lee Masters

Art Meditation

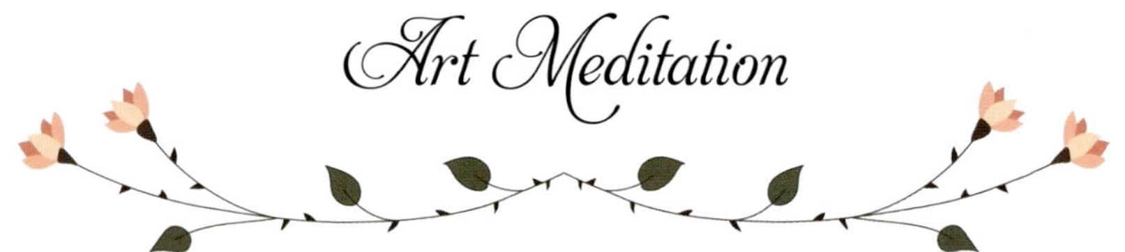

Art can help a busy mind become calm. Mandalas are a great example. Sand mandalas made in some schools of Buddhism are intricately-patterned, circular creations of dyed sands. Completing one is a days-long endeavor that creators use as a method of disciplined meditation. Once complete, the mandala is destroyed as a representation of the impermanence of all things. Some Buddhists make or use painted, drawn, or other permanent mandalas. With these, a person uses their experience of the art as meditation, focusing on the structure, pattern, and symbolism the images contain.

Meditative art is not limited to mandalas. If you're creating something, it can look like anything, and be made with whatever art supplies you like. If you choose to observe art, the art can be anything that draws you in.

Either way, your focus is on what is before you. Give all your attention to what you are doing, seeing, feeling, smelling, or (depending on the art) tasting. This pointed concentration can lead to greater calmness, clarity, and relaxation.

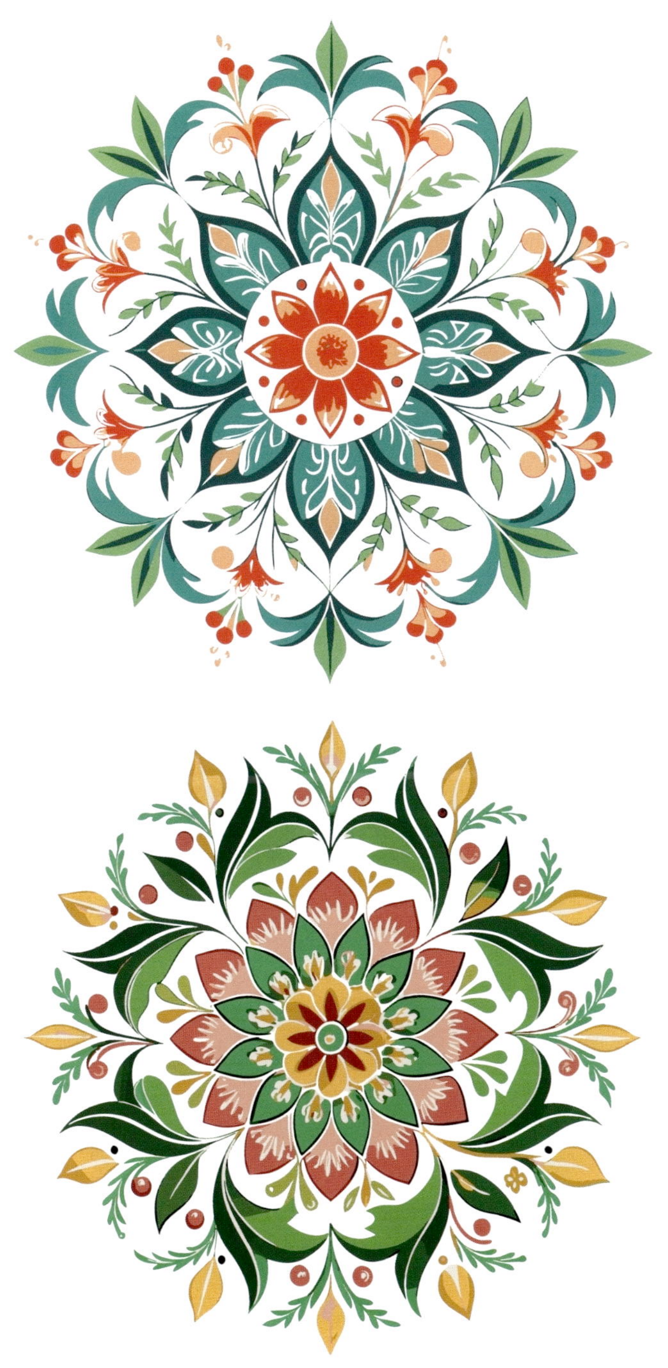

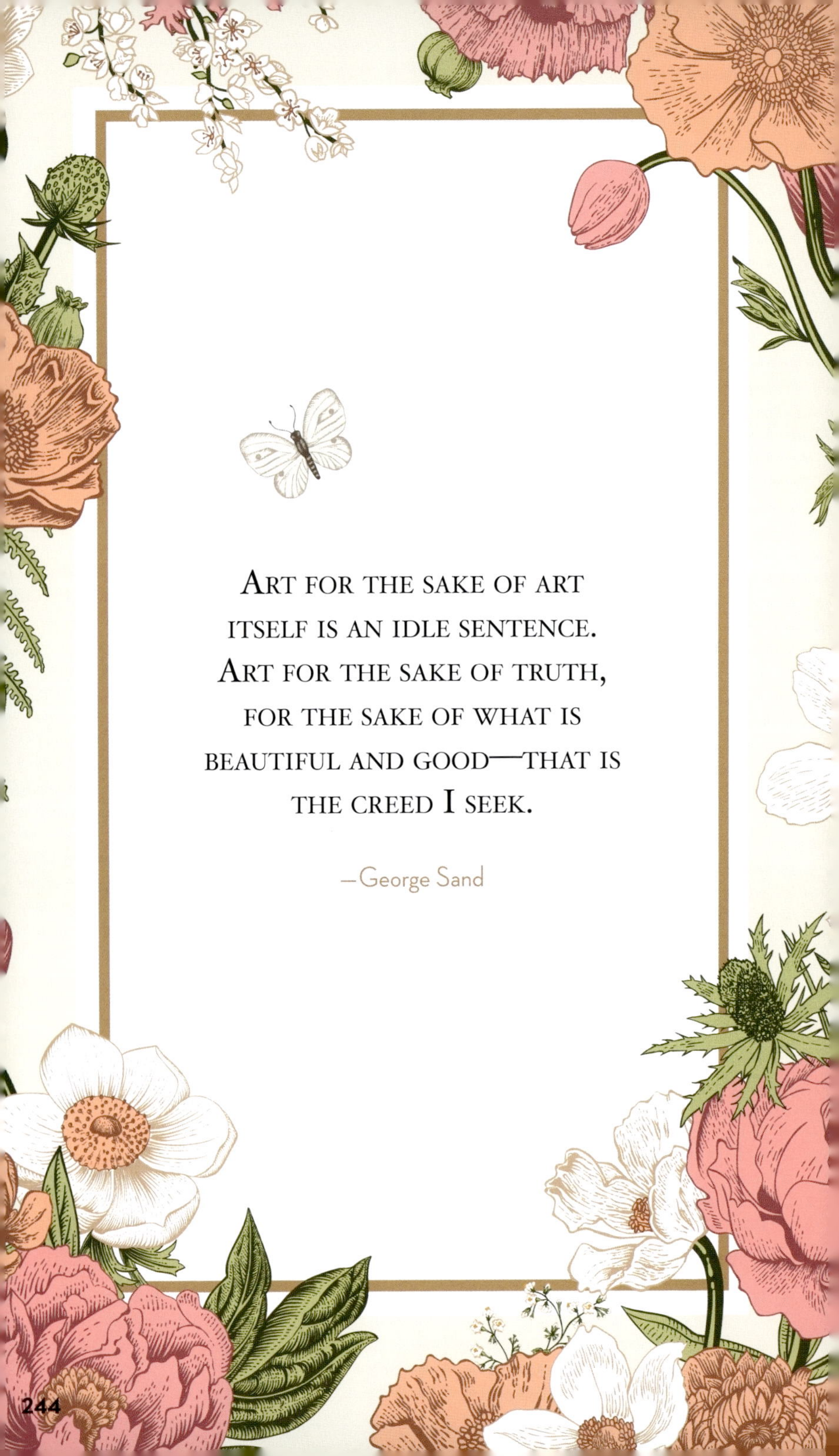

Art for the sake of art itself is an idle sentence. Art for the sake of truth, for the sake of what is beautiful and good—that is the creed I seek.

—George Sand

The work of art must seize upon you, wrap you up in itself, carry you away. It is the means by which the artist conveys his passion; it is the current which he puts forth which sweeps you along in his passion.

—Pierre-Auguste Renoir

Creating Art

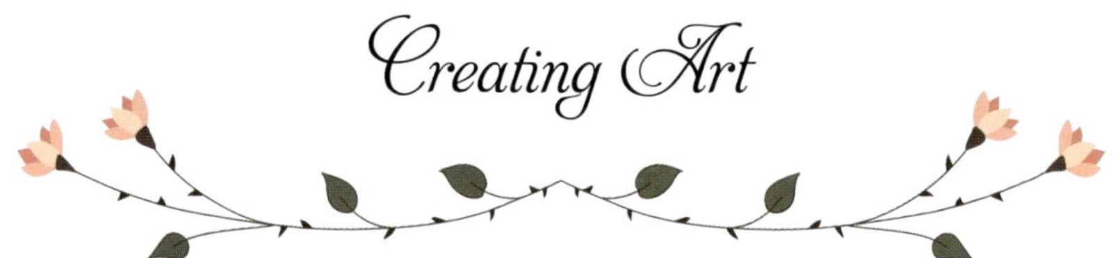

Creating art as part of your meditation is not an exercise in making "good" art. Try to avoid passing judgment on your work. Focus on the process, rather than the product.

You can have a freeform sort of meditation by creating art purely by "feel." Start by taking a moment to simply focus on your breath. When you're ready, begin your creation. Move slowly if that suits you, move faster if that feels right. Focus on what you are doing—choosing a color, drawing a shape—in the moment. What you'll do next doesn't matter yet, and what you did before doesn't matter anymore. As thoughts appear, acknowledge them and let them fade. If following a structure helps, try your hand at a mandala. You don't have to use sand; all you need is a piece of paper and something to draw with.

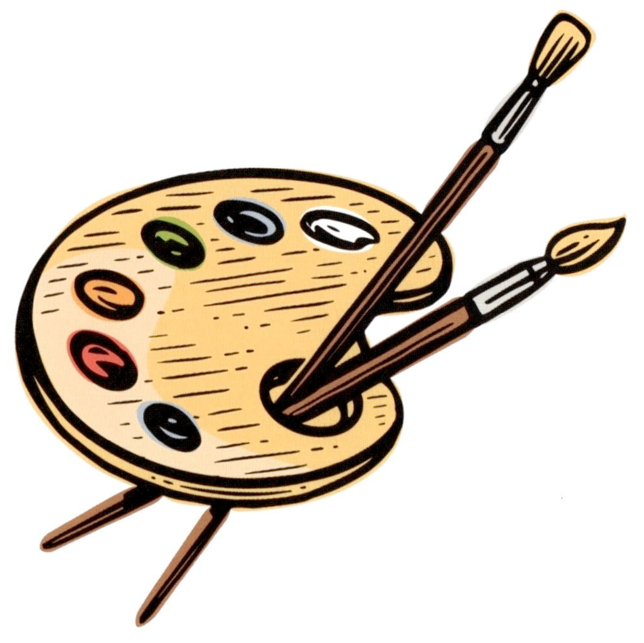

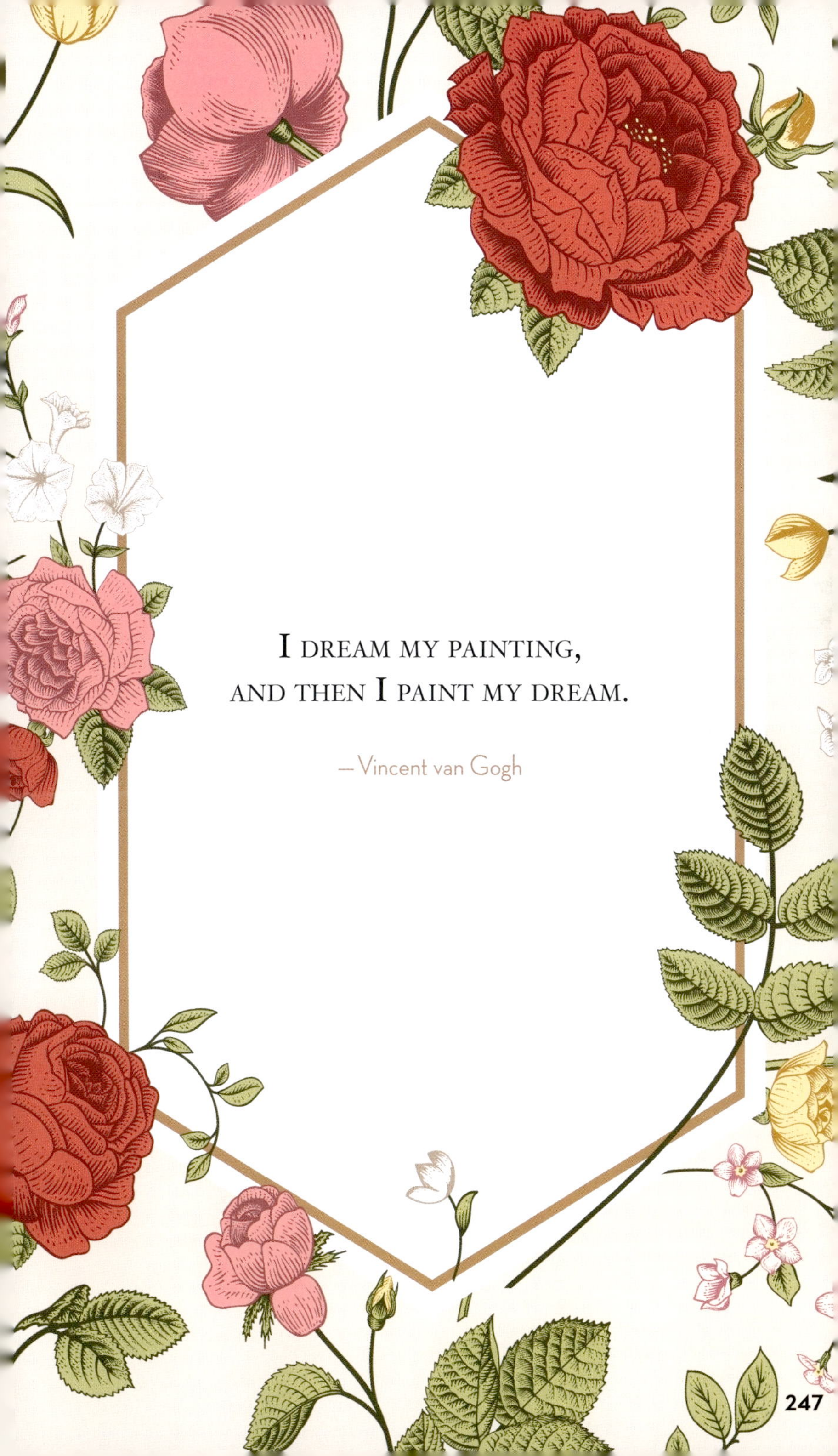

I dream my painting,
and then I paint my dream.

—Vincent van Gogh

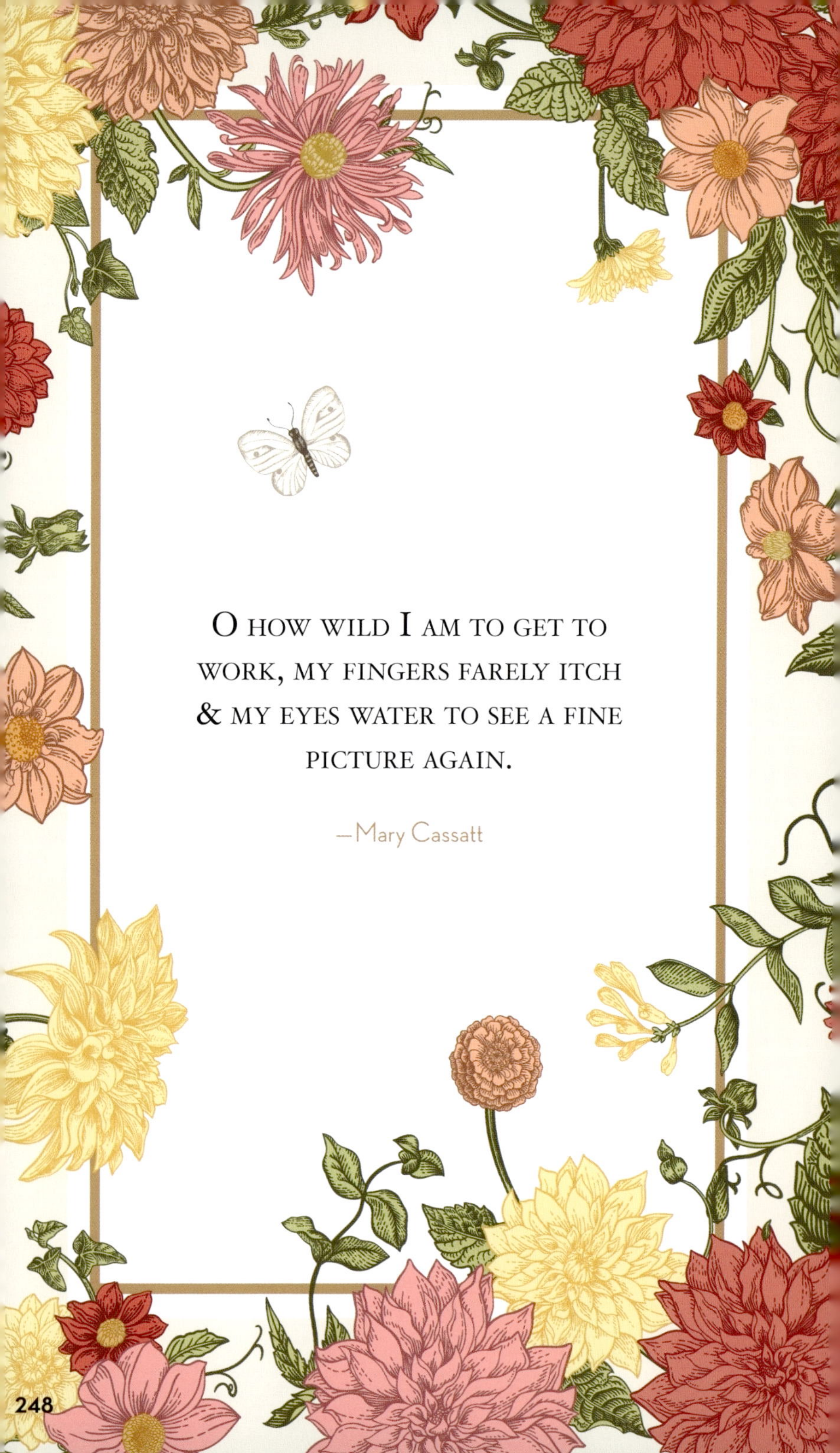

O how wild I am to get to work, my fingers farely itch & my eyes water to see a fine picture again.

—Mary Cassatt

Mandala Exercise

Step 1
Take a few deep breaths to ground yourself. Then return to natural breathing.

Step 2
Draw a small circle, perhaps a centimeter wide, in the center of the paper. This can be freehand or with a compass.

Step 3
Draw a repeating, symmetrical pattern in a ring around the circle. It could be a series of leaves that "grow" from the circle, a ring of dots that encircle it, or anything else. Take your time as you do it, noting the feeling of your hand as it draws, and seeing the shapes you create.

Step 4
Draw a different pattern in a ring around what you have so far. This, too, should be symmetrical, and completely encircle what you have so far.

Step 5
Continue adding rings, changing patterns, until you run out of space on the page.

Step 6 (optional)
You can color in your mandala after you finish drawing.

Experiencing Art

Whether it's a painting, sculpture, photograph, or clay pot, you can incorporate existing art into meditation. In this type of practice, your focus is on the sensations that come as you study the artwork.

Step 1

Close your eyes and take a few deep breaths. Then return to normal breathing.

Step 2

Open your eyes and look at the image as a whole. Note any initial reactions you have to it, any emotions, thoughts, or memories it conjures.

Step 3

Consider the details of the image. What colors do you see? What shapes? What textures? How do objects or elements in the piece of art interact with one another?

Step 4

Imagine yourself becoming part of what you see in the artwork. You're in the setting of the image. Go through your senses. What do you smell, hear, feel, taste? This can work even if the art is abstract. What sensations come to you when you imagine being inside or surrounded by the colors and shapes?

Step 5

When you're ready to end the meditation, close your eyes again and take a few deep breaths.

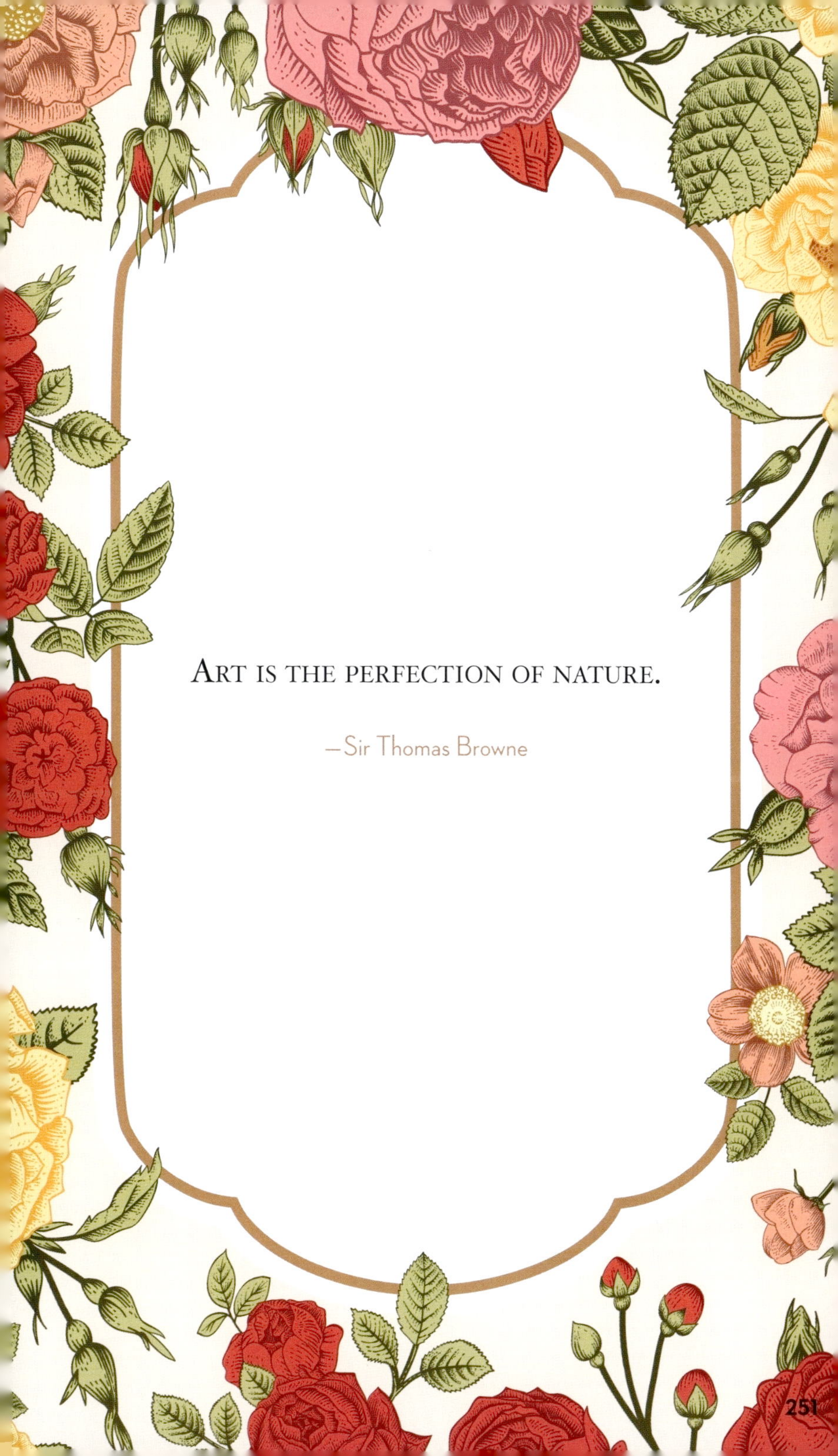

Art is the perfection of nature.

—Sir Thomas Browne

We expect to see art in a museum, captured on a canvas, or cast from bronze. But if we are open, it is everywhere. Today, look for art in unexpected places: it is there in bright graffiti glimpsed from the train. It lives in the koi fish and lilies tattooed on the arm of a passerby. Let us be open to what beauty is, and where it might reside. Let us make a work of art of our own lives!

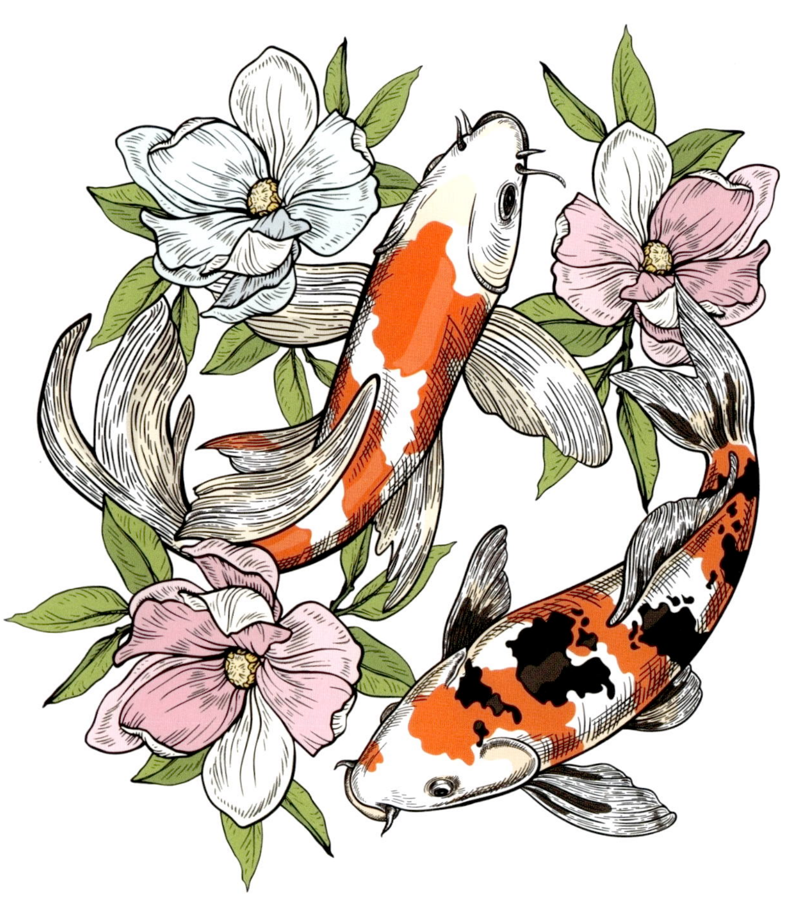

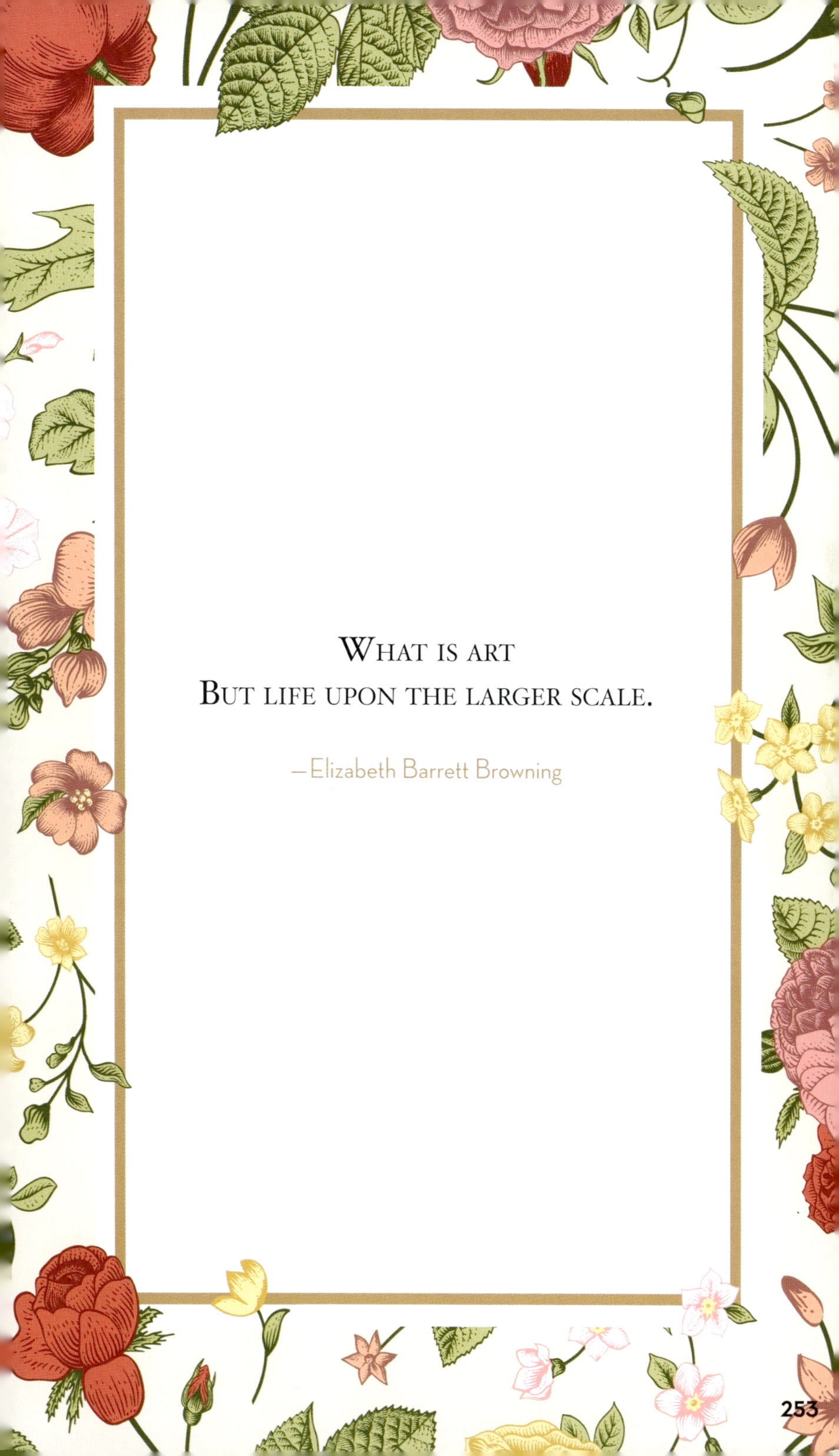

What is art
But life upon the larger scale.

—Elizabeth Barrett Browning

Meditate with your eyes open. Find a beautiful piece of visual art that takes you to another place: a photograph, perhaps, or a richly textured oil painting. Let yourself be absorbed in the details of the imagery as you imagine the artist's vision. Close your eyes and be in that place for a while, simply breathing.

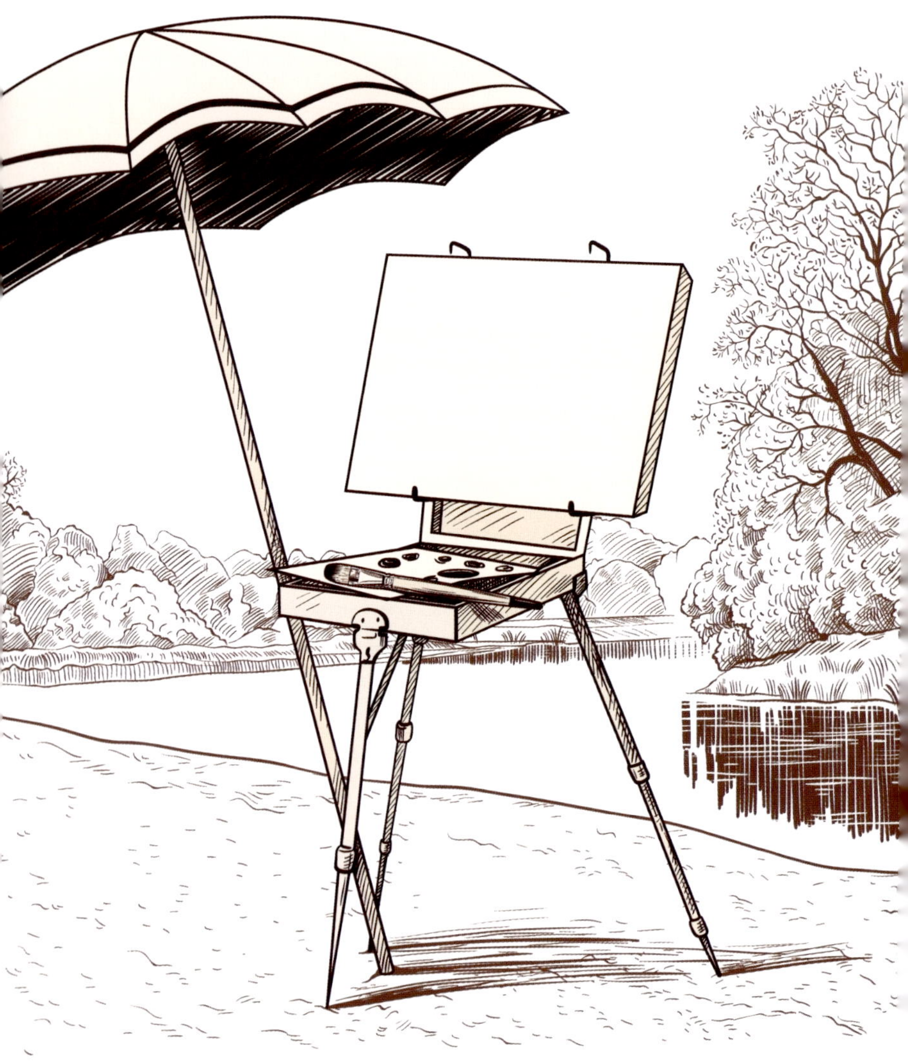

Contemplative Reading

Many religions use contemplative reading or similar practices. The goal is to feel a connection to the divine by way of sacred text. In Christian tradition, it's called Lectio Divina, or divine reading. It involves spending time with a short section of text and considering it outside of any historical or theological context, creating a deeply personal relationship with the words. The driving question is, roughly, "What is the divine saying to me, right now?"

Time

You can spend 10 minutes on the entire process, or 10 or more minutes on each step. Christian monks once practiced by repeating the words six times. A good place to start is with three or four repetitions, then see if you'd like to add more.

Posture

Make sure you're comfortable, and that you can remain so for the length of your practice.

Remember

Your mind will wander, and that's ok. When it wanders, acknowledge that it has. Then gently bring your attention back to the words. Also, try not to consciously assign a meaning to the passage. Focus instead on how you experience and react to the passage.

Step 1
Choose a short section of a sacred text. People often choose something that is one or two sentences long.

Step 2
Read the passage aloud, slowly and deliberately. Listen carefully to the sound of the words. Sit quietly for a few minutes considering what they mean to you.

Step 3
Read the passage aloud again. Try to read it with a different emphasis or rhythm. Sit quietly for a few more minutes.

Step 4
Repeat this process at least once more.

Step 5
Think about how the passage made you feel, any images it sparked in your imagination, and any words or phrases that stuck out to you. Spend several minutes with this process.

Step 6
Focus on a word, phrase, emotion, or vision the passage brought up for you that was very dominant in your mind. Consider what this dominant thought is saying to you, in this moment. Spend several minutes with this process.

Step 7
Let conscious thought fade. Bring your focus to your breath. Breathe naturally.

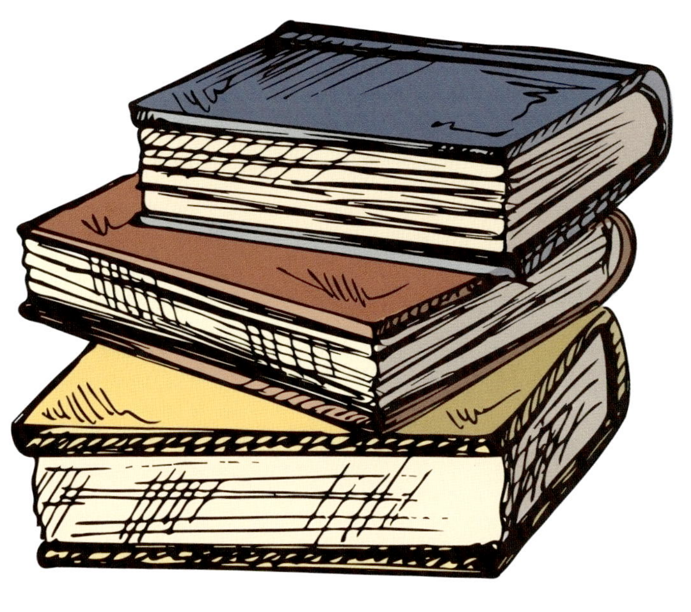

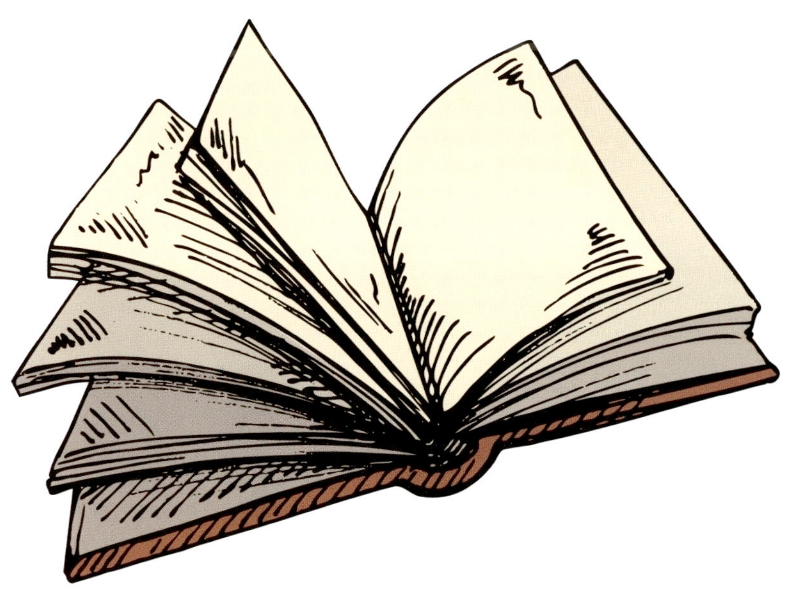

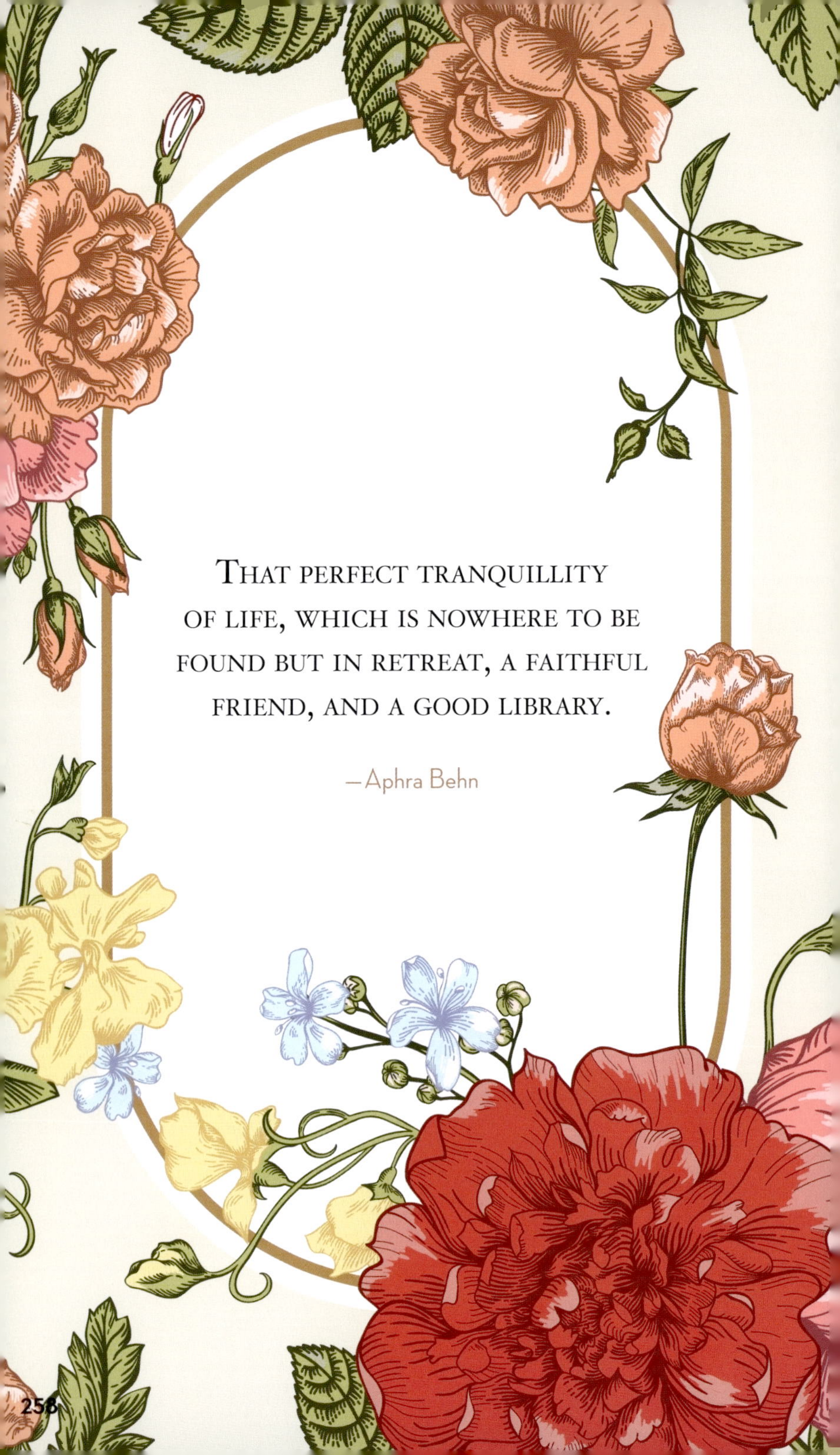

THAT PERFECT TRANQUILLITY OF LIFE, WHICH IS NOWHERE TO BE FOUND BUT IN RETREAT, A FAITHFUL FRIEND, AND A GOOD LIBRARY.

—Aphra Behn

Old books link us to the past. When you crack one open, the dry scent rising from the pages is like a promise of adventure and edification. Even as we read about those who lived long ago, we might see our own desires and joys mirrored back to us. The pages allow us to meditate on our connection to those who have gone before us, and what an intense comfort that can be!

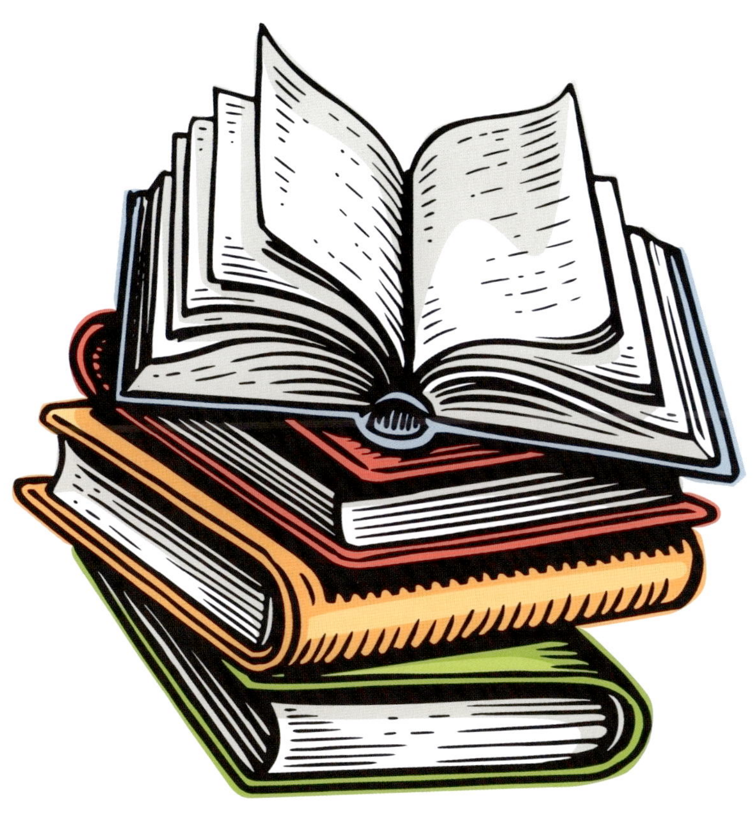

Sharing Calm

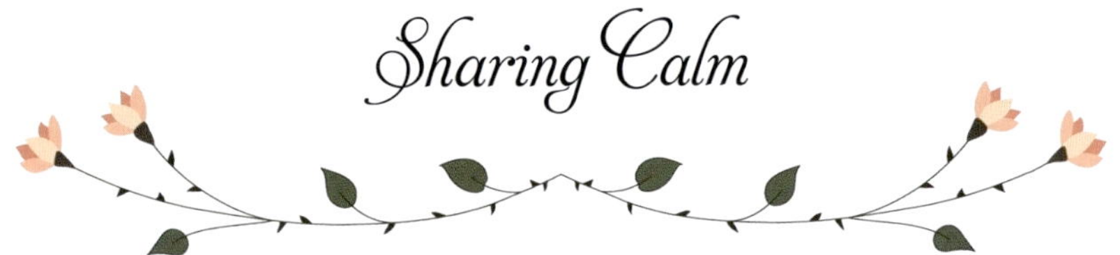

When my daughter occasionally has trouble getting to sleep, I read poetry to her. It's a nice experience to share: I like reading out loud, something I don't do so much anymore, and she enjoys being read to. We are drawn together, and the word rhythms put us both into a good, meditative space. Poetry can calm and uplift.

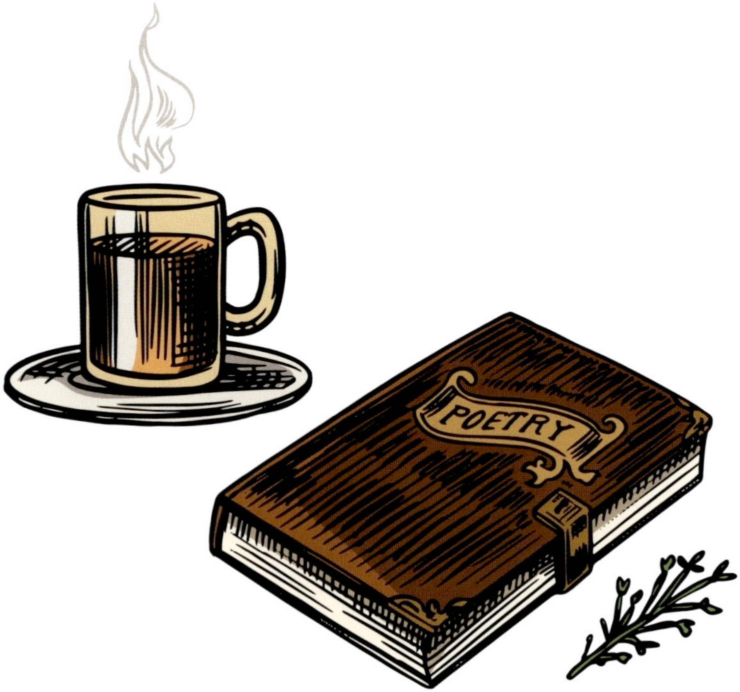

A Brief Escape

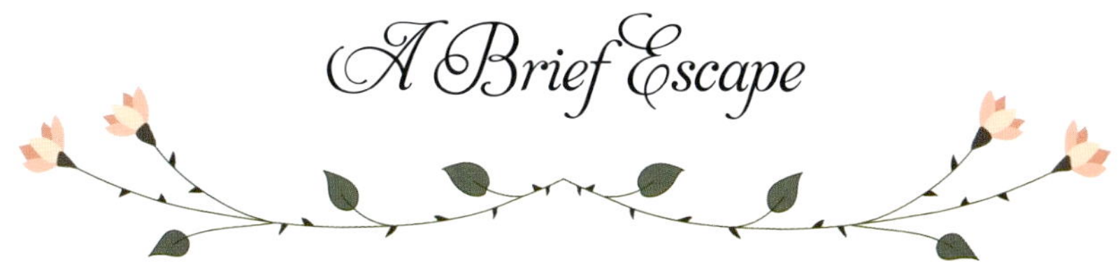

Allow yourself to get caught up in a good book or movie with full presence, immersing yourself in the world of the plot and characters. This is a mindful playtime, letting your imagination run wild and experiencing someone's journey as if it was your own. Being mindful is not restricted to minding your own life, but sometimes escaping into a great novel or show and fully appreciating the entertainment.

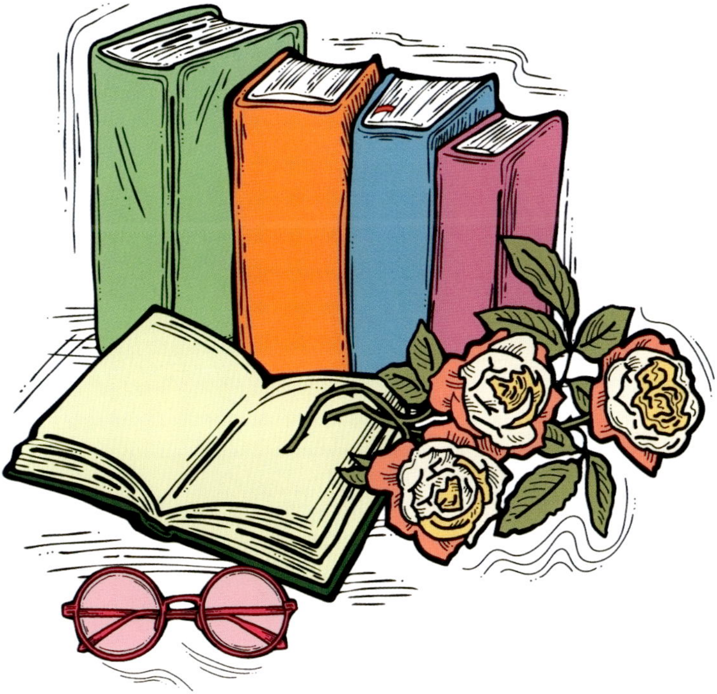

Immersive Writing

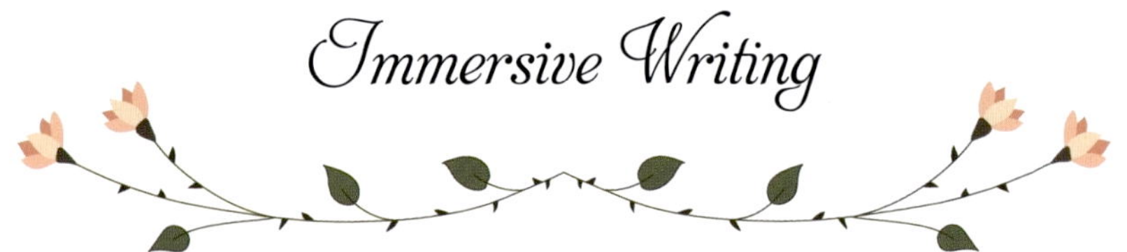

Though I tend to type manuscripts and projects for work, when it comes to personal notes, I write them by hand. I like the scratch of pen against paper, the feel of a writing instrument in my fingers. I like the way ink flows, not always evenly. All my letters aren't formed the same way, and there is beauty and character in this. Longhand has its immersive pleasures.

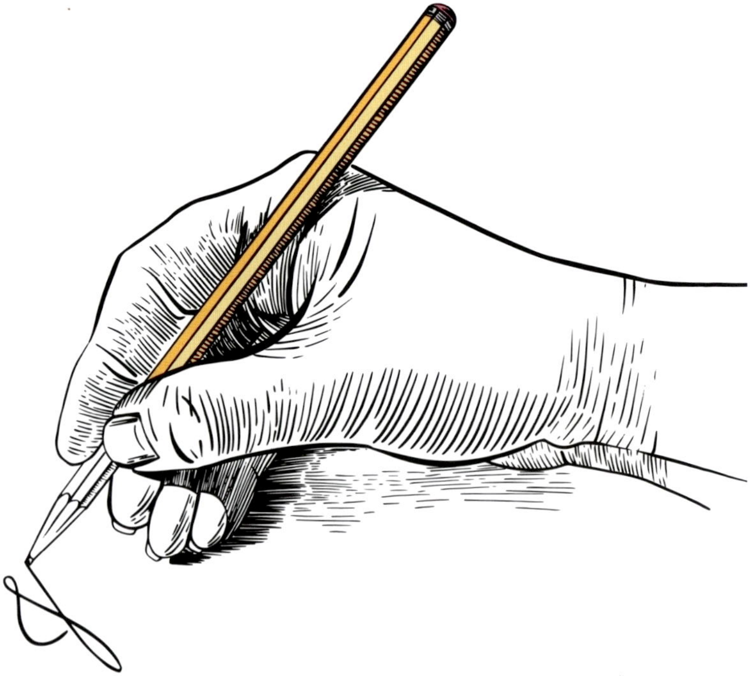

Calming Hands

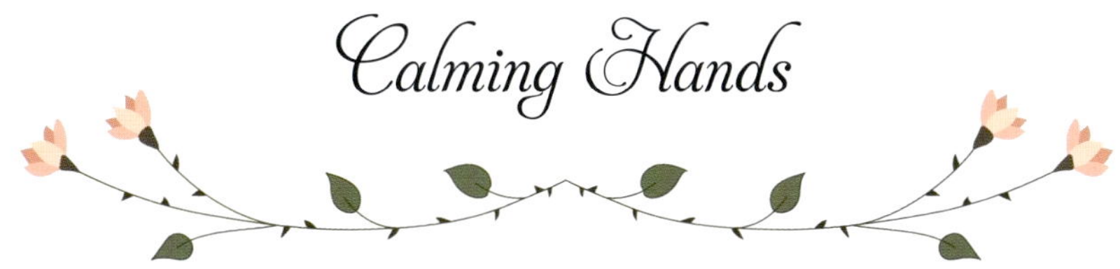

Some people call it "monkey mind": racing thoughts that keep one up at night and increase stress levels during the day. Here's a novel way to calm down and increase focus and patience: try beading, knitting, crocheting, or some other form of crafting. Try something you can do by heart so that you don't have to keep track of a pattern. Keep your project easily accessible so that it can be picked up on a whim, and enjoy the fact that you are creating a calm space in your life and making something beautiful!

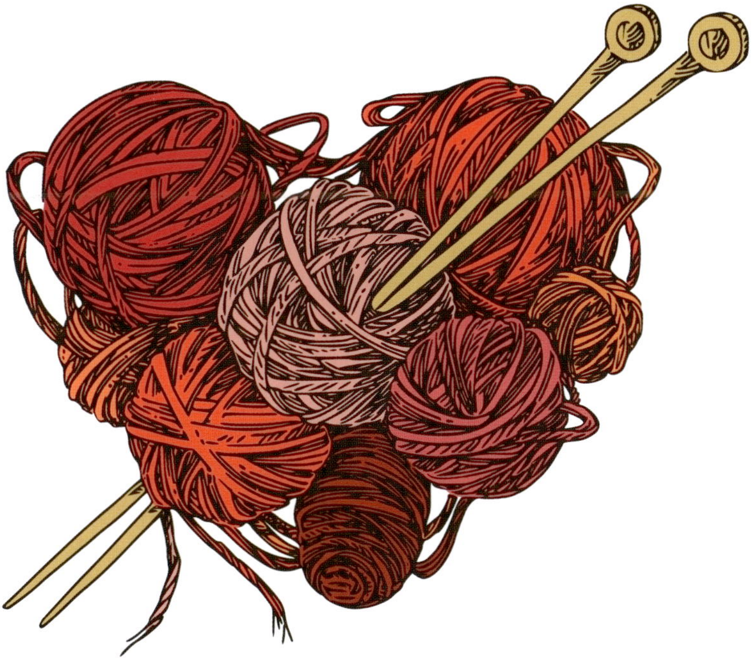

Mindful Cooking

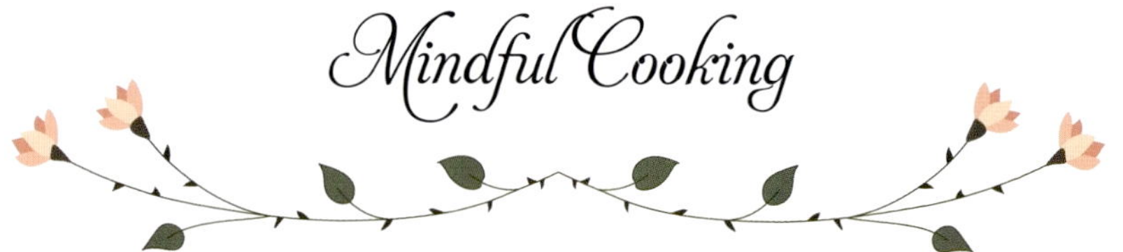

Cooking from scratch can be deeply satisfying. The next time a recipe calls for spices, try grinding them using a mortar and pestle. Take your time. Enjoy the feel of the smooth stone pestle in your hand; breathe in the deep, fresh scent of the spices as you grind them to powder. The very act is mindful and gratifying, and you will add to your meal an indescribable resonance.

Mindful Eating

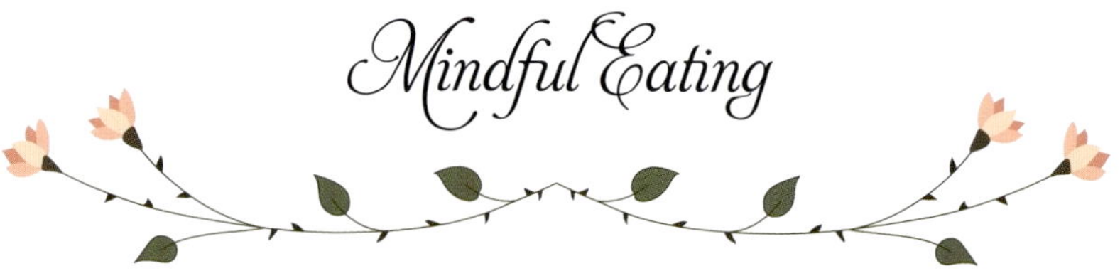

Eat mindfully. Appreciate the smells, the texture, and the taste of your food. Savor each bite.

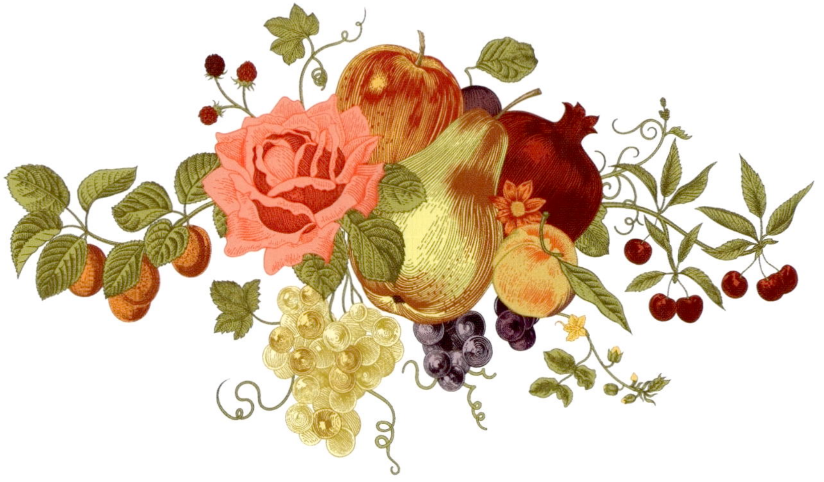

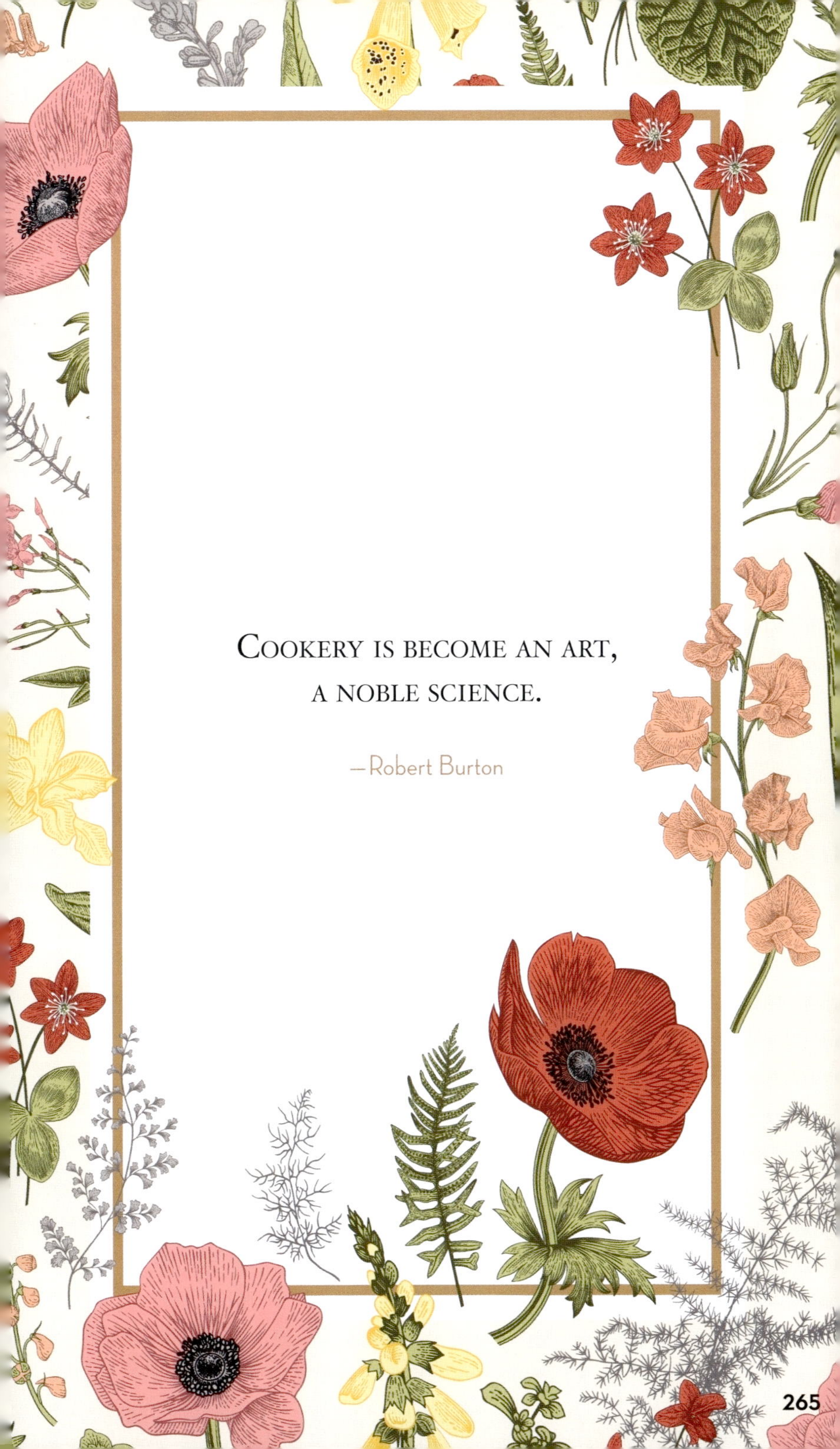

Cookery is become an art,
a noble science.

—Robert Burton

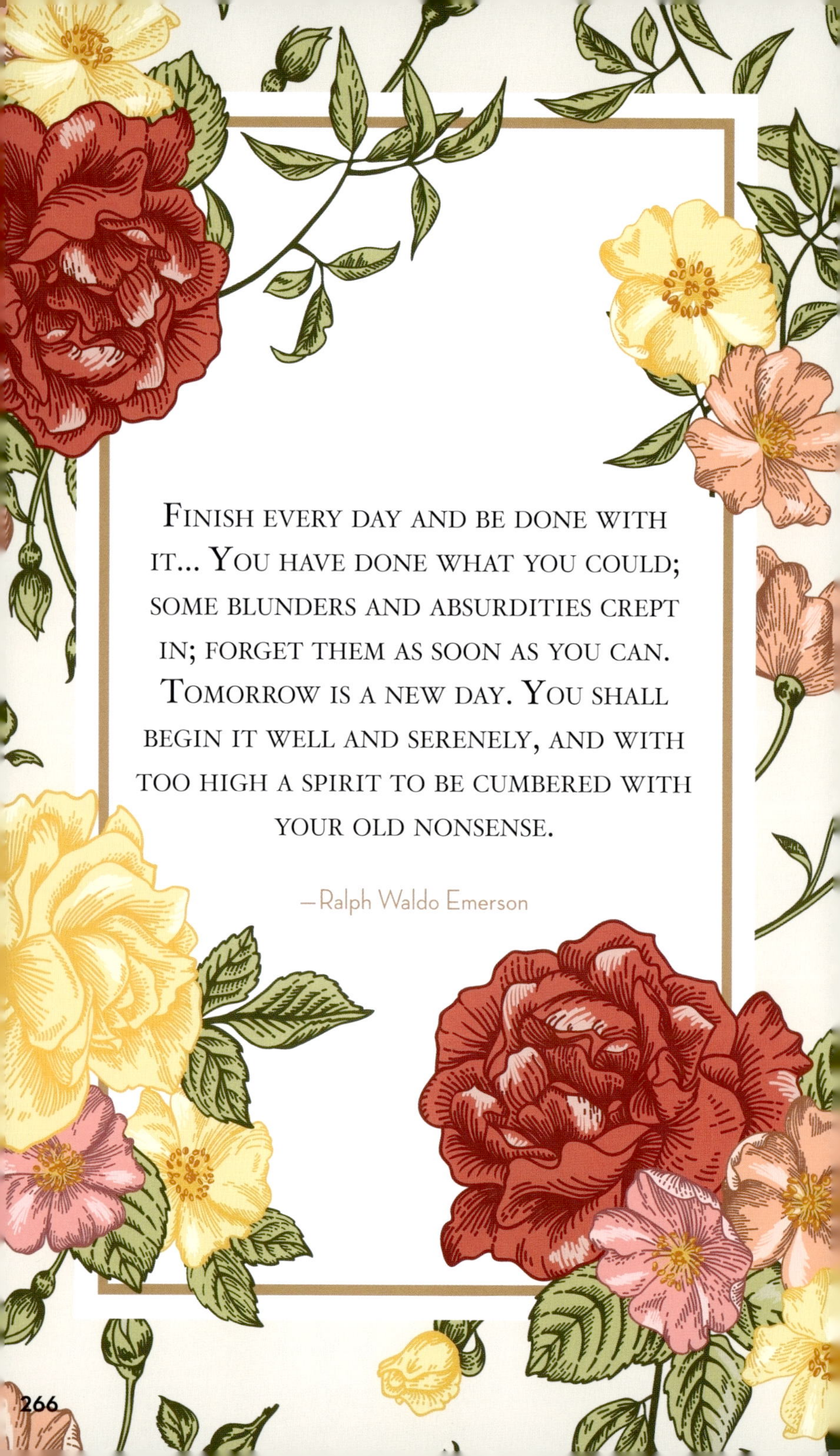

FINISH EVERY DAY AND BE DONE WITH IT... YOU HAVE DONE WHAT YOU COULD; SOME BLUNDERS AND ABSURDITIES CREPT IN; FORGET THEM AS SOON AS YOU CAN. TOMORROW IS A NEW DAY. YOU SHALL BEGIN IT WELL AND SERENELY, AND WITH TOO HIGH A SPIRIT TO BE CUMBERED WITH YOUR OLD NONSENSE.

—Ralph Waldo Emerson

Listen to your heart. Don't let worries grow and fester. Sit in the silence and acknowledge your sensations, your anxieties, and your desires, before rising anew, refreshed.

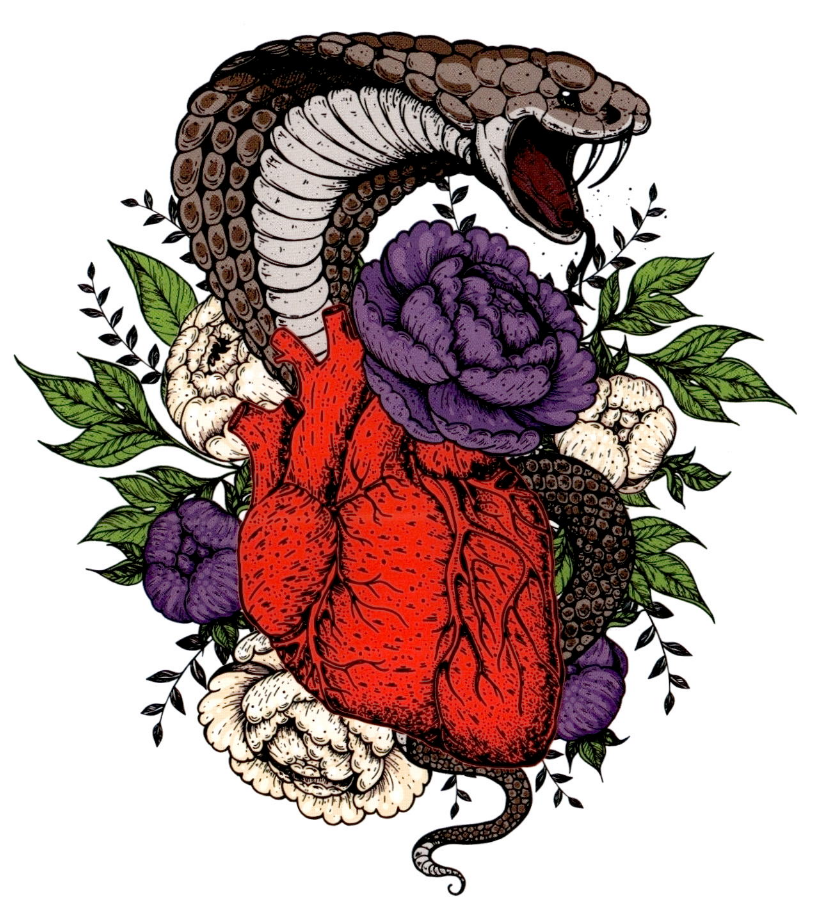

Laughter is mindfulness in action. Notice the next time you laugh, how tuned in and present you are to the moment. Notice how joyful you feel, letting go and responding without hesitation or worry about how you look to others. Laugh often, loudly and fully, from the inside out. Being alive has its hard times, but it is also filled with opportunities to experience the sheer pleasure of a good, life-affirming belly laugh.

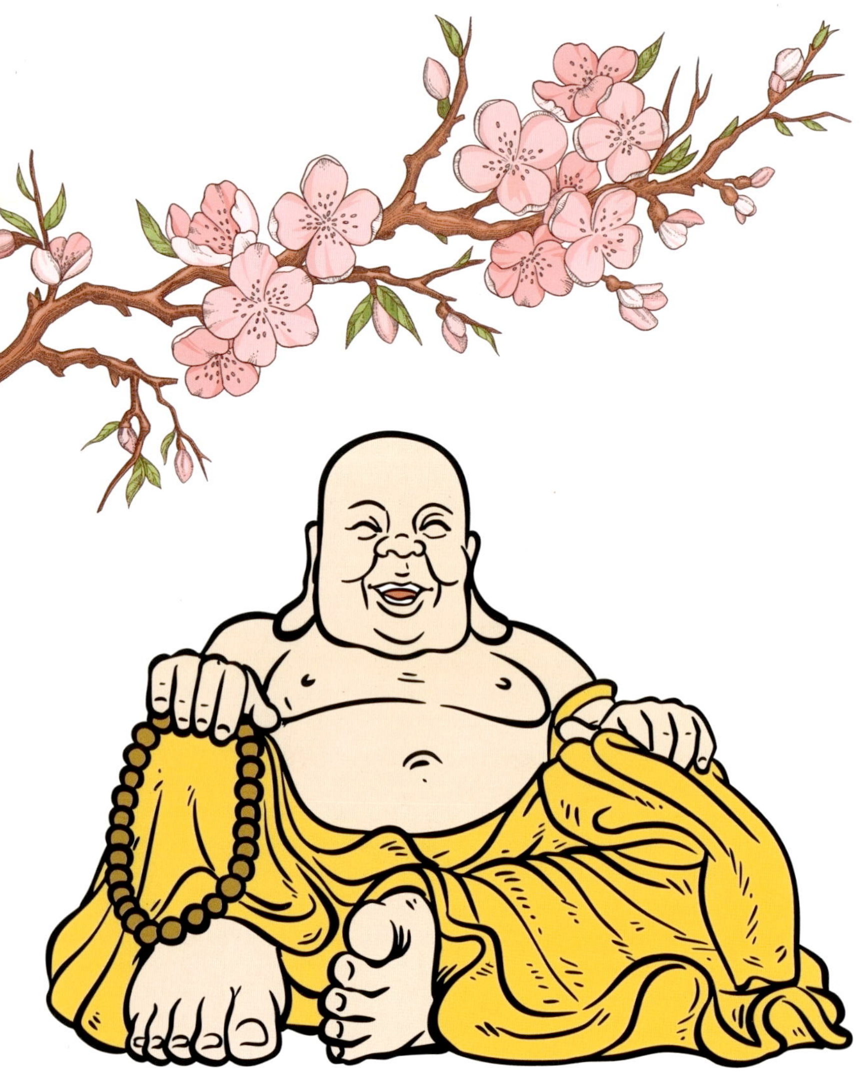